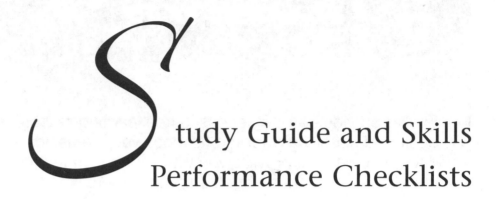

Study Guide and Skills Performance Checklists

for

Fundamentals of Nursing,

Seventh edition

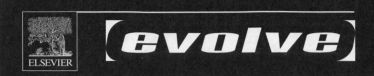

Evolve provides online access to free learning resources and activities designed specifically for the textbook you are using in your class. The resources will provide you with information that enhances the material covered in the book and much more.

⁝• *Visit the Web address listed below to start your learning evolution today!*

http://evolve.elsevier.com/Potter/fundamentals/

Evolve Student Learning Resources for Potter & Perry: Fundamentals of Nursing, 7th edition offer the following features:

- **Audio Summaries** for each chapter are downloadable to an mp3 device or CD.
- **Student Learning Activities** include Match Its and Drag and Drops.
- **Animations** include exciting images related to various chapters in the textbook.
- **Video Clips** demonstrate important steps in various nursing skills throughout the textbook.
- **Weblinks** are an exciting resource that lets you link to hundreds of websites carefully chosen to supplement the content of the textbook.
- **Content updates** include the latest information from the authors of the textbook to help keep you current with recent developments in this area of study.

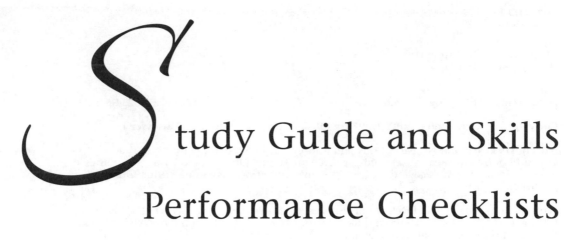

Study Guide and Skills Performance Checklists

for

POTTER/PERRY
Fundamentals of Nursing,
7th edition

Study Guide by
Geralyn Ochs, RN, MSN, BC-ACNP/ANP
Associate Professor of Nursing
St. Louis University School of Nursing
St. Louis, Missouri

Skills Performance Checklists by
Jerrilee LaMar, PhD, RN, BC
Assistant Professor of Nursing
University of Evansville
Evansville, Indiana

Linda Turchin, RN, MSN
Assistant Professor
Fairmont State University
Fairmont, West Virginia

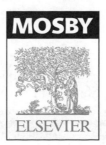

MOSBY

ELSEVIER

MOSBY
ELSEVIER

11830 Westline Industrial Drive
St. Louis, Missouri 63146

Fundamentals of Nursing, 7th Edition   ISBN: 978-0-323-05251-1

Library of Congress Control Number 978-0-323-05251-1

Executive Editor: Susan Epstein
Developmental Editor: Lynda Huenefeld
Publishing Services Manager: John Rogers
Project Manager: Kathleen L. Teal
Design Direction: Amy Buxton

Printed in the United States of America

Last digit is the print number: 9 8 7 6 5

Introduction

The *Study Guide to accompany Fundamentals of Nursing*, 7th edition, has been developed to encourage independent learning for beginning nursing students. As you begin to read the text, you may note a difference in style or format from other books you've used in the past; the terms are new, and the focus of the content is different. You may be wondering, "How will I possibly learn all of the material in this chapter?" The essential objective of this study guide is to assist you in this endeavor, to help you learn *what* you need to know, and then self-test with hundreds of review questions.

This study guide follows the text chapter for chapter. Whatever chapter your instructor assigns, you will use the same chapter number in this study guide. The outline format was designed to help you learn to read nursing content more effectively and with greater understanding. Each chapter of this study guide has the following sections to assist you to comprehend and recall.

The *Preliminary Reading* section is designed to teach prereading strategies. You need to become familiar with the chapter by first reading the chapter title, the key concepts and key terms (found at the end of each chapter), and all headings, as well as reviewing all photographs, drawings, tables, and boxes. This can be done rather quickly and will give you an overall idea of the content of the chapter.

The *Comprehensive Understanding* section is next and is in outline format. This will prove to be a very valuable tool not only as you first read the chapter but also as you review for tests. This outline identifies the topics and main ideas of each chapter as an aid to concentration, comprehension, and retaining textbook information. By completing this outline you will learn to "pull-out" key information in the chapter. As you write the answers in the study guide, you will be reinforcing that content. Once completed, this outline will serve as a review tool for exams.

The *Review Questions* in each chapter provide a valuable means of testing and reinforcing your knowledge of the material read and the answers written in the outline. Each question is multiple choice and written in the NCLEX®-style format. As a further aid for independent learning, each answer requires a rationale (the reason *why* the option you selected is correct). An answer key for the Review Questions and other chapter exercises has been provided to your instructor. If this has been shared with you, it can prove a valuable review tool.

The clinical chapters, Chapters 27 to 31 and 37 to 50, include exercises based on the care plans found in the text. These exercises provide practice in synthesizing nursing process and critical thinking as you, the nurse, care for clients. Taking one aspect of the nursing process, you will be asked to imagine you are the nurse in the case study and to think about what knowledge, experiences, standards, and attitudes might be used in caring for the client. Write your answers in the appropriate boxes.

When you finish answering the review questions and synthesis exercises, take a few minutes for self-evaluation. If you answered a question incorrectly, begin to analyze the thoughts that led you to the wrong answer:

- Did you miss the key word or phrase?
- Did you read into it something that wasn't stated?
- Did you not understand the subject matter?
- Did you use an incorrect rationale for selecting your response?

Each incorrect response is an opportunity to learn. Go back to the text and reread any content that is still unclear. In the long run, it will be a time-saving activity.

NCLEX is a registered trademark of the National Council of State Boards of Nursing, Inc.

A performance checklist is provided for each of the skills presented in the text. The checklists may be used by instructors to evaluate your competence in performing the techniques. You may need to adapt these skills in order to meet a client's special needs or follow the particular policy of an institution.

The learning activities presented in this study guide will assist you in completing the semester with a firm understanding of nursing concepts and process that you can rely on throughout your professional career.

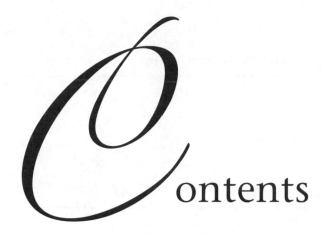

Contents

Unit V   *Psychosocial Basis for Nursing Practice*

Unit VI   *Scientific Basis for Nursing Practice*

Unit VII   *Basic Human Needs*

Unit VIII   *Clients With Special Needs*

Skills Performance Checklists

ix

1

Nursing Today

Preliminary Reading

Chapter 1, pp. 1–14

Comprehensive Understanding

1. Define *nursing* (according to the American Nursing Association [ANA]). _____
_____

Historical Perspective Highlights

2. How did Florence Nightingale see the role of the nurse in the early 1800s? _____
_____

Match the following.

3. _____ Clara Barton
4. _____ Lillian Wald and Mary Brewster
5. _____ Isabel Hampton Robb
6. _____ Mary Mahoney

a. First professionally trained African American nurse
b. Initially founded the Nurses' Associated Alumnae, which later became the ANA
c. Opened the Henry Street Settlement, focusing on the health needs of the poor
d. Founder of the American Red Cross

Societal Influences on Nursing

7. What are the external forces that have affected nursing practice in the twenty-first century?
_____
_____

Influence of Today's Health Care Delivery System

8. Identify some of challenges to our nursing practice today.
_____
_____

Nursing as a Profession

9. What are the five primary characteristics of a profession?

    a. _____

    b. _____

    c. _____

    d. _____

    e. _____

10. What are the ANA Standards of Practice?

    a. _____

    b. _____

    c. _____

    d. _____

    e. _____

11. Identify the ANA Standards of Professional Performance.

    _____

    _____

12. Describe nursing's code of ethics.

    _____

    _____

    _____

Educational Preparation for Nurses

Match the following.

13. _____ Associate degree
14. _____ Baccalaureate degree
15. _____ Master's degree
16. _____ Doctor of Philosophy
17. _____ Doctor of Nursing Practice
18. _____ In-service education
19. _____ Continuing education

a. A practice doctorate
b. Emphasizes research-based clinical practice
c. A 2-year program focusing on basic sciences and theoretical and clinical courses
d. A 4-year program that includes social sciences, arts, and humanities
e. Emphasizes basic research and theory
f. Organized educational programs offered by various institutions
g. Instruction or training provided by agencies

Nursing Practice

20. What is the purpose of Nurse Practice Acts?

    _____

    _____

21. According to Benner, an expert nurse goes through five levels of proficiency. Identify them.

    _____

    _____

Professional Responsibilities and Roles

Match the following.

22. _____ Autonomy
23. _____ Caregiver
24. _____ Advocate
25. _____ Educator
26. _____ Communicator
27. _____ Manager
28. _____ Advanced practice nurse (APN)
29. _____ Clinical nurse specialist (CNS)
30. _____ Nurse practitioner
31. _____ Certified nurse-midwife (CNM)
32. _____ Certified registered nurse anesthetist (CRNA)

a. Investigates problems to improve nursing care and to expand the scope of nursing practice
b. Independent nursing interventions that the nurse initiates without medical orders
c. Is essential for all nursing roles and activities
d. Helps the client regain health and maximum level of independent function
e. Manages client care and the delivery of specific nursing services within a health care agency
f. Has personnel, policy, and budgetary responsibility for a specific nursing unit
g. Explains, demonstrates, reinforces, and evaluates the client's progress in learning
h. Works primarily in schools of nursing and staff development

33. _____ Nurse educator
34. _____ Nursing administrator
35. _____ Nurse researcher
36. _____ Accountability

i. Specializes in a specific disease or a specific field
j. Involves the independent care for women in normal pregnancy, labor, and delivery
k. Detects and manages self-limiting acute and chronic stable medical conditions
l. Provides surgical anesthesia
m. Functions as a clinician, educator, case manager, consultant, and researcher
n. Protects the client's human and legal rights and provides assistance in asserting those rights
o. Responsible professionally and legally for the type of care rendered

Review Questions

Select the appropriate answer and cite the rationale for choosing that particular answer.

37. The factor that best advanced the practice of nursing in the first century was:
    1. Growth of cities
    2. Teachings of Christianity
    3. Better education of nurses
    4. Improved conditions for women

Answer: _____   Rationale: _____
_____
_____

38. The graduate nurse must pass a licensure examination administered by the:
    1. State Boards of Nursing
    2. National League for Nursing
    3. Accredited school of nursing
    4. American Nurses Association

Answer: _____   Rationale: _____
_____
_____

39. A group that lobbies at the state and federal levels for advancement of the nurse's role, economic interest, and health care is the:
    1. State Boards of Nursing
    2. American Nurses Association
    3. American Hospital Association
    4. National Student Nurses Association

Answer: _____   Rationale: _____
_____
_____

2

The Health Care Delivery System

Preliminary Reading

Chapter 2, pp. 15–21

Comprehensive Understanding

Health Care Regulation and Competition

Match the following.

1. _____ Prospective payment system
2. _____ Diagnosis-related groups (DRGs)
3. _____ Capitation
4. _____ Resource utilization groups (RUGs)
5. _____ Managed care
6. _____ Independent practice association (IPA)
7. _____ Medicare
8. _____ Medicaid

a. Providers receive a fixed amount per client
b. Eliminated cost-based reimbursement
c. The organization assumes financial risk in addition to providing client care
d. Fee-for-service and capitated clients
e. Utilized in long-term care
f. Hospitals receive a set dollar amount based on an assigned group
g. Federally funded, state-operated health insurance for low-income families
h. Federally funded health insurance for people 65 years of age and older

Levels of Health Care

Preventive and Primary Health Care Services

9. Explain the difference between primary health care and primary care.

_____

_____

_____

Secondary and Tertiary Care (Acute Care)

10. Because of _____, more services are available on nursing units, thus minimizing the need to transfer clients across multiple areas.

11. In an attempt to contain costs, hospitals utilized this model, _____, which focuses particularly on discharge planning.

12. Explain the role of the nurse in the above model. _____

13. _____ is a centralized, coordinated, multidisciplinary process that ensures that the client has a plan for continuing care after leaving the health care agency.

14. Explain what a critical pathway is.

_____

_____

15. Identify the instructions needed before clients leave health care facilities.

a. _____

b. _____

c. _____

d. _____

e. _____

f. _____

Restorative Care

16. The goal of restorative care is:

_____

_____

Match the following.

21. _____ Assisted living

22. _____ Respite care

23. _____ Adult day care center

24. _____ Hospice

a. Allows clients to retain more independence by living at home

b. Focus of care is palliative, not curative, treatment

c. Provides short-term relief to the family members who care for the client

d. Long-term care setting with greater resident autonomy

Issues in Health Care Delivery

25. Briefly explain evidence-based practice.

_____

_____

26. _____ is a continuous process that focuses on improving the performance of all providers.

27. _____ are client outcomes that are directly related to nursing care.

28. The Picker/Commonwealth Program for Patient-Centered Care identified seven dimensions that cover most of the scope of nursing practice. Identify them.

a. _____

b. _____

c. _____

d. _____

e. _____

f. _____

g. _____

17. Give some examples of home care services.

_____

_____

18. _____ restores a person to the fullest physical, mental, social, vocational, and economic potential possible.

19. At skilled nursing facilities clients receive:

_____

20. The Resident Assessment Instrument (RAI) consists of _____, _____, and _____

Review Questions

Select the appropriate answer and cite the rationale for choosing that particular answer.

29. Health promotion activities are designed to help clients:
    1. Reduce the risk of illness
    2. Maintain maximal function
    3. Promote habits related to health care
    4. All of the above

Answer: _____   Rationale: _____

_____

_____

30. Rehabilitation services begin:
    1. When the client enters the health care system
    2. After the client's physical condition stabilizes
    3. After the client requests rehabilitation services
    4. When the client is discharged from the hospital

Answer: _____   Rationale: _____

_____

_____

31. An example of an extended care facility is a:
    1. Home care agency
    2. Skilled nursing facility
    3. Suicide prevention center
    4. State-owned psychiatric hospital

Answer: _____   Rationale: _____

_____

_____

32. A client and his or her family facing the end stages of a terminal illness might best be served by a:
    1. Hospice
    2. Rehabilitation center
    3. Extended care facility
    4. Crisis intervention center

Answer: _____   Rationale: _____

_____

_____

3

Community-Based Nursing Practice

Preliminary Reading

Chapter 3, pp. 32–43

Comprehensive Understanding

Community-Based Health Care

1. Community-based health care focuses on: _____

Achieving Healthy Populations and Communities

2. Give some examples of comprehensive community assessments. _____

Community Health Nursing

3. Briefly describe the differences between:
    a. Public health nursing focus: _____
    _____

    b. Community health nursing focus: _____
    _____

Community-Based Nursing

4. Community-based nursing care takes place in: _____

5. Identify the four social interaction units.
    a. _____
    b. _____
    c. _____
    d. _____

Vulnerable Populations

6. Vulnerable populations are those clients who:
    a. _____
    b. _____
    c. _____

Identify the risk factors for the following vulnerable groups.

7. Immigrant population: _____

8. Poor and homeless persons: _____

9. Abused clients: _____

10. Substance abusers: _____

11. Severely mentally ill: _____

12. Older adults: _____

Competency in Community-Based Nursing

A nurse in a community-based practice must have a variety of skills and talents in assisting clients within the community. Briefly explain the competencies the nurse needs in the following roles.

13. Caregiver: _____

14. Case manager: _____

15. Change agent: _____

16. Client advocate: _____

17. Collaborator: _____

18. Counselor: _____

19. Educator: _____

20. Epidemiologist: _____

Community Assessment

21. There are three components of a community that need to be assessed. Identify them, and give an example.

    a. _____

    b. _____

    c. _____

Review Questions

Select the appropriate answer and cite the rationale for choosing that particular answer.

22. Among the communication skills needed to provide nursing care to community clients is the ability to:
    1. Speak the client's language or dialects
    2. Manage generational interfamilial conflict
    3. Clarify client values and care expectations
    4. Follow medical prescriptions in many settings

    Answer: _____ Rationale: _____

    _____

    _____

23. Which of the following is an example of an intrinsic risk factor for homelessness?
    1. Severe anxiety disorders
    2. Psychotic mental disorders
    3. Living below the poverty line
    4. Progressive chronic alcoholism

    Answer: _____ Rationale: _____

    _____

    _____

24. When the community health nurse refers clients to appropriate resources and monitors and coordinates the extent and adequacy of services to meet family health care needs, the nurse is functioning in the role of:
    1. Advocate
    2. Counselor
    3. Collaborator
    4. Case manager

    Answer: _____ Rationale: _____

    _____

    _____

25. The first step in community assessment is determining the community's:
    1. Goals
    2. Set factors
    3. Boundaries
    4. Throughputs

Answer:_____ Rationale: _____

_____

_____

4

Theoretical Foundations of Nursing Practice

Preliminary Readings

Chapter 4, pp. 44–52

Comprehensive Understanding

Domain of Nursing

Match the following.

1. _____ Domain
2. _____ Paradigm
3. _____ Nursing paradigm
4. _____ Person
5. _____ Environment
6. _____ Nursing

a. All possible conditions affecting the client and the setting of health care delivery
b. The diagnosis and treatment of human responses to actual or potential health problems
c. Perspective of a profession
d. Links science, philosophy, and theories accepted and applied by the discipline
e. Includes four linkages—the person, health, environment, and nursing
f. Is the recipient of nursing care

Theory

Match the following concepts that relate to theories.

7. _____ Nursing theories
8. _____ Theory
9. _____ Phenomenon
10. _____ Concepts
11. _____ Definitions
12. _____ Assumptions
13. _____ Grand theories
14. _____ Middle-range theories
15. _____ Descriptive theories
16. _____ Prescriptive theories

a. Aspect of reality that people consciously sense or experience
b. Action oriented and test the validity and predictability of nursing interventions
c. Address specific phenomena and reflect practice
d. Ideas and mental images
e. View client situations, organize data, analyze and interpret information
f. Concepts, definitions, and assumptions or propositions
g. Describe, speculate, and describe consequences of phenomena
h. Activity necessary to measure the concepts, relationships, or variables
i. "Taken for granted" statements
j. Structural framework for broad, abstract ideas about nursing

Interdisciplinary Theories

17. Give an example of an interdisciplinary theory.

_____

_____

18. Give an example of a systems theory.

_____

_____

19. List the five levels of Maslow's hierarchy of human needs.
    a. _____
    b. _____
    c. _____
    d. _____
    e. _____

Selected Nursing Theories

Match the following nursing theories.

20. _____ Nightingale's
21. _____ Peplau's
22. _____ Henderson's
23. _____ Rogers'
24. _____ Orem's
25. _____ Leininger's
26. _____ Roy's
27. _____ Watson's
28. _____ Benner and Wrubel's

a. Personal concern as an inherent feature of nursing practice
b. Transcultural
c. Client's self-care needs
d. The environment was the focus of nursing care
e. Nurse-client relationship
f. The goal is to help the client adapt
g. Help client perform 14 basic needs
h. Philosophy of transpersonal caring
i. The "unitary human being"

Review Questions

Select the appropriate answer and cite the rationale for choosing that particular answer.

29. Which of the following conceptual models views the person and the environment as energy fields coexisting with the universe?
    1. Roy's adaptation model
    2. Orem's model of self-care
    3. King's model of personal, interpersonal, and social systems
    4. Rogers' life process interactive person-environmental model

Answer: _____   Rationale: _____

_____

_____

30. Who is considered to have been the first nursing theorist?
    1. Linda Richards
    2. Mary Adelaide Nutting
    3. Virginia Henderson
    4. Florence Nightingale

Answer: _____   Rationale: _____

_____

_____

31. How would you distinguish between theories and assumptions?
    1. Assumptions are tested, and theories are not.
    2. Theories organize reality, but assumptions are not real.
    3. Assumptions are assumed to be true, but theories are not.
    4. Theories test hypotheses, but assumptions need no scientific proof.

Answer: _____   Rationale: _____

_____

_____

32. The development of nursing knowledge depends on:
    1. Logic and reasoning
    2. Science and philosophy
    3. Definitions and hypothesis
    4. Observation and verification

Answer: _____   Rationale: _____

_____

_____

5

Evidence-Based Practice

Preliminary Reading

Chapter 5, pp. 53–67

Comprehensive Understanding

A Case for Evidence

1. Define *evidence-based practice*. _____

2. Identify the five steps of evidence-based practice.

   a. _____

   b. _____

   c. _____

   d. _____

   e. _____

3. Identify the four elements of a PICO question.

   a. _____

   b. _____

   c. _____

   d. _____

4. Identify the sources where you can find the evidence.

   _____

   _____

5. A peer-reviewed article is a: _____

6. What are clinical guidelines? _____

7. Explain why there may be a bias in how studies are conducted.

   _____

   _____

Critiquing the Evidence

Briefly explain the following elements of evidence-based articles that will need to be critiqued.

 8. Abstract: _____

 9. Introduction: _____

10. Literature review: _____

11. Manuscript narrative:
    a. Clinical studies: _____
    b. Research studies: _____

12. Results:
    a. Clinical studies: _____
    b. Research studies: _____

13. Implications: _____

14. Explain how you can integrate the evidence. _____

Nursing Research

15. Define *nursing research*. _____

16. Define *outcomes research*. _____

Scientific Method

17. Define *scientific* method. _____

18. List the five characteristics of scientific research.
    a. _____
    b. _____
    c. _____
    d. _____
    e. _____

Nursing and the Scientific Approach
Briefly describe the following quantitative methods.

19. Experimental: _____

20. Surveys: _____

21. Evaluation: _____

22. Qualitative research is: _____

23. Define the following design strategies that are used with qualitative research.
    a. Ethnography: _____
    b. Phenomenology: _____
    c. Grounded theory: _____

Research Process

24. The research process consists of phases or steps. Briefly explain each of the following.
    a. Problem identification: _____
    b. Study design: _____
    c. Conducting the study: _____
    d. Data analysis: _____
    e. Use of the findings: _____

Quality and Performance Improvement

25. Define *quality improvement*. _____

26. Define *performance improvement*. _____

Review Questions

Select the appropriate answer and cite the rationale for choosing that particular answer.

27. Research studies can most easily be identified by:
    1. Examining the contents of the report
    2. Looking for the study only in research journals
    3. Reading the abstract and conclusion of the report
    4. Looking for the word *research* in the title of the report

Answer: _____   Rationale: _____

_____

_____

28. A research report includes all of the following except:
    1. The researcher's interpretation of the study results
    2. A description of methods used to conduct the study
    3. A summary of other research studies with the same results
    4. A summary of literature used to identify the research problem

Answer: _____   Rationale: _____

_____

_____

29. Practice guidelines for the treatment of adults with low back pain is an example of:
    1. Clinical guidelines
    2. Quantitative nursing research
    3. Outcomes management research
    4. A randomized controlled trial (RCT)

Answer: _____   Rationale: _____

_____

_____

6

Health and Wellness

Preliminary Reading

Chapter 6, pp. 68–83

Comprehensive Understanding

1. Define *illness behavior*. _____

Healthy People Documents

2. Goals for *Healthy People 2010* include:
   a. _____
   b. _____

3. The four focus areas of *Healthy People 2010* are:
   a. _____
   b. _____
   c. _____
   d. _____

Definition of Health

4. Define *health*. _____
   _____

Models of Health and Illness

5. Identify some practices of each health behavior.
   a. Positive health behavior: _____
   b. Negative health behavior: _____

6. Describe the three components of the health belief model.
   a. _____
   b. _____
   c. _____

7. The health promotion model focuses on three areas. They are:

   a. _____

   b. _____

   c. _____

8. Define the main concepts of the holistic health model. _____

   _____

   _____

Variables Influencing Health and Health Beliefs and Practices

9. Briefly describe the following internal variables.

   a. Developmental stage:

      _____

      _____

   b. Intellectual background:

      _____

      _____

   c. Perception of functioning:

      _____

      _____

   d. Emotional factors:

      _____

      _____

   e. Spiritual factors:

      _____

      _____

10. Briefly describe the following external variables.

   a. Family practices:

      _____

      _____

   b. Socioeconomic factors:

      _____

      _____

   c. Cultural background:

      _____

      _____

Health Promotion, Wellness, and Illness Prevention

11. Define *health promotion*.

    _____

    _____

12. Define *wellness*.

    _____

    _____

13. Define *illness prevention*.

    _____

    _____

14. Identify the differences between the following strategies for health promotion.

    a. Passive strategies:

       _____

       _____

    b. Active strategies:

       _____

       _____

       _____

15. Identify the health activities of each of the following levels of preventive care.

    a. Primary:

       _____

       _____

    b. Secondary:

       _____

       _____

    c. Tertiary:

       _____

       _____

Risk Factors

16. Define *risk factor*.

    _____

    _____

    _____

17. Identify at least two risk factors for each of the following categories.

    a. Genetic and physiological factors:

    _____

    _____

    b. Age:

    _____

    _____

    c. Environment:

    _____

    _____

    d. Lifestyle:

    _____

    _____

Risk Factor Modification and Changing Health Behaviors

18. Briefly explain the five stages of health behavior change.

    a. Precontemplation:

    _____

    _____

    b. Contemplation:

    _____

    _____

    c. Preparation:

    _____

    _____

    d. Action:

    _____

    _____

    e. Maintenance:

    _____

    _____

Illness

19. Define *illness*. _____

20. Explain the two general classifications of illness.

    a. Acute illness:

    _____

    _____

    b. Chronic illness:

    _____

    _____

21. Illness behavior involves:

    _____

    _____

22. Give examples of the following variables that influence illness.

    a. Internal variables:

    _____

    _____

    b. External variables:

    _____

    _____

Impact of Illness on the Client and Family

23. The client and family commonly experience the following. Briefly explain each one.

    a. Behavioral and emotional changes:

    _____

    _____

    b. Impact on body image:

    _____

    _____

    c. Impact on self-concept:

    _____

    _____

    d. Impact on family roles:

    _____

    _____

    e. Impact on family dynamics:

    _____

    _____

Review Questions

Select the appropriate answer and cite the rationale for choosing that particular answer.

24. Internal variables influencing health beliefs and practices include:
    1. Developmental stage
    2. Intellectual background
    3. Emotional and spiritual factors
    4. All of the above

    Answer: _____   Rationale: _____

    _____

    _____

25. Any variable increasing the vulnerability of an individual or a group to an illness or accident is a (an):
    1. Risk factor
    2. Illness behavior
    3. Lifestyle determinant
    4. Negative health behavior

    Answer: _____   Rationale: _____

    _____

    _____

26. All of the following characterize illness behavior except:
    1. Calling a health care provider
    2. Ignoring a physical symptom
    3. Interpreting physical symptoms
    4. Withdrawing from work activities

    Answer: _____   Rationale: _____

    _____

    _____

27. Marsha states, "My chubby size runs in our family. It's a glandular condition. Exercise and diet won't change things much." The nurse determines that this is an example of Marsha's:
    1. Health beliefs
    2. Active strategy
    3. Acute situation
    4. Positive health behavior

    Answer: _____   Rationale: _____

    _____

    _____

7

Caring for the Cancer Survivor

Preliminary Reading

Chapter 7, pp. 84–94

Comprehensive Understanding

The Effects of Cancer on Quality of Life

1. A cancer survivor is at risk for a wide range of treatment-related problems. Briefly explain the following.
   a. Second cancer: _____
   b. Late effects of chemotherapy: _____
   c. Neuropathy: _____
   d. Fatigue:_____
   e. Cognitive changes: _____

2. Identify the persistent symptoms that may occur after either a lumpectomy or
   a. Mastectomy. _____

3. Explain the following psychosocial effects of cancer.
   a. Distress: _____
   b. Posttraumatic stress disorder:_____
   c. Disrupted interpersonal relationships:

      _____

4. Identify the social impact that cancer causes across the life span.
   a. Adolescents and young adults: _____
   b. Adults (30 to 59 years): _____
   c. Older adults: _____

5. Cancer survivors most at risk for spiritual distress are those with:
   a. _____
   b. _____
   c. _____
   d. _____
   e. _____

Cancer and Families

6. Identify some of the reasons that caring for a client with cancer causes family distress.

_____

_____

Implications for Nursing

7. List the type of questions that you may use to assess the cancer survivor.

_____

_____

8. The nurse's responsibilities with client education for the client initially diagnosed with cancer are:

_____

_____

Components of Survivorship Care

9. The four essential components of survivorship care are:

   a. _____

   b. _____

   c. _____

   d. _____

Review Questions

Select the appropriate answer and cite the rationale for choosing that particular answer.

10. Many cancer survivors report attention problems, loss of memory, and difficulty recognizing and solving problems. This is an example of impaired:
    1. Social well-being
    2. Physical well-being
    3. Spiritual well-being
    4. Psychological well-being

Answer: _____ Rationale: _____

_____

_____

11. All of the following are the numerous social concerns that older adults are faced with as a result of cancer except:
    1. Retirement
    2. Fixed income
    3. Isolation from social supports
    4. Ample medical insurance coverage

Answer: _____ Rationale: _____

_____

_____

12. The essential components of survivorship are all of the following except:
    1. Surveillance for cancer spread
    2. Care for the client by oncologists only
    3. Intervention for consequences of cancer
    4. Prevention and detection of new cancers and recurrent cancer

Answer: _____ Rationale: _____

_____

_____

8

Caring in Nursing Practice

Preliminary Reading

Chapter 8, pp. 95–105

Comprehensive Understanding

Theoretical Views on Caring

1. Define *caring*. _____

2. Explain Leininger's concept of care from a transcultural perspective.

_____

_____

3. Summarize Watson's transpersonal caring.

_____

_____

4. What does Watson mean by "transformative model"?

_____

_____

5. Swanson's theory of caring consists of five categories. Explain each.
   a. Knowing:

   _____

   _____

   b. Being with:

   _____

   _____

   c. Doing for:

   _____

   _____

   d. Enabling:

   _____

   _____

   e. Maintaining belief:

   _____

   _____

Ethics of Care

6. Identify the nurse's responsibilities in relation to the ethic of care.

   _____

   _____

Caring in Nursing Practice

7. Summarize the concept of presence.

   _____

   _____

8. The use of touch is one comforting approach. Explain the differences between the three categories of touch.

   a. Task-oriented:

   _____

   b. Caring:

   _____

   c. Protective:

   _____

9. Describe what listening involves.

   _____

   _____

10. When a caring relationship is established, the client and nurse come to know one another so that both move toward a healing relationship by:

    a. _____

    b. _____

    c. _____

    d. _____

11. List the 11 caring behaviors that are perceived by families.

    a. _____

    b. _____

    c. _____

    d. _____

    e. _____

    f. _____

    g. _____

    h. _____

    i. _____

    j. _____

    k. _____

The Challenge of Caring

12. Summarize the challenges facing nursing in today's health care system.

    _____

    _____

Review Questions

Select the appropriate answer and cite the rationale for choosing that particular answer.

13. Leininger's care theory states that the client's caring values and behaviors are derived largely from:
    1. Gender
    2. Culture
    3. Experience
    4. Religious beliefs

    Answer: _____   Rationale: _____

    _____

    _____

14. The central common theme of the caring theories is:
    1. Maintenance of client homeostasis
    2. Compensation for client disabilities
    3. Pathophysiology and self-care abilities
    4. The nurse-client relationship and psychosocial aspects of care

Answer: _____ Rationale: _____

_____

_____

15. In order for the nurse to effectively listen to the client, he or she needs to:
    1. Lean back in the chair
    2. Sit with the legs crossed
    3. Maintain good eye contact
    4. Respond quickly with appropriate answers to the client

Answer: _____ Rationale: _____

_____

_____

16. The nurse demonstrates caring by:
    1. Maintaining professionalism at all costs
    2. Doing all the necessary tasks for the client
    3. Following all of the health care provider's orders accurately
    4. Helping family members become active participants in the care of the client

Answer: _____ Rationale: _____

_____

_____

9

Culture and Ethnicity

Preliminary Reading

Chapter 9, pp. 106–120

Comprehensive Understanding

Match the following.

1. _____ Culture
2. _____ Sikh
3. _____ Subcultures
4. _____ Ethnicity
5. _____ Emic worldview
6. _____ Etic worldview
7. _____ Enculturation
8. _____ Acculturation
9. _____ Biculturalism
10. _____ Cultural backlash
11. _____ Transcultural nursing
12. _____ Culturally congruent care
13. _____ Ethnocentrism

a. A tendency to hold one's own life as superior to others
b. Study of cultures to understand the similarities and differences across human groups
c. Thoughts, communications, actions, customs, and beliefs of racial, ethnic, and religious groups
d. Insider or native perspective
e. A man who wears visible artifacts, which symbolize allegiance to Sikhism
f. Shared identity related to social and cultural heritage
g. Care that fits the person's valued life patterns and set of meanings
h. Represent various ethnic, religious, and other groups with distinct characteristics from the dominant culture
i. An outsider's perspective
j. When an individual identifies equally with two or more cultures
k. Individual rejects a new culture due to a negative experience
l. Socialization into one's own culture
m. Adapting to and adopting a new culture

14. Foster identified two distinct categories of cross-cultural healers. Explain each one.

a. Naturalistic practitioners:

_____

_____

b. Personalistic practitioners:

_____

_____

Match the following.

15. _____ Chinese and Southeast Asians
16. _____ Asian Indians
17. _____ Native Americans
18. _____ African Americans
19. _____ Hispanics

a. Combination of prayers, chanting, and herbs to treat illness caused by supernatural factors
b. Old lady "granny midwife" as their healer
c. Use of products that restore the balance between yin and yang
d. *Curandero* as their healer
e. Naturalistic therapies to prevent and treat illness

Cultural Assessment

20. Cultural assessment is:

_____
_____
_____

21. The aim of asking questions in the cultural assessment is to:

_____
_____
_____

Selected Components of Cultural Assessment
Explain the following components of a cultural assessment.

22. Ethnic heritage and ethnohistory:

_____
_____
_____

23. Biocultural history:

_____
_____
_____

24. Social organization:

_____
_____
_____

25. Religious and spiritual beliefs:

_____
_____
_____

26. Communication patterns:

_____
_____
_____

27. Time orientation:

_____
_____
_____

28. Caring beliefs and practices:

_____
_____
_____

29. List the recurrent caring constructs identified in both Western and non-Western cultures.
    a. _____
    b. _____
    c. _____
    d. _____
    e. _____
    f. _____
    g. _____
    h. _____
    i. _____
    j. _____
    k. _____

Nursing Assessment

30. Briefly explain the three nursing decision and action modes to achieve culturally congruent care.
    a. Cultural care preservation or maintenance:

    _____
    _____

    b. Cultural care accommodation or negotiation:

    _____
    _____

    c. Cultural care repatterning or restructuring:

    _____
    _____

Review Questions

Select the appropriate answer and cite the rationale for choosing that particular answer.

31. Which of the following is not included in evaluating the degree of heritage consistency in a client?
    1. Gender
    2. Culture
    3. Ethnicity
    4. Religion

Answer: _____   Rationale: _____

_____

_____

32. When providing care to clients with varied cultural backgrounds, it is imperative for the nurse to recognize that:
    1. Cultural considerations must be put aside if basic needs are in jeopardy
    2. Generalizations about the behavior of a particular group may be inaccurate
    3. Current health standards should determine the acceptability of cultural practices
    4. Similar reactions to stress will occur when individuals have the same cultural background

Answer: _____   Rationale: _____

_____

_____

33. To be effective in meeting various ethnic needs, the nurse should:
    1. Treat all clients alike
    2. Be aware of clients' cultural differences
    3. Act as if he or she is comfortable with the client's behavior
    4. Avoid asking questions about the client's cultural background

Answer: _____   Rationale: _____

_____

_____

34. The most important factor in providing nursing care to clients in a specific ethnic group is:
    1. Communication
    2. Time orientation
    3. Biological variation
    4. Environmental control

Answer: _____   Rationale: _____

_____

_____

10

Caring for Families

Preliminary Reading

Chapter 10 pp. 121–135

Comprehensive Understanding

The Family

Define the three important attributes that characterize contemporary families.

1. Durability: _____

_____

2. Resiliency: _____

_____

3. Diversity: _____

_____

4. A family is defined as: _____

_____

Current Trends and New Family Forms

Summarize the various family forms.

5. Nuclear family:

_____

_____

6. Extended family:

_____

_____

7. Single-parent family:

_____

_____

8. Blended family:

_____

_____

9. Alternative patterns of relationships:

_____

_____

Explain the following threats and concerns facing the family.

10. Changing economic status:

_____

_____

11. Homelessness:

_____

_____

12. Familyviolence:

_____

_____

13. Acute or chronic illness:

_____

_____

Explain how the following examples impact the family.

14. Trauma:

_____

_____

15. Human immunodeficiency virus (HIV):

_____

_____

16. End of life:

_____

_____

Theoretical Approaches: An Overview

Summarize the following general perspectives when working with or studying families.

17. Family health system:

_____

_____

18. Developmental stages:

_____

_____

Attributes of Families

19. Structure may enhance or detract from the family's ability to respond to stressors. Briefly explain each of the following.

   a. Rigid structure:

   _____

   _____

   b. Open structure:

   _____

   _____

20. Family functioning focuses on the processes used by the family to achieve its goals. Identify these processes.

_____

_____

21. Identify the variables that affect the structure, function, and health of a family.

_____

_____

22. Explain the following attributes of healthy families.
    a. Hardiness:

    _____

    _____

    b. Resiliency:

    _____

    _____

Family Nursing

Identify the three levels and focuses proposed for family nursing practice. Briefly explain each.

23. Family as context:

    _____

    _____

24. Family as client:

    _____

    _____

25. Family as system:

    _____

    _____

Nursing Process for the Family

26. Three factors underlie the family approach to the nursing process. Name them.
    a. _____
    b. _____
    c. _____

27. Identify areas to include in the family assessment.

    _____

    _____

28. Summarize the challenges for family nursing in relation to each of the following.
    a. Discharge planning:

    _____

    _____

    b. Cultural diversity:

    _____

    _____

29. When implementing family-centered care, the following need to be addressed. Briefly explain.
    a. Health promotion:

    _____

    _____

    b. Family strengths:

    _____

    _____

    c. Acute care:

    _____

    _____

    d. Restorative care:

    _____

    _____

30. Identify the conflicts that affect the "sandwich generation."

    _____

    _____

    _____

Review Questions

Select the appropriate answer and cite the rationale for choosing that particular answer.

31. Family structure can best be described as:
    1. A complex set of relationships
    2. A basic pattern of predictable stages
    3. The pattern of relationships and ongoing membership
    4. Flexible patterns that contribute to adequate functioning

Answer: _____   Rationale: _____

_____

_____

32. When planning care for a client and using the concept of family as client, the nurse:
    1. Includes only the client and his or her significant other
    2. Considers the developmental stage of the client and not the family
    3. Understands that the client's family will always be a help to the client's health goals

4. Realizes that cultural background is an important variable when assessing the family

Answer: _____   Rationale: _____

_____

_____

33. Interventions used by the nurse when providing care to a rigidly structured family include:
    1. Attempting to change the family structure
    2. Providing solutions for problems as they arise
    3. Exploring with the family the benefits of moving toward more flexible modes of action
    4. Administering nursing care in a manner that provides minimal opportunity for change

Answer: _____   Rationale: _____

_____

_____

11

Developmental Theories

Preliminary Reading

Chapter 11. pp. 136–147

Comprehensive Understanding

Growth and Development

1. Briefly explain the following processes that affect growth and development.
   a. Biologic processes:_____
   _____
   _____

   b. Cognitive processes: _____
   _____
   _____

   c. Socioemotional processes:_____
   _____
   _____

Developmental Theories

2. Briefly summarize Gesell's theory of development.
   _____
   _____

3. Explain the five psychosexual developmental stages of Freud's theory.
   a. Stage 1: Oral:_____
   _____
   _____

   b. Stage 2: Anal:_____
   _____
   _____

   c. Stage 3: Phallic: _____
   _____
   _____

d. Stage 4: Latency: _____

e. Stage 5: Genital: _____

Match the following stages of Erickson (psychosocial development) to those of Piaget (cognitive/moral development).

4. _____ Trust versus mistrust
5. _____ Autonomy versus shame
6. _____ Initiative versus guilt
7. _____ Industry versus inferiority
8. _____ Identity versus role confusion

a. Use of symbols; egocentric
b. Sensorimotor period
c. Formal operations period
d. Preoperational period
e. Concrete operations period

9. Define *temperament*.

_____

_____

Gould's research supports stage theory in adult development with a set of themes. Briefly explain the five themes identified.

10. First theme:

_____

_____

11. Second theme:

_____

_____

12. Third theme:

_____

_____

13. Fourth theme:

_____

_____

14. Fifth theme:

_____

_____

15. Contemporary life-events approach considers:

_____

_____

16. Explain the two stages of Piaget's moral development theory.

a. Heteronomous morality: _____

_____

_____

b. Autonomous morality:_____

_____

_____

Kohlberg identified six stages of moral development under three levels. Briefly explain each.

17. Level I: Preconventional level:

_____

Stage 1:

_____

Stage 2:

_____

18. Level II: Conventional level:

_____

Stage 3:

_____

Stage 4:

_____

_____

19. Level III: Postconventional level:

_____

Stage 5:

_____

Stage 6:

_____

_____

Review Questions

Select the appropriate answer and cite the rationale for choosing that particular answer.

20. According to Piaget, the school-age child is in the third stage of cognitive development, which is characterized by:
    1. Concrete operations
    2. Conventional thought
    3. Postconventional thought
    4. Identity versus role diffusion

    Answer: _____ Rationale: _____
    _____
    _____

21. According to Erickson, the developmental task of adolescence is:
    1. Industry versus inferiority
    2. Identity versus role confusion
    3. Autonomy versus shame and doubt
    4. Role acceptance versus role confusion

    Answer: _____ Rationale: _____
    _____
    _____

22. According to Erickson's developmental theory, the primary developmental task of the middle years is to:
    1. Achieve intimacy
    2. Achieve generativity
    3. Establish a set of personal values
    4. Establish a sense of personal identity

    Answer: _____ Rationale: _____
    _____
    _____

23. According to Kohlberg, children develop moral reasoning as they mature. Which of the following is most characteristic of a preschooler's stage of moral development?
    1. The rules of correct behavior are obeyed.
    2. Behavior that pleases others is considered good.
    3. Showing respect for authority is important behavior.
    4. Actions are determined as good or bad in terms of their consequences.

    Answer: _____ Rationale: _____
    _____
    _____

12

Conception Through Adolescence

Preliminary Reading

Chapter 12 pp. 148–176

Comprehensive Understanding

Selecting a Developmental Framework for Nursing

Conception

Match the following terms that address intrauterine and extrauterine life.

1. _____ Nagele's rule
2. _____ Fertilization
3. _____ Germinal period
4. _____ Zygote
5. _____ Embryonic period
6. _____ Fetal period
7. _____ Teratogens
8. _____ Prematurity

a. The beginning of the third week through the eighth week after conception
b. Sperm penetrates the ovum
c. Ninth week after conception; ends with birth
d. Factors that are capable of producing functional or structural damage to the fetus
e. Newly formed organism with its full genetic complement
f. Infant between 20 and 37 weeks' gestation
g. First 2 weeks after conception
h. Computes the length of pregnancy

Newborn

Match the following terms that address the newborn.

9. _____ Neonatal period
10. _____ Molding
11. _____ Fontanels
12. _____ Cognitive development
13. _____ Hyperbilirubinemia
14. _____ Inborn errors of metabolism
15. _____ Circumcision
16. _____ Safety concerns

a. Car seats and cribs
b. Genetic disorders caused by the absence or deficiency of a substance essential to cellular metabolism
c. Overlapping of the soft skull bones
d. First month of life
e. Innate behavior, reflexes, and sensory functions
f. Excessive amount of bilirubin in the blood
g. Benefits include prevention of penile cancer and urinary tract infections (UTIs)
h. Diamond and triangular shapes between the unfused bones of the skull

The Infant

17. Infancy is the period from _____ to _____.

18. Summarize the physical changes that occur in the infant.

    _____

    _____

19. Describe the cognitive changes that occur in the infant.

    _____

    _____

20. Identify the language development in the infant and how to help parents further develop the infant's language.

    _____

    _____

21. Explain the following psychosocial changes that occur.
    a. Separation and individuation:

    _____

    _____

    b. Play:

    _____

    _____

22. Explain the following in relation to health risks of the infant.
    a. Injury prevention:

    _____

    _____

    b. Child maltreatment:

    _____

    _____

23. Briefly explain health concerns related to the following.
    a. Nutrition:

    _____

    _____

    b. Immunizations:

    _____

    _____

    c. Sleep:

    _____

    _____

The Toddler

24. Toddlerhood ranges from _____ to _____.

25. Describe language ability at this stage.

    _____

    _____

26. Describe the moral development of a toddler.

_____

_____

27. Identify the health risks of a toddler.

_____

_____

The Preschooler

28. The preschool period ranges from _____ to _____.

29. Describe the cognitive changes that occur with the preschooler.

_____

_____

30. Explain the following.
    a. Moral development:

    _____

    _____

    b. Language:

    _____

    _____

31. Describe the concept of play for the preschooler.

_____

_____

32. Explain health concerns related to the following for this group.
    a. Nutrition:

    _____

    _____

    b. Sleep:

    _____

    _____

    c. Vision:

    _____

    _____

The School-Age Child

33. The school-age years range from _____ to _____.

34. Define the cognitive skills that develop in the school-age child.

_____

_____

35. Summarize psychosocial development in relation to the following.
    a. Moral development:

    _____

    _____

  b. Peer relationships:

  _____

  _____

  c. Sexual identity:

  _____

  _____

  d. Stress:

  _____

  _____

36. Identify the health risks for the school-age child.

  _____

  _____

37. Give an example of a health promotion intervention that is appropriate for the school-age child.

  a. Nutrition:

  _____

  _____

  b. Oral hygiene:

  _____

  _____

  c. Infections:

  _____

  _____

  d. Drug use:

  _____

  _____

  e. Sexuality:

  _____

  _____

The Adolescent

38. The adolescent period ranges from _____ to _____.

39. List the four major physical changes that occur.

  a. _____

  _____

  b. _____

  _____

  c. _____

  _____

  d. _____

  _____

40. Menarche is:

  _____

41. Briefly explain the cognitive abilities of this group.

_____

_____

42. Identify some hints for communicating with the adolescent.

_____

_____

43. Explain the following components of total identity.

   a. Sexual identity:

_____

_____

   b. Group identity:

_____

_____

   c. Family identity:

_____

_____

   d. Vocational identity:

_____

_____

   e. Moral identity:

_____

_____

   f. Health identity:

_____

_____

44. Identify the leading causes of death for adolescents.

   a. _____

   b. _____

   c. _____

45. List the six warning signs of suicide for adolescents.

   a. _____

_____

   b. _____

_____

   c. _____

_____

   d. _____

_____

   e. _____

_____

   f. _____

_____

46. Define the two eating disorders that follow.

    a. Anorexia nervosa:

    _____

    _____

    b. Bulimia nervosa:

    _____

    _____

47. Identify health promotion interventions for the adolescent in regard to the following.

    a. Unintentional injuries:

    _____

    _____

    b. Substance abuse:

    _____

    _____

    c. Sexual activity:

    _____

    _____

    d. Firearms:

    _____

    _____

48. Identify the concerns of rural adolescents.

    _____

    _____

49. Identify the concerns of minority adolescents.

    _____

    _____

Review Questions

Select the appropriate answer and cite the rationale for choosing that particular answer.

50. The mother of a 2-year-old expresses concern that her son's appetite has diminished and that he seems to prefer milk to other solid foods. Which response by the nurse reflects knowledge of principles of communication and nutrition?
    1. "Have you considered feeding him when he doesn't seem interested in feeding himself?"
    2. "Oh, I wouldn't be too worried; children tend to eat when they're hungry. I just wouldn't give him dessert unless he eats his meal."
    3. "That is not uncommon in toddlers. You might consider increasing his milk to 2 quarts per day to be sure he gets enough nutrients."
    4. "A toddler's rate of growth normally slows down. It's common to see a toddler's appetite diminish in response to decreased calorie needs."

Answer: _____ Rationale: _____

_____

_____

51. To stimulate cognitive and psychosocial development of the toddler, it is important for parents to:
    1. Set firm and consistent limits
    2. Foster sharing of toys with playmates and siblings
    3. Provide clarification about what is right and wrong
    4. Limit confusion by restricting exploration of the environment

    Answer: _____   Rationale: _____

    _____

    _____

52. Which of the following is true of the developmental behaviors of school-age children?
    1. Fears center on the loss of self-control.
    2. Positive feedback from parents and teachers is crucial to development.
    3. Formal and informal peer group membership is the key in forming self-esteem.
    4. A full range of defense mechanisms is used, including rationalization and intellectualization.

    Answer: _____   Rationale: _____

    _____

    _____

53. Adolescents have mastered age-appropriate sexuality when they feel comfortable with their sexual:
    1. Choices
    2. Behaviors
    3. Relationships
    4. All of the above

    Answer: _____   Rationale: _____

    _____

    _____

13

Young to Middle Adult

Preliminary Reading

Chapter 13, pp. 177–190

Comprehensive Understanding

The Young Adult

1. Young adulthood is the period from _____ to _____.

2. Identify the personal lifestyle assessment of a young adult.

   _____

   _____

3. Briefly explain the cognitive development of the period in relation to educational, life, and occupational experiences.

   _____

   _____

4. Explain the psychosocial patterns of the following age-groups.
   a. 23 to 28 years:

   _____

   _____

   b. 29 to 34 years:

   _____

   _____

   c. 35 to 43 years:

   _____

   _____

5. The young adult must make decisions concerning a career, marriage, and parenthood. Briefly explain the general principles involved.
   a. Lifestyle:

   _____

   _____

   b. Career:

   _____

   _____

   c. Sexuality:

   _____

   _____

   d. Childbearing cycle:

   _____

   _____

6. Describe the following types of families.
   a. Singlehood:

   _____

   _____

   b. Parenthood:

   _____

   _____

   c. Alternative parenting:

   _____

   _____

Briefly explain the risk factors for young adults in regard to the following.
7. Family history:

   _____

   _____

8. Personal hygiene habits:

   _____

   _____

9. Violent death and injury:

   _____

   _____

10. Substance abuse:

   _____

   _____

11. Unplanned pregnancies:

   _____

   _____

12. Sexually transmitted diseases:

   _____

   _____

13. Environmental and occupational risks:

   _____

   _____

Identify a health promotion activity for the following.
14. Infertility:

   _____

   _____

15. Exercise:

   _____

   _____

16. Routine health screening:

   _____

   _____

17. Psychosocial health:

_____

_____

Explain the physiological changes that occur to the pregnant woman and the childbearing family.
18. Prenatal care:

_____

_____

19. Braxton Hicks contractions:

_____

_____

20. Puerperium:

_____

_____

21. Lactation:

_____

_____

The Middle Adult

22. Middle adulthood is the period from _____ to _____.

23. Identify the major physiological changes that occur between 40 and 65 years of age.

_____

_____

24. Define the following.
    a. *Perimenopause:*

    _____

    b. *Menopause:*

    _____

    c. *Climacteric:*

    _____

Summarize the psychosocial development of the middle adult in the following areas.
25. "Sandwich generation":

_____

_____

26. Career transition:

_____

_____

27. Sexuality:

_____

_____

28. Singlehood:

_____

_____

29. Marital changes:

_____

_____

30. Family transitions:

_____

_____

The following are health concerns for the middle adult. Briefly explain each one.

31. Stress and stress reduction:

_____

_____

32. Obesity:

_____

_____

33. Summarize two psychosocial concerns of the middle adult.

    a. Anxiety:

_____

_____

    b. Depression:

_____

_____

Review Questions

Select the appropriate answer and cite the rationale for choosing that particular answer.

34. The greatest cause of illness and death in the young adult population is:
    1. Violence
    2. Substance abuse
    3. Cardiovascular disease
    4. Sexually transmitted disease

Answer: _____ Rationale: _____

_____

_____

35. Which physiological change would be a normal assessment finding in a middle adult?
    1. Increased breast size
    2. Reduced auditory acuity
    3. Thickening of the waistline
    4. Increased anteroposterior diameter of the thorax

Answer: _____ Rationale: _____

_____

_____

36. In planning client education for Mrs. Smith, a 45-year-old woman who had an ovarian cyst removed, which of the following facts is true about the sexuality of the middle-age adult?
    1. Menstruation ceases after menopause.
    2. Estrogen is produced after menopause.
    3. With removal of the ovarian cyst, pregnancy cannot occur.
    4. After reaching climacteric, a male is unable to father a child.

Answer: _____ Rationale: _____

_____

_____

14

Older Adult

Preliminary Reading

Chapter 14, pp. 191–214

Comprehensive Understanding

1. Older adults are persons age _____ and over.

Match the following terms.

2. _____ Geriatrics
3. _____ Gerontology
4. _____ Gerontological nursing
5. _____ Gerontic nursing

a. Concerned with the assessment of the health and functional status of older adults
b. Nursing care of older adults considered to be the art and practice of nurturing and caring rather than treatment of disease
c. Study of all aspects of the aging process and its consequences
d. Branch of medicine dealing with the diagnosis and treatment of diseases that affect the older adult

Myths and Stereotypes

6. Identify four myths and/or stereotypes regarding the older adult.

   a. _____
   b. _____
   c. _____
   d. _____

Theories of Aging

Give a brief description of the following biological theories.

7. Stochastic theories:

   _____

   _____

8. Nonstochastic theories:

   _____

   _____

9. Describe the three classic psychosocial theories of aging.
   a. Disengagement theory:

   _____

   _____

   b. Activity theory:

   _____

   _____

   c. Continuity theory:

   _____

   _____

Developmental Tasks of Older Adults

10. List the seven developmental tasks of the older adult.
    a. _____
    b. _____
    c. _____
    d. _____
    e. _____
    f. _____
    g. _____

Community-Based and Institutional Health Care Services

11. Identify the six aspects of quality to consider when selecting a nursing home.
    a. _____
    b. _____
    c. _____
    d. _____
    e. _____
    f. _____

Assessing the Needs of Older Adults

Nurses need to take into account five key points to ensure an age-specific approach.

12. _____

   _____

13. _____

   _____

14. _____

   _____

15. _____

   _____

16. _____

   _____

17. Identify the early indicators of an acute illness.
    a. _____
    b. _____
    c. _____
    d. _____
    e. _____
    f. _____
    g. _____

Match the following common physiological changes to the system.

18. _____ Integumentary
19. _____ Respiratory
20. _____ Cardiovascular
21. _____ Gastrointestinal
22. _____ Musculoskeletal
23. _____ Neurological
24. _____ Sensory
25. _____ Genitourinary
26. _____ Reproductive
27. _____ Endocrine

a. Decreased estrogen production, atrophy of vagina, uterus, and breasts
b. Decrease in saliva, gastric secretions, and pancreatic enzymes
c. Decreased ability to respond to stress
d. Pigmentation changes, glandular atrophy, thinning hair
e. 50% decrease in renal blood flow, decreased bladder capacity
f. Decreased cough reflex and vital capacity, increased airway resistance
g. Lower cardiac output, decreased baroreceptor sensitivity
h. Presbyopia, presbycusis, decreased proprioception
i. Decalcification of bones, degenerative changes, dehydration of intervertebral disks
j. Degeneration of nerve cells, decrease in neurotransmitters

28. Functional status in the older adult refers to:

_____

_____

29. Explain the three common conditions that affect cognition.

   a. Delirium:

   _____

   _____

   b. Dementia:

   _____

   _____

   c. Depression:

   _____

   _____

30. Identify the psychosocial changes that occur in the older adult.

   a. _____

   b. _____

   c. _____

   d. _____

   e. _____

Addressing the Health Concerns of Older Adults

31. List the frequent causes of death in the older adult.

   a. _____

   b. _____

   c. _____

   d. _____

   e. _____

   f. _____

   g. _____

   h. _____

32. List general preventative measures to recommend to the older adult.

   a. _____

   b. _____

   c. _____

   d. _____

   e. _____

   f. _____

   g. _____

Match the following health concerns.

33. _____ Heart disease
34. _____ Cancer
35. _____ Stroke
36. _____ Smoking
37. _____ Alcohol abuse
38. _____ Nutrition
39. _____ Dental problems
40. _____ Exercise
41. _____ Arthritis
42. _____ Falls
43. _____ Sensory impairments
44. _____ Pain
45. _____ Medication use

a. Mobility depends on the extent of the disease and joints affected
b. Changes in vision, hearing, taste, and smell
c. Leading cause of death
e. Third leading cause of death
d. Consequences include depression, sleep difficulties, changes in mobility, decreased socialization
f. Risk factors: impaired vision, arthritis, incontinence, medication reactions
g. Risk factor in the four most common causes of death
h. Second most common cause of death
i. Level of activity and clinical conditions affect older adults' needs
j. Polypharmacy
k. Due to depression, loneliness, and lack of social support
l. Caries, gingivitis, and ill-fitting dentures
m. Maintains and strengthens functional ability and promotes well-being

Match the following interventions used to maintain the psychosocial health of the older adult.

46. _____ Therapeutic communication
47. _____ Touch
48. _____ Reality orientation

a. Assisting with grooming and hygiene
b. An alternative approach to communication with a confused adult
c. Nurse expresses attitudes of concern, kindness, and compassion

49. _____ Validation therapy
50. _____ Reminiscence
51. _____ Body image

d. Technique to make the older adult aware of time, place, and person
e. Can significantly lower agitation levels in demented older adults
f. Recalling the past

Older Adults and the Acute Care Setting

Explain why the older adult is at risk for each of the following.

52. Transient urinary incontinence: _____

_____

_____

53. Skin breakdown: _____

_____

_____

54. Falls: _____

_____

_____

Older Adults and Restorative Care

55. Summarize the two types of ongoing care for the older adult.

a. _____

_____

b. _____

_____

Review Questions

Select the appropriate answer and cite the rationale for choosing that particular answer.

56. Which statement describing delirium is correct?
   1. Symptoms of delirium are irreversible.
   2. The onset of delirium is slow and insidious.
   3. Symptoms of delirium are stable and unchanging.
   4. Causes include electrolyte imbalances and cerebral anoxia.

Answer: _____   Rationale: _____

_____

_____

57. Nutritional needs of the older adult:
   1. Include increased proteins and carbohydrates
   2. Are exactly the same as those of young and middle adults
   3. Include increased amounts of vitamin C, vitamin A, and calcium
   4. Include increased kilocalories to support metabolism and activity

Answer: _____   Rationale: _____

_____

_____

58. Ms. Dale states that she does not need the TV turned on because she cannot see very well. Normal visual changes in older adults include all of the following except:
   1. Double vision
   2. Sensitivity to glare
   3. Decreased visual acuity
   4. Decreased accommodation to darkness

Answer: _____   Rationale: _____

_____

_____

59. Mr. DeLone states that he is worried about his parents' plans to retire. All of the following would be appropriate responses regarding retirement of the older adult except:
   1. Retirement may affect an individual's physical and psychological functioning
   2. Positive adjustment is often related to how much a person planned for the retirement
   3. Reactions to retirement are influenced by the importance that has been attached to the work role
   4. Retirement for most persons represents a sudden shock that is irreversibly damaging to self-image and self-esteem

Answer: _____   Rationale: _____

_____

_____

15

Critical Thinking in Nursing Practice

Preliminary Reading

Chapter 15, pp. 215–229

Comprehensive Understanding

Critical Thinking Defined

1. Define *critical thinking*.

_____

_____

2. Define *evidenced-based knowledge*.

_____

_____

3. Identify the concepts and behaviors of a critical thinker.
   a. Truth seeking:

   _____

   _____

   b. Open-mindedness:

   _____

   _____

   c. Analyticity:

   _____

   _____

   d. Systematicity:

   _____

   _____

   e. Self-confidence:

   _____

   _____

   f. Inquisitiveness:

   _____

   _____

   g. Maturity:

   _____

   _____

Levels of Critical Thinking in Nursing

4. Three levels of critical thinking in nursing have been identified. Briefly describe each.

   a. Basic:

   _____

   _____

   b. Complex:

   _____

   _____

   c. Commitment:

   _____

   _____

Critical Thinking Competencies

Match the following cognitive processes to critical thinking competencies.

5. _____ Scientific method
6. _____ Problem solving
7. _____ Decision making
8. _____ Diagnostic reasoning
9. _____ Inference
10. _____ Clinical decision making
11. _____ Nursing process

a. Focuses on problem resolution
b. Process of drawing conclusions from related pieces of evidence
c. Systematic, ordered approach to gathering data and solving problems
d. Evaluating the solution over time to make sure it is effective
e. Five-step clinical decision-making approach
f. Careful reasoning so that the best options are chosen for the best outcomes
g. Determining a client's health status after you have assigned meaning to the behaviors and symptoms presented

Critical Thinking Model for Clinical Decision Making

12. List the five components of critical thinking.

    a. _____

    b. _____

    c. _____

    d. _____

    e. _____

Match the following attitudes with the appropriate application to practice.

13. _____ Confidence
14. _____ Thinking independently
15. _____ Fairness
16. _____ Responsibility
17. _____ Risk taking
18. _____ Discipline
19. _____ Perseverance
20. _____ Creativity
21. _____ Curiosity
22. _____ Integrity
23. _____ Humility

a. Refer to policy and procedure manual to review steps of a skill
b. Explore and learn more about a client to make appropriate clinical judgments
c. Speak with conviction and always be prepared to perform care safely
d. Be cautious of an easy answer; look for a pattern and find a solution
e. Be willing to recommend alternative approaches to nursing care
f. Look for different approaches if interventions are not working
g. Read the nursing literature
h. Take time to be thorough, and manage your time effectively
i. Do not compromise nursing standards or honesty in delivering nursing care
j. Listen to both sides in any discussion
k. Recognize when you need more information to make a decision

24. Explain the two standards used in the critical thinking model.

    a. Intellectual:

    _____

    b. Professional:

    _____

    _____

Developing Critical Thinking Skills

25. Define *reflective journaling*.

    _____

    _____

26. Define *concept mapping*.

    _____

    _____

Review Questions

Select the appropriate answer and cite the rationale for choosing that particular answer.

27. Clinical decision making requires the nurse to:
    1. Improve a client's health
    2. Standardize care for the client
    3. Follow the health care provider's orders for client care
    4. Establish and weigh criteria in deciding the best choice of therapy for a client

Answer: _____ Rationale: _____

_____

28. Which of the following is not one of the five steps of the nursing process?
    1. Planning
    2. Evaluation
    3. Assessment
    4. Hypothesis testing

Answer: _____ Rationale: _____

_____

29. Gathering, verifying, and communicating data about the client to establish a database is an example of which component of the nursing process?
    1. Planning
    2. Evaluation
    3. Assessment
    4. Implementation
    5. Nursing diagnosis

Answer: _____ Rationale: _____

_____

30. Completing nursing actions necessary for accomplishing a care plan is an example of which component of the nursing process?
    1. Planning
    2. Evaluation
    3. Assessment
    4. Implementation
    5. Nursing diagnosis

Answer: _____ Rationale: _____

_____

16

Nursing Assessment

Preliminary Reading

Chapter 16, pp. 230–246

Comprehensive Understanding

A Critical Thinking Approach to Assessment

Match the following terms.

1. _____ Nursing process
2. _____ Assessment
3. _____ Database
4. _____ Cue
5. _____ Inference

a. Your judgment or interpretation of cues
b. The client's perceived needs, health problems, and responses
c. Information that was obtained through the use of the senses
d. Approach to identify, diagnose, and treat human responses to health and illness
e. Collection, verification, and analysis of data

List Gordon's 11 functional health patterns.

6. _____

7. _____

8. _____

9. _____

10. _____

11. _____

12. _____

13. _____

14. _____

15. _____

16. _____

17. Define the two primary sources of data.

   a. *Subjective data:*

   _____

   _____

   b. *Objective data:*

   _____

   _____

18. Identify the variety of sources where data can be obtained.

    a. _____
    b. _____
    c. _____
    d. _____
    e. _____

19. During the initial interviewing process, nurses have the opportunity to:

    a. _____
    b. _____
    c. _____
    d. _____
    e. _____

20. Protected health information includes demographic data that relates to:

    a. _____
    b. _____
    c. _____

21. Nursing health history includes:

    _____
    _____

22. During an interview, the following are utilized. Briefly explain.

    a. Open-ended questions:

    _____
    _____

    b. Back channeling:

    _____
    _____

    c. Closed-ended questions:

    _____
    _____

Match the following basic components of the health history.

23. _____ Biographical information
24. _____ Reasons for seeking health care
25. _____ Client expectations
26. _____ Present illness/health concerns
27. _____ Health history
28. _____ Family history
29. _____ Environmental history
30. _____ Psychosocial history
31. _____ Spiritual history
32. _____ Review of systems

a. Represents the totality of one's being
b. Reveals the client's support systems, coping mechanisms
c. Data about the immediate and blood relatives
d. Systematic method for collecting data from all body systems
e. What is important to the client
f. Factual demographic data about the client
g. Client's perception
h. Essential and relevant data about the nature and onset of symptoms
i. Health care experiences and current health habits and lifestyle patterns
j. Client's home and work, focusing on determining the client's safety

Define the following terms related to the physical examination.

33. *Data validation:*

    _____
    _____

34. *Data analysis:*

    _____
    _____

35. Identify some common practices related to documentation, the last part of a complete assessment.

    _____
    _____

Review Questions

Select the appropriate answer and cite the rationale for choosing that particular answer.

36. The interview technique that is most effective in strengthening the nurse-client relationship by demonstrating the nurse's willingness to hear the client's thoughts is:
    1. Direct question
    2. Problem-solving
    3. Problem-seeking
    4. Open-ended question

    Answer: _____   Rationale: _____
    _____
    _____

37. While obtaining a health history, the nurse asks Mr. Jones if he has noted any change in his activity tolerance. This is an example of which interview technique?
    1. Direct question
    2. Problem-solving
    3. Problem-seeking
    4. Open-ended question

    Answer: _____   Rationale: _____
    _____
    _____

38. Mr. Davis tells the nurse that he has been experiencing more frequent episodes of indigestion. The nurse asks if the indigestion is associated with meals or a reclining position and asks what relieves the indigestion. This is an example of which interview technique?
    1. Direct question
    2. Problem-solving
    3. Problem-seeking
    4. Open-ended question

    Answer: _____   Rationale: _____
    _____
    _____

39. The information obtained in a review of systems (ROS) is:
    1. Objective
    2. Subjective
    3. Based on the nurse's perspective
    4. Based on physical examination findings

    Answer: _____   Rationale: _____
    _____
    _____

17

Nursing Diagnosis

Preliminary Reading

Chapter 17, pp. 247–260

Comprehensive Understanding

Critical Thinking and the Nursing Diagnostic Process

Match the following terms that relate to diagnostic conclusions.

1. _____ Medical diagnosis
2. _____ Collaborative problem
3. _____ Client-centered problems
4. _____ Defining characteristics
5. _____ Actual nursing diagnosis
6. _____ Risk nursing diagnosis
7. _____ Wellness nursing diagnosis

a. You select this type of diagnosis when the client wishes to or has achieved an optimal level of health
b. The clinical criteria or assessment findings that support an actual nursing diagnosis
c. Human responses to health conditions or life processes
d. Identification of a disease condition
e. Actual or potential physiological complication that is monitored in collaboration with others
f. Nursing interventions are defined in terms of clients' problems
g. Human responses to health conditions that may possibly develop due to risk factors

Define the following components of the nursing process.

8. *Diagnostic label:* _____

9. *Related factor:* _____

10. *Etiology:* _____

11. *Definition:* zx _____

12. *Risk factors:* _____

_____

_____

13. Identify the purpose of concept mapping.

_____

_____

Sources of Diagnostic Errors

List the practice tips that are essential in avoiding data collection errors.

14. _____

15. _____

16. _____

17. _____

18. _____

Identify steps to take to avoid the following diagnostic errors.

19. Errors in interpretation and analysis of data:

_____

_____

20. Errors in data clustering:

_____

_____

21. Errors in the diagnostic statement:

_____

_____

Review Questions

Select the appropriate answer and cite the rationale for choosing that particular answer.

22. A nursing diagnosis:
    1. Identifies nursing problems
    2. Is not changed during the course of a client's hospitalization
    3. Is derived from the physician's history and physical examination
    4. Is a statement of a client response to a health problem that requires nursing intervention

    Answer: _____   Rationale: _____

    _____

    _____

23. The first part of the nursing diagnosis statement:
    1. May be stated as a medical diagnosis
    2. Identifies the cause of the client problem
    3. Identifies appropriate nursing interventions
    4. Identifies an actual or potential health problem

    Answer: _____   Rationale: _____

    _____

    _____

24. The second part of the nursing diagnosis statement:
    1. Is usually stated as a medical diagnosis
    2. Identifies the expected outcomes of nursing care
    3. Identifies the probable cause of the client problem
    4. Is connected to the first part of the statement with the phrase "related to"

    Answer: _____   Rationale: _____

    _____

    _____

25. Which of the following is the correctly stated nursing diagnosis?
    1. Needs to be fed related to broken right arm
    2. Impaired skin integrity related to fecal incontinence
    3. Abnormal breath sounds caused by weak cough reflex
    4. Impaired physical mobility related to rheumatoid arthritis

    Answer: _____   Rationale: _____

    _____

    _____

18

Planning Nursing Care

Preliminary Reading

Chapter 18, pp. 261–277

Comprehensive Understanding

Establishing Priorities

1. Nurses establish priorities in relation to importance and time. Briefly explain the following.
   a. High: _____
   _____
   b. Intermediate: _____
   _____
   c. Low: _____
   _____

Critical Thinking in Establishing Goals and Expected Outcomes

Match the following.

2. _____ Goal
3. _____ Client-centered goal
4. _____ Short-term goal
5. _____ Long-term goal
6. _____ Expected outcome
7. _____ Nursing-sensitive client outcome

a. An individual, family, or community state, behavior, or perception that is measurable in response to a nursing intervention
b. Specific and measurable behavior or response that reflects a client's highest possible level of wellness
c. Objective behavior that is expected over a long period
d. An aim, intent, or end in a client's condition or behavior
e. Objective behavior that you expect the client will achieve in a short time
f. Specific measurable change in a client's status that you expect to occur

Guidelines for Writing Goals and Expected Outcomes

There are seven guidelines to follow when writing goals and expected outcomes. Describe each of them.

8. Client-centered: _____
_____

9. Singular goal or outcome: _____
    _____

10. Observable: _____
    _____

11. Measurable: _____
    _____

12. Time-limited: _____
    _____

13. Mutual: _____
    _____

14. Realistic: _____
    _____

Critical Thinking in Planning Nursing Care

There are three categories of interventions, and category selection is based on the client's needs. Define and give an example of each.

15. *Independent nursing interventions:*
    _____
    _____

16. *Dependent nursing interventions:*
    _____
    _____

17. *Collaborative interventions:*
    _____
    _____

18. Identify the six factors the nurse uses to select nursing interventions for a specific client.
    a. _____
    b. _____
    c. _____
    d. _____
    e. _____
    f. _____

Planning Nursing Care

19. Define the purposes of the nursing care plan.
    _____
    _____

Briefly explain the following types of care plans.

20. Student care plans:
    _____
    _____

21. Institutional care plans:

_____

_____

22. Computerized care plans:

_____

_____

23. Critical pathways:

_____

_____

Identify the nine steps in preparing for concept mapping.

24. _____

_____

25. _____

_____

26. _____

_____

27. _____

_____

28. _____

_____

29. _____

_____

30. _____

_____

31. _____

_____

32. _____

_____

Consulting Other Health Care Professionals

33. Consultation is a process in which:

_____

_____

34. List the six responsibilities of the nurse when seeking consultation.

a. _____

b. _____

c. _____

d. _____

e. _____

f. _____

Review Questions

Select the appropriate answer and cite the rationale for choosing that particular answer.

35. The following statement appears on the nursing care plan for an immunosuppressed client: The client will remain free from infection throughout hospitalization. This statement is an example of a (an):
1. Long-term goal
2. Short-term goal
3. Nursing diagnosis
4. Expected outcome

Answer: _____ Rationale: _____

_____

_____

36. The following statements appear on a nursing care plan for a client after a mastectomy: Incision site approximated; absence of drainage or prolonged erythema at incision site; and client remains afebrile. These statements are examples of:
1. Long-term goals
2. Short-term goals
3. Nursing diagnosis
4. Expected outcomes

Answer: _____ Rationale: _____

_____

_____

37. The planning step of the nursing process includes which of the following activities?
    1. Assessing and diagnosing
    2. Evaluating goal achievement
    3. Setting goals and selecting interventions
    4. Performing nursing actions and documenting them

Answer: _____ Rationale: _____

_____

_____

19

Implementing Nursing Care

Preliminary Reading

Chapter 19, pp. 278–289

Comprehensive Understanding

1. Define the following terms related to implementation.
   a. *Nursing intervention:*

   _____

   b. *Direct care:*

   _____

   c. *Indirect care:*

   _____

Critical Thinking in Implementation

2. Identify the factors that should be considered when making decisions about implementation.
   a. _____
   b. _____
   c. _____
   d. _____

Standard Nursing Interventions

Define the following terms:

3. *Clinical guideline:*

   _____

4. *Standing orders:*

   _____

5. *Nursing Interventions Classification (NIC) interventions:*

   _____

Implementation Process

Briefly explain the five preparatory activites for implementation of safe and effective nursing care.

6. Reassessing the client:

   _____

7. Reviewing and revising the existing nursing care plan:

   _____

8. Organizing resources and care delivery:

   _____

9. Anticipating and preventing complications:

   _____

10. Implementation skills:

    _____

Direct Care

11. Define *activities of daily living (ADLs)*.

    _____

    _____

12. Instrumental activities of daily living include:

    _____

    _____

13. Physical care techniques include:

    _____

    _____

14. Counseling is:

    _____

    _____

15. The focus of teaching is:

    _____

    _____

16. An adverse reaction is:

    _____

    _____

17. Preventive nursing actions are:

    _____

    _____

Indirect Care

18. Define interdisciplinary care plan.

    _____

    _____

19. Briefly explain the responsibility of the nurse for delegating and supervising others.

    _____

    _____

Achieving Client Goals

20. Client adherence is:

_____

_____

Review Questions

Select the appropriate answer and cite the rationale for choosing that particular answer.

21. Which of the following is not true of standing orders?
    1. Standing orders are commonly found in critical care and community health settings.
    2. Standing orders are approved and signed by the health care provider in charge of care before implementation.
    3. With standing orders, nurses have the legal protection to intervene appropriately in the client's best interest.
    4. With standing orders, the nurse relies on the health care provider's judgment to determine if the intervention is appropriate.

Answer: _____ Rationale: _____

_____

_____

22. The nursing care plan calls for the client, a 300-pound woman, to be turned every 2 hours. The client is unable to assist with turning. The nurse knows that she may hurt her back if she attempts to turn the client by herself. The nurse should:
    1. Turn the client by herself
    2. Ask another nurse to help her turn the client
    3. Rewrite the care plan to eliminate the need for turning
    4. Ignore the intervention related to turning in the care plan

Answer: _____ Rationale: _____

_____

_____

23. Mrs. Kay comes to the family clinic for birth control. The nurse obtains a health history and performs a pelvic examination and Pap smear. The nurse is functioning according to:
    1. Protocol
    2. Standing order
    3. Nursing care plan
    4. Intervention strategy

Answer: _____ Rationale: _____

_____

_____

24. Mary Jones is a newly diagnosed diabetic client. The nurse shows Mary how to administer an injection. This intervention activity is:
    1. Teaching
    2. Managing
    3. Counseling
    4. Communicating

Answer: _____ Rationale: _____

_____

_____

20

Evaluation

Preliminary Reading

Chapter 20, pp. 290–300

Comprehensive Understanding

Critical Thinking and Evaluation

1. The purpose of conducting evaluative measures is:

   _____

   _____

2. Identify the five elements of the evaluation process.

   a. _____

   b. _____

   c. _____

   d. _____

   e. _____

3. To objectively evaluate the success in achieving outcomes of care, the nurse should use the following steps.

   a. _____

   b. _____

   c. _____

   d. _____

   e. _____

Briefly explain the following parts of the evaluative process.

4. Care plan revision:

   _____

   _____

5. Discontinuing a care plan:

   _____

   _____

6. Modifying a care plan:

   _____

   _____

7. Goals and expected outcomes:

   _____

   _____

8. Interventions:

   _____

   _____

Quality Improvement

Define the following terms.

9. *Quality improvement:*

   _____

   _____

10. *Outcomes management:*

    _____

    _____

Review Questions

Select the appropriate answer and cite the rationale for choosing that particular answer.

11. Measuring the client's response to nursing interventions and his or her progress toward achieving goals occurs during which phase of the nursing process?
    1. Planning
    2. Evaluation
    3. Assessment
    4. Nursing diagnosis

Answer: _____ Rationale: _____

_____

_____

12. Evaluation is:
    1. Only necessary if the health care provider orders it
    2. An integrated, ongoing nursing care activity
    3. Begun immediately before the client's discharge
    4. Performed primarily by nurses in the quality assurance department

Answer: _____ Rationale: _____

_____

_____

13. The criteria used to determine the effectiveness of a nursing action are based on the:
    1. Nursing diagnosis
    2. Expected outcomes
    3. Client's satisfaction
    4. Nursing interventions

Answer: _____ Rationale: _____

_____

_____

14. When a client-centered goal has not been met in the projected time frame, the most appropriate action by the nurse would be to:
    1. Rewrite the plan using different interventions
    2. Continue with the same plan until the goal is met
    3. Repeat the entire sequence of the nursing process to discover needed changes
    4. Conclude that the goal was inappropriate or unrealistic and eliminate it from the plan

Answer: _____ Rationale: _____

_____

_____

21

Managing Client Care

Preliminary Reading

Chapter 21, pp. 301–312

Comprehensive Understanding

Building a Nursing Team

Match the following terms.

1. _____ Magnet recognition
2. _____ Team nursing
3. _____ Total patient care
4. _____ Primary nursing
5. _____ Case management
6. _____ Decentralized management
7. _____ Responsibility
8. _____ Autonomy
9. _____ Authority
10. _____ Accountability

a. Places registered nurses (RNs) at the bedside and improves accountability for client outcomes and professional relationships
b. RN is responsible for all aspects of patient care for one or more clients
c. Decision making is moved down to the level of the staff; managers and staff are more actively involved
d. American Nurses Credentialing Center (ANCC) recognizes excellence in nursing service and quality
e. RN leads the team that is made up of other RNs, licensed practical nurses (LPNs), and technicians
f. Duties and activities that an individual is employed to perform
g. Accepting the commitment to provide excellent care and the responsibility for the outcomes of the actions
h. Freedom of choice and responsibility for choices
i. Legitimate power to give commands and make final decisions specific to a given position
j. Approach that coordinates and links health care services to clients, streamlining costs and maintaining quality

Identify the five approaches the nurse manager utilizes to support staff involvement.

11. _____

12. _____

13. _____

14. _____

15. _____

Leadership Skills for Nursing Students

Identify the leadership skills a student nurse may develop, and summarize each.

16. Clinical decisions:

_____
_____

17. Priority setting:

_____
_____

18. Organizational skills:

_____
_____

19. Use of resources:

_____
_____

20. Time management:

_____
_____

21. Evaluation:

_____
_____

22. Team communication:

_____
_____

23. Identify the five rights of delegation.
    a. _____
    b. _____
    c. _____
    d. _____
    e. _____

24. Summarize the requirements for appropriate delegation.
    a. _____
    b. _____
    c. _____
    d. _____
    e. _____

Review Questions

Select the appropriate answer and cite the rationale for choosing that particular answer.

25. A student nurse practicing primary leadership skills would demonstrate all of the following except:
    1. Being sensitive to the group's feelings
    2. Recognizing others for their contribution
    3. Developing listening skills and being aware of personal motivation
    4. Assuming primary responsibility for planning, implementation, follow-up, and evaluation

Answer: _____ Rationale: _____

_____
_____

22

Ethics and Values

Preliminary Reading

Chapter 22, pp. 313–324

Comprehensive Understanding

Match the following terms in health ethics.

1. _____ Autonomy
2. _____ Beneficence
3. _____ Nonmaleficence
4. _____ Justice
5. _____ Fidelity

a. An obligation to follow through with care offered to clients
b. The best interests of the client remain more important than self-interest
c. Fairness
d. Commitment to include clients in decisions about care
e. Avoidance of harm or hurt

Professional Nursing Code of Ethics

6. Identify the four basic principles of the code of ethics.

   a. _____

   b. _____

   c. _____

   d. _____

Values

Define the following terms related to values.

7. *Value:*

   _____

8. *Value formation:*

   _____

9. *Values clarification:*

   _____

Ethics and Philosophy
Briefly explain the following philosophical constructs in relation to ethical systems.

10. Deontology:

   _____

11. Utilitarianism:

   _____

12. Feminist ethics:

_____
_____
_____

13. Ethic of care:

_____
_____
_____

How to Process an Ethical Dilemma

To distinguish an ethical problem from other kinds of problems, the nurse must decide whether the problem has one or more of the following characteristics.

14. _____

15. _____

16. _____

17. Identify the seven guidelines for ethical processing and decision making.

  a. _____
  _____

  b. _____
  _____

  c. _____
  _____

  d. _____
  _____

  e. _____
  _____

  f. _____
  _____

  g. _____
  _____

18. Identify the purposes of the ethics committee.

_____
_____

Issues in Bioethics

Briefly describe the following issues that are common in health care settings.

19. Quality of life:

_____
_____

20. Genetic screening:

_____
_____

21. Futile care:

_____
_____

Review Questions

Select the appropriate answer and cite the rationale for choosing that particular answer.

22. A health care issue often becomes an ethical dilemma because:
  1. Decisions must be made based on value systems
  2. The choices involved do not appear to be clearly right or wrong
  3. Decisions must be made quickly, often under stressful conditions
  4. A client's legal rights coexist with a health professional's obligations

Answer: _____ Rationale: _____
_____
_____

23. Which statement about an institutional ethics committee is correct?
  1. The ethics committee would be the first option in addressing an ethical dilemma.
  2. The ethics committee replaces decision making by the client and health care providers.
  3. The ethics committee relieves health care professionals from dealing with ethical issues.
  4. The ethics committee provides education, policy recommendations, and case consultation.

Answer: _____ Rationale: _____
_____
_____

24. The nurse is working with parents of a seriously ill newborn. Surgery has been proposed for the infant, but the chances of success are unclear. In helping the parents resolve this ethical conflict, the nurse knows that the first step is:
  1. Exploring reasonable courses of action
  2. Identifying people who can solve the difficulty
  3. Clarifying values related to the cause of the dilemma
  4. Collecting all available information about the situation.

Answer: _____ Rationale: _____
_____
_____

23

Legal Implications in Nursing Practice

Preliminary Reading

Chapter 23, pp. 325–338

Comprehensive Understanding

Legal Limits of Nursing

Match the following key terms.

1. _____ Nurse Practice Acts
2. _____ Regulatory law
3. _____ Common law
4. _____ Criminal laws
5. _____ Felony
6. _____ Misdemeanor
7. _____ Civil laws
8. _____ Standards of care

a. Are the legal guidelines for nursing practice and provide the minimum acceptable nursing care
b. Prevent harm to society and provide punishment for crimes
c. Is a crime of serious nature that has a penalty of imprisonment for greater then a year or even death
d. Protect the rights of individual persons within our society and encourage fair and equitable treatment
e. Describe and define the legal boundaries of nursing practice within each state
f. Judicial decisions made in courts when individual legal cases are decided
g. Less serious crime that has a penalty of a fine or imprisonment for less than a year
h. Reflects decisions made by administrative bodies

Federal Statutory Issues in Nursing Practice

Briefly explain the following.

9. Americans With Disabilities Act:

_____

_____

10. Emergency Medical Treatment and Active Labor Act (EMTALA):

_____

_____

11. Mental Health Parity Act:

_____

_____

12. Patient Self-Determination Act:

_____

_____

13. Living wills:

_____
_____

14. Durable Power of Attorney for Health Care:

_____
_____

15. Uniform Anatomical Gift Act:

_____
_____

16. Health Insurance Portability and Accountability Act of 1996 (HIPAA):

_____
_____

17. The Joint Commission (TJC) specific guidelines for the use of restraints are:

a. _____
   _____

b. _____
   _____

c. _____
   _____

State Statutory Issues in Nursing Practice

Explain the following issues that affect nursing practice on a state level.

18. Licensure:

_____
_____

19. Good Samaritan laws:

_____
_____

20. Public health laws:

_____
_____

21. Uniform Determination of Death Act:

_____
_____

22. Physician-assisted suicide:

_____
_____

Civil and Common Law Issues in Nursing Practice

Match the following terms.

23. _____ Tort
24. _____ Assault
25. _____ Battery
26. _____ False imprisonment
27. _____ Malice
28. _____ Slander
29. _____ Libel
30. _____ Negligence
31. _____ Malpractice
32. _____ Informed consent

a. Person's agreement to allow something to happen, based on disclosure of risks, benefits, and alternatives
b. Referred to as professional negligence, below the standard of care
c. One verbalizes the false statement
d. Civil wrong made against a person or property
e. Any intentional touching without consent
f. Written defamation of character
g. Any intentional threat to bring about harmful or offensive contact
h. Unjustified restraining of a person without legal warrant
i. Person publishing information knows it is false
j. Conduct that falls below the standard of care

Legal Relationships in Nursing Practice

33. Briefly explain the process that a nurse needs to follow when a staffing assignment is unreasonable.

_____
_____
_____
_____
_____

34. Identify what the nurse's responsibility is when he or she "floats" to another nursing unit.

_____
_____
_____
_____
_____

35. What is the nurse's responsibility with physicians' orders?

_____
_____
_____
_____
_____
_____

Risk Management

36. Risk management is:

_____
_____

37. Identify the purpose of the incident report.

_____
_____

Review Questions

Select the appropriate answer and cite the rationale for choosing that particular answer.

38. The scope of nursing practice is legally defined by:
    1. State Nurse Practice Acts
    2. Professional nursing organizations
    3. Hospital policy and procedure manuals
    4. Health care providers in the employing institutions

Answer: _____   Rationale: _____
_____
_____

39. A student nurse who is employed as a nursing assistant may perform any functions that:
    1. Have been learned in school
    2. Are expected of a nurse at that level
    3. Are identified in the position's job description
    4. Require technical rather than professional skill

Answer: _____   Rationale: _____
_____
_____

40. A confused client who fell out of bed because side rails were not used is an example of which type of liability?
    1. Felony
    2. Battery
    3. Assault
    4. Negligence

Answer: _____   Rationale: _____
_____
_____

41. The nurse puts a restraint jacket on a client without the client's permission and without a physician's order. The nurse may be guilty of:
    1. Battery
    2. Assault
    3. Neglect
    4. Invasion of privacy

Answer: _____   Rationale: _____
_____
_____

42. In a situation in which there is insufficient staff to implement competent care, a nurse should:
    1. Organize a strike
    2. Refuse the assignment
    3. Inform the clients of the situation
    4. Accept the assignment but make a protest in writing to the administration

Answer: _____   Rationale: _____
_____
_____

24

Communication

Chapter 24, pp. 339–360

Comprehensive Understanding

Communication and Nursing Practice

1. Define *communication*.

   a. _____

   b. _____

2. Identify the two bases for an individual's perceptions.

   a. _____

   b. _____

Levels of Communication

Match the following levels of communication.

3. _____ Intrapersonal
4. _____ Interpersonal
5. _____ Transpersonal
6. _____ Small-group
7. _____ Public

a. Interaction with an audience
b. Interaction that occurs within a person's spiritual domain
c. Occurs within an individual
d. One-to-one interaction between the nurse and the other person
e. Interaction that occurs with a small number of persons

Basic Elements of the Communication Process

Match the following terms that address communication.

8. _____ Referent
9. _____ Sender
10. _____ Receiver
11. _____ Message
12. _____ Channels
13. _____ Feedback
14. _____ Interpersonal variables
15. _____ Environment
16. _____ Verbal communication

a. Factors within both the sender and the receiver that influence communication
b. Code that conveys specific meaning through the combination of words
c. Person who encodes and delivers the message
d. Refers to all factors (verbal and nonverbal) that influence communication
e. Art and music are utilized to enhance understanding and promote healing
f. Person who decodes the message
g. Motivates one person to communicate with another
h. Setting for the sender-receiver interaction
i. Interpretation of a word's meaning influenced by the thoughts and feelings that people have about the word

17. _____ Connotative meaning
18. _____ Intonation
19. _____ Timing
20. _____ Symbolic
21. _____ Metacommunication

j. Content of the communication
k. Often provides information about the person's emotional state or energy level
l. Means of conveying and receiving messages through the senses
m. Indicates whether the receiver understood the meaning of the sender's message
n. When a client expresses an interest in communicating

22. Identify the four zones of personal space.
    a. _____
    b. _____
    c. _____
    d. _____

23. Identify the four zones of touch.
    a. _____
    b. _____
    c. _____
    d. _____

Professional Nursing Relationships

The nurse-client relationship is characterized by four goal-directed phases. Briefly explain the phases.

24. Preinteraction phase:

25. Orientation phase:

26. Working phase:

27. Termination phase:

Explain the Focus of the Following Relationships.

28. Nurse-family:

29. Nurse–health care team:

30. Nurse-community:

Elements of Professional Communication

31. List the elements of professional communication.
    a. _____
    b. _____
    c. _____
    d. _____
    e. _____

Communication Within the Nursing Process

Assessment

32. List the contextual factors that influence communication.
    a. _____
    b. _____

c. _____

d. _____

e. _____

33. Gender influences communication. Explain how communication differs in regard to gender.

a. Male:

_____

_____

b. Female:

_____

_____

Nursing Diagnosis

34. The primary diagnosis used to describe the client with limited or no ability to communicate is:

_____

_____

_____

_____

_____

Implementation

Match the following therapeutic communication techniques.

38. _____ Active listening
39. _____ Sharing observations
40. _____ Sharing empathy
41. _____ Sharing hope
42. _____ Sharing humor
43. _____ Sharing feelings
44. _____ Using touch
45. _____ Using silence
46. _____ Providing information
47. _____ Clarifying
48. _____ Focusing
49. _____ Paraphrasing
50. _____ Asking relevant questions
51. _____ Summarizing
52. _____ Self-disclosure
53. _____ Confrontation

35. Identify the defining characteristics of the diagnosis above.

_____

_____

_____

_____

_____

36. Identify the related factors that contribute to the above diagnosis.

_____

_____

_____

_____

_____

Planning

37. List the goals and outcomes for the client with the above diagnosis.

a. _____

b. _____

c. _____

d. _____

a. Helping clients by making observations, acknowledging feelings, encouraging communication
b. Used to center on key elements or concepts of the message
c. Concise review of key aspects of an interaction
d. Subjectively true, personal experiences about self that are intentionally revealed to another
e. Being attentive to what the client is saying both verbally and nonverbally
f. The goal is to bring hope and joy to the situation
g. Helps the client communicate without the need for extensive questioning
h. Helping the client become aware of inconsistencies in his or her feelings, attitudes, beliefs, and behaviors
i. Seeking information needed for decision making
j. Restating another's message more briefly using one's own words
k. Restating an unclear or ambiguous message
l. Clients have the right to know about their health status and what is happening in their environment
m. Ability to understand and accept another person's reality
n. Useful when people are confronted with decisions that require much thought
o. Sharing a vision of the future and resources
p. Most potent form of communication

Match the following nontherapeutic communication techniques with the appropriate responses.

54. _____ Asking personal questions
55. _____ Giving personal opinions

a. "No one here would intentionally lie to you."
b. "How can you say you didn't sleep a wink? You were snoring all night long."

56. _____ Changing the subject
57. _____ Autonomic responses
58. _____ False reassurance
59. _____ Sympathy
60. _____ Asking for explanations
61. _____ Approval or disapproval
62. _____ Defensive responses
63. _____ Passive responses
64. _____ Arguing

c. "I'm so sorry about your mastectomy; it must be terrible to lose a breast."
d. "You shouldn't even think about assisted suicide; it is not right."
e. "Why are you so anxious?"
f. "Older adults are always confused."
g. "Why don't you and John get married?"
h. "Don't worry, everything will be all right."
i. "Things are bad, and there's nothing I can do about it."
j. "Let's not talk about your problems with the insurance company. It's time for your walk."
k. "If I were you, I'd put your mother in a nursing home."

Briefly identify the communication techniques to use with the client with special needs.

65. Cannot speak clearly:

_____

_____

66. Cognitively impaired:

_____

_____

67. Hearing impaired:

_____

_____

68. Visually impaired:

_____

_____

69. Unresponsive:

_____

_____

70. Does not speak English:

_____

_____

Evaluation

Identify what the process recording analysis reveals.

71. _____

72. _____

73. _____

74. _____

75. _____

76. _____

77. _____

Review Questions

Select the appropriate answer and cite the rationale for choosing that particular answer.

78. In demonstrating the method for deep breathing exercises, the nurse places his or her hands on the client's abdomen to explain diaphragmatic movement. This technique involves the use of which communication element?
    1. Referent
    2. Message
    3. Feedback
    4. Tactile channel

Answer: _____ Rationale: _____

_____

_____

79. Which statement about nonverbal communication is correct?
    1. The nurse's verbal messages should be reinforced by nonverbal cues.
    2. It is easy for a nurse to judge the meaning of a client's facial expression.
    3. The physical appearance of the nurse rarely influences nurse-client interaction.
    4. Words convey meanings that are usually more significant than nonverbal communication.

Answer: _____ Rationale: _____

_____

_____

80. The term referring to the sender's attitude toward the self, the message, and the listener is:
    1. Denotative meaning
    2. Metacommunication
    3. Connotative meaning
    4. Nonverbal communication

Answer: _____   Rationale: _____

_____

_____

81. The referent in the communication process is:
    1. Information shared by the sender
    2. The means of conveying messages
    3. That which motivates the communication
    4. The person who initiates the communication

Answer: _____   Rationale: _____

_____

_____

82. The nurse is conducting an admission interview with the client. To maintain the client's territoriality and maximize communication, the nurse should sit:
    1. 4 to 12 feet from the client
    2. 0 to 18 inches from the client
    3. 12 feet or more from the client
    4. 18 inches to 4 feet from the client

Answer: _____   Rationale: _____

_____

_____

25

Client Education

Preliminary Reading

Chapter 25, pp. 361–383

Comprehensive Understanding

Purposes of Client Education

Briefly explain client education in each phase of health care.

1. Maintenance and promotion of health and illness prevention:

_____

_____

2. Restoration of health:

_____

_____

3. Coping with impaired functions:

_____

_____

Teaching and Learning

Match the following terms.

4. _____ Teaching	a.	The mental state that allows the learner to focus on and comprehend a learning activity
5. _____ Learning	b.	A person's perceived ability to successfully complete a task
6. _____ Learning objective	c.	Interactive process that promotes learning
7. _____ Cognitive learning	d.	Force that acts on or within a person, causing the person to behave in a particular way
8. _____ Affective learning		
9. _____ Psychomotor learning	e.	Integration of mental and muscular activity, ranging from perception to origination
10. _____ Attentional set		
11. _____ Motivation	f.	Describes what the learner will be able to do after successful instruction
12. _____ Self-efficacy	g.	Receiving, responding, valuing, organizing, characterizing
	h.	Acquisition of new knowledge, behaviors, and skills
	i.	Knowledge, comprehension, application analysis, synthesis, evaluation

13. List the five stages of adaptation to illness and grief.
    a. _____
    b. _____
    c. _____
    d. _____
    e. _____

Summarize how each of the following influences the ability to learn.

14. Learning in children:
    _____
    _____

15. Adult learning:
    _____
    _____

16. Physical capability:
    _____
    _____

Integrating the Nursing and Teaching Processes

17. Explain how the nursing process and the teaching process differ.
    a. The nursing process requires:
    _____
    _____
    b. The teaching process focuses on:
    _____
    _____

Assessment

Success in teaching the client requires the nurse to assess the following factors. List the elements of each factor.

18. Learning needs:
    a. _____
    b. _____
    c. _____

19. Motivation to learn:
    a. _____
    b. _____
    c. _____
    d. _____
    e. _____
    f. _____
    g. _____

20. Ability to learn:
    a. _____
    b. _____
    c. _____
    d. _____
    e. _____
    f. _____

21. Teaching environment:
    a. _____
    b. _____
    c. _____

22. Resources for learning:
    a. _____
    b. _____
    c. _____
    d. _____
    e. _____

23. Define *functional illiteracy*.
    _____
    _____

Nursing Diagnosis

24. Describe how the nurse would define the problem.
    _____
    _____
    _____
    _____
    _____

Planning

The principles of teaching are techniques that incorporate the principles of learning. Explain the following principles.

25. Setting priorities:
    _____
    _____
    _____
    _____
    _____

26. Timing:
    _____
    _____
    _____
    _____

27. Organizing teaching material: _____

_____   _____

_____   _____

Implementation

Match the following teaching approaches.

28. _____ Telling
29. _____ Participating
30. _____ Entrusting
31. _____ Reinforcement
32. _____ One-on-one instruction
33. _____ Group instruction
34. _____ Return demonstration
35. _____ Analogies
36. _____ Role play
37. _____ Simulation

a. Economical way to teach clients in groups that often involves both lecture and discussion
b. The nurse poses a pertinent problem or situation for clients to solve, which provides an opportunity to identify mistakes
c. The nurse outlines the task the client will perform and gives explicit instructions
d. Supplement verbal instruction with familiar images
e. The nurse and client set objectives and become involved in the learning process together
f. People play themselves or someone else
g. The chance to practice the skill
h. Most common method of instruction
i. Provides the client the opportunity to manage self-care
j. Using a stimulus that increases the probability for a response

Evaluation

38. Identify the nurse's responsibility in evaluating the outcomes of the teaching learning process.

_____

_____

Review Questions

Select the appropriate answer and cite the rationale for choosing that particular answer.

39. An internal impulse that causes a person to take action is:
    1. Anxiety
    2. Motivation
    3. Adaptation
    4. Compliance

Answer: _____   Rationale: _____

_____

_____

40. Demonstration of the principles of body mechanics used when transferring clients from bed to chair would be classified under which domain of learning?
    1. Social
    2. Affective
    3. Cognitive
    4. Psychomotor

Answer: _____   Rationale: _____

_____

_____

41. Which of the following clients is most ready to begin a client-teaching session?
    1. Ms. Hernandez, who is unwilling to accept that her back injury may result in permanent paralysis
    2. Mr. Frank, a newly diagnosed diabetic, who is complaining that he was awake all night because of his noisy roommate
    3. Mrs. Brown, a client with irritable bowel syndrome, who has just returned from a morning of testing in the gastrointestinal (GI) laboratory
    4. Mr. Jones, a client who had a heart attack 4 days ago and now seems somewhat anxious about how this will affect his future

Answer: _____   Rationale: _____

_____

_____

42. The nurse works with pediatric clients who have diabetes. Which is the youngest age-group to which the nurse can effectively teach psychomotor skills such as insulin administration?
    1. Toddler
    2. Preschool
    3. School-age
    4. Adolescent

Answer: _____   Rationale: _____

_____

_____

43. Which of the following is an appropriately stated learning objective for Mr. Ryan, a newly diagnosed diabetic?
    1. Mr. Ryan will understand diabetes.
    2. Mr. Ryan will be taught self-administration of insulin by 5/2.
    3. Mr. Ryan will know the signs and symptoms of low blood sugar by 5/5.
    4. Mr. Ryan will perform blood glucose monitoring with the EZ-Check Monitor by the time of discharge.

Answer: _____   Rationale: _____

_____

_____

26

Documentation and Informatics

Preliminary Reading

Chapter 26, pp. 384–409

Comprehensive Understanding

Define the following terms.

1. *Documentation:* _____

2. *Accreditation:* _____

3. *Diagnosis-related group (DRG):* _____

Confidentiality

4. Explain the new rights for clients related to the Health Insurance Portability and Accountability Act (HIPAA).

    a. _____

    b. _____

    c. _____

    d. _____

Standards

5. The standards of documentation by The Joint Commission require:

_____

Multidisciplinary Communication Within the Health Care Team

Define the following.

6. *Client record:* _____

7. *Reports:* _____

8. *Consultations:* _____

9. *Referrals:* _____

Purposes of Records

Match the following purposes of a record.

10. _____ Communication
11. _____ Legal documentation
12. _____ Financial billing
13. _____ Education
14. _____ Research
15. _____ Auditing

a. Objective, ongoing reviews to determine the degree to which quality improvement standards are met
b. Learning the nature of an illness and the individual client's responses
c. Means by which client needs and progress, individual therapies, client education, and discharge planning are conveyed to others in the health care team
d. Gathering of statistical data of clinical disorders, complications, therapies, recovery, and deaths
e. One of the best defenses for legal claims
f. To determine the accurate and timely reimbursement

Guidelines for Quality Documentation and Reporting

Five important guidelines must be followed to ensure quality documentation and reporting. Explain each one.

16. Factual: _____

17. Accurate: _____

18. Complete: _____

19. Current: _____

20. Organized: _____

Methods of Recording

Match the following documentation systems used for recording client data.

21. _____ Narrative notes
22. _____ Problem-oriented medical record (POMR)
23. _____ SOAP
24. _____ SOAPIE
25. _____ PIE
26. _____ Focus charting
27. _____ Source record
28. _____ Charting by exception
29. _____ Case management
30. _____ Critical pathways

a. Incorporates a multidisciplinary approach to documenting care
b. Focuses on deviations from the established norm or abnormal findings; highlights trends or changes
c. Database, problem list, care plan, and progress notes
d. Multidisciplinary care plans that include client problems, key interventions, and expected outcomes
e. Separate section for each discipline
f. SOAP with intervention and evaluation added
g. Involves the use of data, action, and response
h. Problem, intervention, and evaluation
i. Subjective, objective, assessment, and plan

Common Record-Keeping Forms

Match the following formats used for record keeping.

31. _____ Admission nursing history forms
32. _____ Flow sheets
33. _____ Kardex
34. _____ Acuity records
35. _____ Standardized care plans
36. _____ Discharge summary forms

a. Determine the hours of care and staff required for a given group of clients
b. Has activity, treatment, nursing care plan sections that organize information for quick reference
c. Provide baseline data to compare with changes in the client's condition
d. Emphasize previous learning by the client and the care that should be continued
e. Data entry of assessments such as vital signs, hygiene measures, ambulation, restraint checks
f. Preprinted, established guidelines used to care for the client

Reporting

Change-of-Shift Reports
Identify the nine major areas to include in a change-of-shift report.

37. _____
38. _____
39. _____
40. _____
41. _____
42. _____
43. _____
44. _____
45. _____

46. List the information that needs to be documented with telephone reports.

_____

_____

47. List the guidelines the nurse should follow when receiving telephone orders from health care providers.
    a. _____
    b. _____
    c. _____
    d. _____
    e. _____
    f. _____

48. List the nine major information areas in a transfer report.
    a. _____
    b. _____
    c. _____
    d. _____
    e. _____
    f. _____
    g. _____
    h. _____
    i. _____

Review Questions

Select the appropriate answer and cite the rationale for choosing that particular answer.

49. The primary purpose of a client's medical record is to:
    1. Provide validation for hospital charges
    2. Satisfy requirements of accreditation agencies
    3. Provide the nurse with a defense against malpractice
    4. Communicate accurate, timely information about the client

Answer: _____ Rationale: _____

_____

_____

50. Which of the following is correctly charted according to the six guidelines for quality recording?
    1. "Was depressed today."
    2. "Respirations rapid; lung sounds clear."
    3. "Had a good day. Up and about in room."
    4. "Crying. States she doesn't want visitors to see her like this."

Answer: _____ Rationale: _____
_____
_____

51. During a change-of-shift report:
    1. Two or more nurses always visit all clients to review their plan of care
    2. The nurse should identify nursing diagnoses and clarify client priorities
    3. Nurses should exchange judgments they have made about client attitudes
    4. Client information is communicated from a nurse on a sending unit to a nurse on a receiving unit

Answer: _____ Rationale: _____
_____
_____

52. An incident report is:
    1. A legal claim against a nurse for negligent nursing care
    2. A summary report of all falls occurring on a nursing unit
    3. A report of an event inconsistent with the routine care of a client
    4. A report of a nurse's behavior submitted to the hospital administration

Answer: _____ Rationale: _____
_____
_____

53. If an error is made while recording, the nurse should:
    1. Erase it or scratch it out
    2. Leave a blank space in the note
    3. Draw a single line through the error and initial it
    4. Obtain a new nurse's note and rewrite the entries

Answer: _____ Rationale: _____
_____
_____

27

Self-Concept

Preliminary Reading

Chapter 27, pp. 410–425

Comprehensive Understanding

1. Define *self-concept.* _____

Nursing Knowledge Base

Development of Self-Concept

2. Self-concept is a dynamic perception that is based on the following.

   a. _____

   b. _____

   c. _____

   d. _____

   e. _____

   f. _____

   g. _____

   h. _____

   i. _____

Components and Interrelated Terms of Self-Concept

Match the following terms.

3. _____ Identity
4. _____ Body image
5. _____ Role performance
6. _____ Reinforcement-extinction
7. _____ Inhibition
8. _____ Substitution
9. _____ Imitation
10. _____ Identification
11. _____ Self-esteem

a. Individual replaces one behavior with another, providing the same gratification

b. Certain behaviors become common or are avoided, depending on whether they are approved and reinforced or discouraged and punished

c. Individual's overall feeling of self-worth

d. Individual internalizes the beliefs, behaviors, and values of role models into a personal, unique expression of self

e. The way in which individuals perceive their ability to carry out significant roles

f. Includes physical appearance, structure, or function of the body

g. Individual learns to refrain from behaviors, even when tempted to engage in them

h. Individual acquires knowledge, skills, or behaviors from members of the social group

i. Internal sense of individuality, wholeness, and consistency of a person over time and in different situations

Stressors Affecting Self-Concept

12. A self-concept stressor is any:

_____

_____

Match the following stressors that affect self-concept.

13. _____ Identity
14. _____ Body image
15. _____ Role performance
16. _____ Role conflict
17. _____ Role ambiguity
18. _____ Role strain
19. _____ Role overload

a. Example: perceived inability to meet parental expectations, harsh criticism, and inconsistent discipline
b. Example: providing care to a family member with Alzheimer's disease
c. Example: a middle-age woman with teenage children assuming responsibility for the care of her older parents
d. Amputation, facial disfigurement, or scars from burns
e. Unsuccessfully attempting to meet the demands of work and family while carving out some personal time
f. Situational transitions
g. An adolescent attempting to adjust to the physical, emotional, and mental changes of increasing maturity
h. Common in adolescents and employment situations

The Nurse's Effect on the Client's Self-Concept

List five areas the nurse must clarify and assess about himself or herself in order to promote a positive self-concept in clients.

21. _____
22. _____
23. _____
24. _____
25. _____

Self-Concept and the Nursing Process

Assessment

26. Identify the focus of assessing both self-concept and self-esteem.

_____
_____

Nursing Diagnosis

27. List the defining characteristics for situational low self-esteem.

_____
_____

Planning

28. State the expected outcomes for the nursing diagnosis *situational low self-esteem related to a recent job layoff.*

_____
_____

Implementation

29. List some healthy lifestyle measures that contribute to a healthy self-concept.

_____
_____

Evaluation

30. Identify the expected outcomes for a self-concept disturbance.

_____

_____

Review Questions

Select the appropriate answer and cite the rationale for choosing that particular answer.

31. Which developmental stage is particularly crucial for identity development?
    1. Infancy
    2. Young adult
    3. Adolescence
    4. Preschool age

Answer: _____   Rationale: _____

_____

_____

32. Which of the following statements about body image is correct?
    1. Body image refers only to the external appearance of a person's body.
    2. Physical changes are quickly incorporated into a person's body image.
    3. Perceptions by other persons have no influence on a person's body image.
    4. Body image is a combination of a person's actual and perceived (ideal) body.

Answer: _____   Rationale: _____

_____

_____

33. Robert, who is 2 years old, is praised for using his potty instead of wetting his pants. This is an example of learning a behavior by:
    1. Imitation
    2. Substitution
    3. Identification
    4. Reinforcement-extinction

Answer: _____   Rationale: _____

_____

_____

34. Mrs. Watson has just undergone a radical mastectomy. The nurse is aware that Mrs. Watson will probably have considerable anxiety over:
    1. Self-esteem
    2. Body image
    3. Self-identity
    4. Role performance

Answer: _____   Rationale: _____

_____

_____

Critical Thinking Model for Nursing Care Plan for Situational Low Self-Esteem

35. Imagine that you are the student nurse, Susan, in the care plan on page 421 of your text. Complete the *Assessment phase* of the critical thinking model by writing your answers in the appropriate boxes of the model shown. Think about the following.

- In developing Mrs. Johnson's plan of care, what knowledge did Susan apply?

- In what way might Susan's previous experience apply in this case?

- What intellectual or professional standards were applied to Mrs. Johnson?

- What critical thinking attitudes did you use in assessing Mrs. Johnson?

- As you review your assessment, what key areas did you cover?

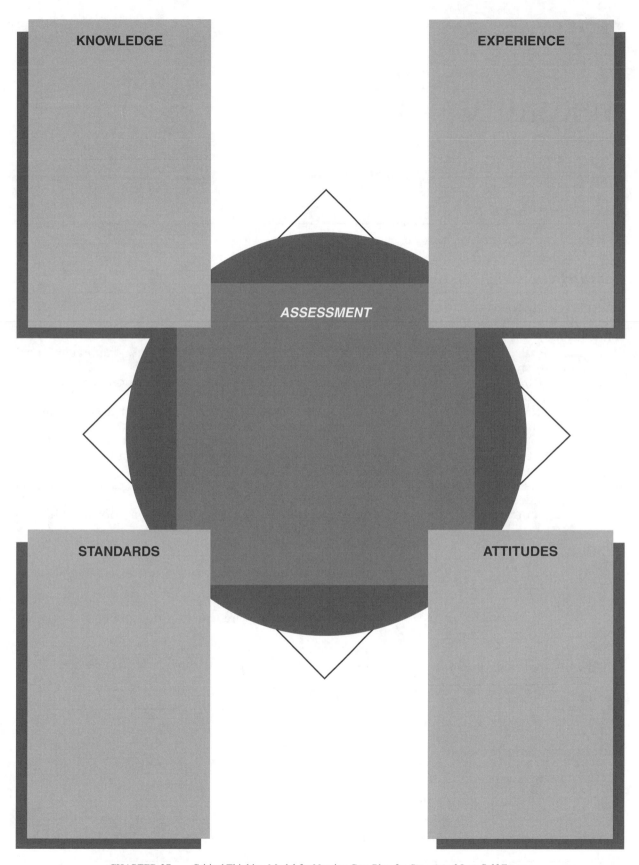

KNOWLEDGE

EXPERIENCE

ASSESSMENT

STANDARDS

ATTITUDES

CHAPTER 27   Critical Thinking Model for Nursing Care Plan for *Situational Low Self-Esteem*

28

Sexuality

Preliminary Reading

Chapter 28, pp. 426–442

Comprehensive Understanding

Scientific Knowledge Base

Match the following terms to the appropriate responses.

1. _____ Sexuality
2. _____ Intercourse
3. _____ Gender roles
4. _____ Gender identity
5. _____ School-age children
6. _____ Adolescents
7. _____ Homosexual
8. _____ Heterosexual
9. _____ Young adulthood
10. _____ Middle adulthood
11. _____ Older adulthood
12. _____ Contraceptive options

a. Pill, intrauterine device (IUD), condoms, diaphragm, tubal ligation, vasectomy
b. Changes in physical appearance lead to concerns about sexual attractiveness
c. Factors include present health status, past and present life satisfaction, status of intimate relationships
d. Need accurate information on sexual activity, emotional responses with relationships, sexually transmitted diseases (STDs), contraception, and pregnancy
e. Have general questions regarding the physical and emotional aspects of sex
f. Part of a person's personality and important for overall health
g. Influenced by culture
h. Sexual functioning
i. The first 3 years are crucial for its development
j. Many adolescents will have at least one experience with an individual or in a group
k. Male and female relationship
l. Intimacy and sexuality are issues for this group

13. Identify the primary routes of human immunodeficiency virus (HIV) transmission.

_____

_____

Nursing Knowledge Base

14. Identify two sociocultural dimensions of sexuality.

a. _____

b. _____

15. Identify three decisional issues regarding sexuality.

a. _____

b. _____

c. _____

16. Identify four alterations in sexual health.
    a. _____
    b. _____
    c. _____
    d. _____

Sexuality and the Nursing Process

Assessment

17. What factors that may affect sexuality would the nurse assess?
    a. _____
    b. _____
    c. _____
    d. _____
    e. _____
    f. _____

18. The PLISSIT assessment of sexuality is:

    _____

    _____

Nursing Diagnosis

19. Identify assessment data that may signal risk for or an actual nursing diagnosis related to sexuality.
    a. _____
    b. _____
    c. _____
    d. _____

Planning

20. The expected outcomes for the nursing diagnosis *sexual dysfunction related to decreased sexual drive* are:
    a. _____
    b. _____
    c. _____

Implementation

21. List the sexual health issues that you would include when educating your client.
    a. _____
    b. _____
    c. _____
    d. _____
    e. _____

Identify strategies that enhance sexual functioning.
22. _____
23. _____
24. _____
25. _____
26. _____
27. _____
28. _____

Acute Care

29. Identify the stressors that may affect a person's sexuality during illness.

    _____

    _____

Evaluation

30. Identify the follow-up discussions to determine whether the goals and outcomes were achieved.
    a. _____
    b. _____

Review Questions

Select the appropriate answer and cite the rationale for choosing that particular answer.

31. At what developmental stage is it particularly important for children reared in single-parent families to be exposed to same-sex adults?
    1. Infancy
    2. School-age
    3. Adolescence
    4. Toddlerhood and preschool years

    Answer: _____ Rationale: _____

    _____

    _____

32. Which statement about sexual response in the older adult is correct?
    1. The resolution phase is slower.
    2. The orgasm phase is prolonged.
    3. The refractory phase is more rapid.
    4. Both genders experience a reduced availability of sex hormones.

    Answer: _____ Rationale: _____

    _____

    _____

33. The only 100% effective method to avoid contracting a disease through sex is:
    1. Abstinence
    2. Using condoms
    3. Avoiding sex with partners at risk
    4. Knowing the sexual partner's health history

Answer: _____   Rationale: _____
_____
_____

Critical Thinking Model for Nursing Care Plan for Sexual Dysfunction

34. Imagine that you are the nurse in the care plan on page 437 of your text. Complete the *Assessment phase* of the critical thinking model by writing your answers in the appropriate boxes of the model shown. Think about the following.
    - In developing Mr. Clements' plan of care, what knowledge did the nurse apply?

- In what way might the nurse's previous experience assist in this case?

- What intellectual or professional standards were applied to Mr. Clements?

- What critical thinking attitudes did you use in assessing Mr. Clements?

- As you review your assessment, what key areas did you cover?

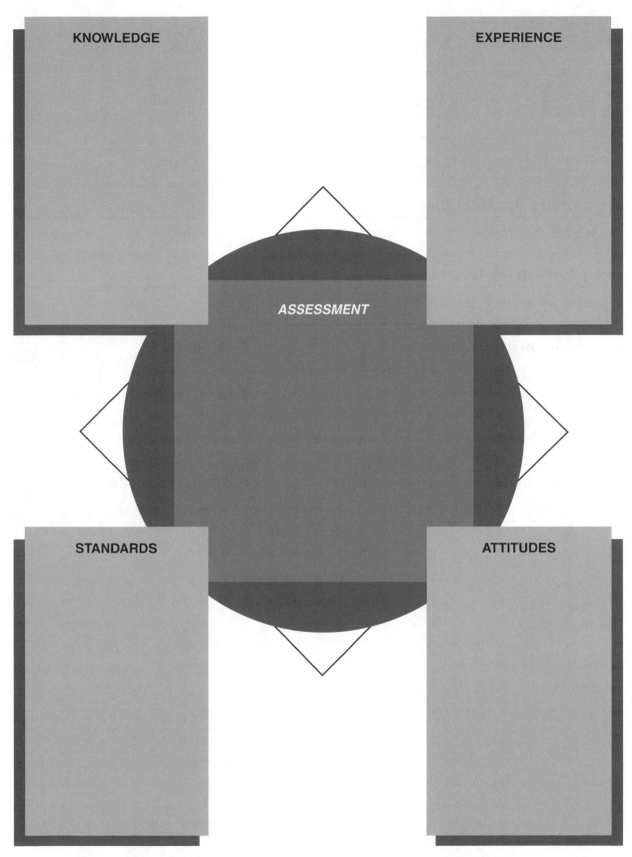

CHAPTER 28   Critical Thinking Model for Nursing Care Plan for *Sexual Dysfunction*

29

Spiritual Health

Preliminary Reading

Chapter 29, pp. 443–460

Comprehensive Understanding

1. Define *spirituality*. _____

Nursing Knowledge Base

Match the following terms.

2. _____ Self-transcendence

3. _____ Connectedness

4. _____ Atheist

5. _____ Agnostic

6. _____ Spiritual well-being

7. _____ Faith

8. _____ Religion

9. _____ Hope

10. _____ Spiritual distress

a. A person has the attitude of something to live for and look forward to

b. Belief that there is no known ultimate reality

c. A relationship with a divinity, higher power

d. Does not believe in the existence of God

e. There is a force outside of and greater than the person

f. Intrapersonally, interpersonally, and transpersonally

g. Having a vertical and horizontal dimension

h. The system of organized beliefs and worship that a person practices

i. Impaired ability to experience and integrate meaning and purpose in life

11. Briefly explain each of the following causes of spiritual distress.

a. Acute illness:

_____

_____

b. Chronic illness:

_____

_____

c. Terminal illness:

_____

_____

d. Near-death experience:

_____

_____

Critical Thinking

Assessment

12. The acronym B-E-L-I-E-F stands for:

_____

_____

Various tools are available to assess a client's spiritual well-being. Briefly summarize the following dimensions.

13. Faith/belief:

_____

_____

14. Life/self-responsibility:

_____

_____

15. Connectedness:

_____

_____

16. Life satisfaction:

_____

_____

17. Culture:

_____

_____

18. Fellowship and community:

_____

_____

19. Ritual and practice:

_____

_____

20. Vocation:

_____

_____

Nursing Diagnosis

List the three nursing diagnoses that pertain to spirituality and their defining characteristics.

21. _____

_____

_____

22. _____

_____

_____

23. _____

_____

_____

Planning

24. Identify the three outcomes for the client to achieve personal harmony.

a. _____

b. _____

c. _____

Implementation

Health Promotion

25. Identify behaviors that establish the nurse's presence.

_____

_____

26. Identify the factors that are evident when a healing relationship develops between a nurse and client.

a. _____

b. _____

c. _____

Acute Care and Restorative and Continuing Care

Explain how the following interventions are helpful in the client's therapeutic plan.

27. Support systems:

_____

_____

28. Diet therapies:

_____

_____

29. Supporting rituals:

_____

_____

30. Prayer:

_____

_____

31. Meditation:

_____

_____

32. Supporting grief work:

_____

_____

Evaluation

33. Identify the successful outcomes of spiritual health.

_____

_____

Review Questions

Select the appropriate answer and cite the rationale for choosing that particular answer.

34. When planning care to include spiritual needs for a client of Islamic faith, the religious practices the nurse should understand include all of the following except:
    1. Strength is gained through group prayer
    2. Family members are a source of comfort
    3. A priest must be present to conduct rituals
    4. Faith healing provides psychological support

Answer: _____   Rationale: _____

_____

_____

35. When consulting with the dietary department regarding meals for a client of the Hindu religion, which of the following dietary items would not be included on the meal trays?
    1. Fruits
    2. Meats
    3. Dairy products
    4. Vegetable entrees

Answer: _____   Rationale: _____

_____

_____

36. If an Islamic client dies, the nurse should be aware of what religious practice?
    1. Last rites are mandatory.
    2. The body is always cremated.
    3. Only relatives and friends may touch the body.
    4. Members of a ritual burial society cleanse the body.

Answer: _____   Rationale: _____

_____

_____

37. If a nurse were to use a nursing diagnosis to relate concerns about spiritual health, which of the following would be used?
    1. Lack of faith
    2. Spiritual distress
    3. Inability to adjust
    4. Religious dilemma

Answer: _____   Rationale: _____

_____

_____

38. Mr. Phillips was recently diagnosed with a malignant tumor. The staff had observed him crying on several occasions, and now he cries as he reads from his Bible. Interventions to help Mr. Phillips cope with his illness would include:
    1. Praying with Mr. Phillips as often as possible
    2. Asking the hospital chaplain to visit him daily
    3. Supporting his use of inner resources by providing time for meditation
    4. Engaging Mr. Phillips in diversional activities to reduce feelings of hopelessness

Answer: _____   Rationale: _____

_____

_____

*Critical Thinking Model for Nursing
Care Plan for Spiritual Distress
Related to Terminal Illness*

39. Imagine that you are Leah, the nurse in the care plan on page 454 of your text. Complete the *Planning phase* of the critical thinking model by writing your answers in the appropriate boxes of the model shown. Think about the following.

- In developing Jose's plan of care, what knowledge did Leah apply?

- In what way might Leah's previous experience assist in developing a plan of care for Jose?

- When developing a plan of care, what intellectual and professional standards were applied?

- What critical thinking attitudes might have been applied to developing Jose's plan?

- How will Leah accomplish the goals?

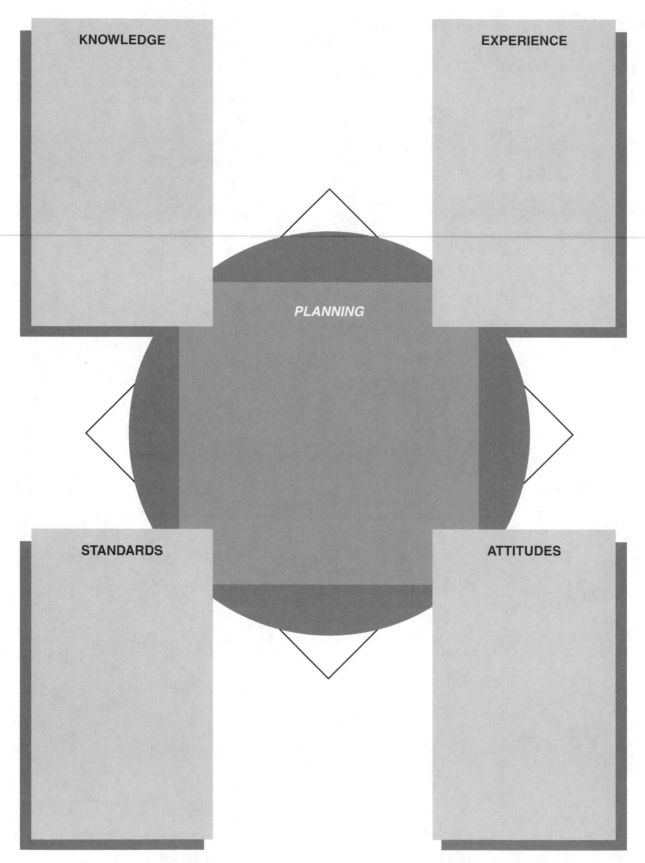

KNOWLEDGE

EXPERIENCE

PLANNING

STANDARDS

ATTITUDES

CHAPTER 29   Critical Thinking Model for Nursing Care Plan for *Spiritual Distress Related to Terminal Illness*

30

The Experience of Loss, Death, and Grief

Preliminary Reading

Chapter 30, pp. 461–484

Comprehensive Understanding

Match the following terms.

1. _____ Maturational losses
2. _____ Situational loss
3. _____ Actual loss
4. _____ Perceived losses
5. _____ Grief
6. _____ Mourning
7. _____ Bereavement
8. _____ Normal grief
9. _____ Complicated grief
10. _____ Chronic grief
11. _____ Delayed grief
12. _____ Excessive grief
13. _____ Exaggerated grief
14. _____ Concomitant grief
15. _____ Anticipatory grief

a. The unconscious process of disengaging before the actual loss or death occurs
b. Captures both grief and mourning, emotional responses and outward behaviors for a person experiencing loss
c. Relationship to the deceased person is not socially sanctioned
d. Very intense emotions of grief
e. Prolonged grief, an inability to move forward after a loss
f. Several significant losses in close succession
g. Emotional response to a loss, which is unique to the individual
h. Distorted grief, usually occurs in individual who has underlying mental illness
i. Suppressing or postponing normal grief responses
j. Dysfunctional, the grieving person has a prolonged or significant time moving forward after a loss
k. Uncomplicated grief, has a known cause and poses no significant disruption in self-concept
l. Culturally influenced rituals that are learned behaviors
m. Form of necessary loss, include all normally expected life changes across the life span
n. Can no longer feel, hear, or know a person or object
o. Sudden, unpredictable external event
p. Are uniquely defined by the person experiencing loss and are less obvious to other people
q. Disenfranchised grief

16. List the phases of the grieving process proposed by each of the theories listed below.

17. Kübler-Ross' five stages of dying:

    a. _____

    b. _____

    c. _____

    d. _____

    e. _____

18. Bowlby's attachment theory, four phases of mourning:

    a. _____

    b. _____

    c. _____

    d. _____

19. Worden's four tasks of mourning:

    a. _____

    b. _____

    c. _____

    d. _____

20. R process model for mourning:

    a. _____

    b. _____

    c. _____

    d. _____

    e. _____

Nursing Knowledge Base

21. Identify the factors that influence loss and grief.

    a. _____

    b. _____

    c. _____

    d. _____

    e. _____

    f. _____

    g. _____

    h. _____

The Nursing Process and Grief

22. Identify the important areas of assessment.

    _____

    _____

Nursing Diagnosis

23. List the nursing diagnoses that pertain to the client experiencing grief, loss, or death.

    a. _____

    b. _____

    c. _____

    d. _____

    e. _____

    f. _____

    g. _____

Planning

24. List three outcomes appropriate for a client who has the nursing diagnosis *powerlessness related to planned cancer therapy secondary to breast cancer.*

    a. _____

    b. _____

    c. _____

Implementation

25. Define *palliative care.* _____

    _____

    _____

    _____

26. List the primary obligations of the collaborative team offering palliative care.

    a. _____

    b. _____

    c. _____

    d. _____

    e. _____

    f. _____

    g. _____

27. Identify the psychosocial care and symptom management that the nurse provides.

    a. _____

    b. _____

    c. _____

    d. _____

    e. _____

    f. _____

    g. _____

    h. _____

    i. _____

Identify the nursing strategies for the family members to facilitate mourning.

28. _____

29. _____

30. _____

31. _____

32. _____

33. _____

34. _____

35. Identify the components of hospice care.

_____

_____

Define the following terms that relate to the care of the client after death.

36. *Organ and tissue donation:*

_____

_____

37. *Autopsy:*

_____

_____

38. *Postmortem care:*

_____

_____

Evaluation

Identify the short- and long-term outcomes that signal a family's recovery from a loss.

39. Short-term:

_____

_____

40. Long-term:

_____

_____

Review Questions

Select the appropriate answer and cite the rationale for choosing that particular answer.

41. Which statement about loss is accurate?
    1. Loss may be maturational, situational, or both.
    2. The degree of stress experienced is unrelated to the type of loss.
    3. Loss is only experienced when there is an actual absence of something valued.
    4. The more an individual has invested in what is lost, the less the feeling of loss.

Answer: _____   Rationale: _____

_____

_____

42. A hospice program emphasizes:
    1. Prolongation of life
    2. Hospital-based care
    3. Palliative treatment and control of symptoms
    4. Curative treatment and alleviation of symptoms

Answer: _____   Rationale: _____

_____

_____

43. Trying questionable and experimental forms of therapy is a behavior that is characteristic of which stage of dying?
    1. Anger
    2. Bargaining
    3. Depression
    4. Acceptance

Answer: _____   Rationale: _____

_____

_____

44. All of the following are crucial needs of the dying client except:
    1. Control of pain
    2. Love and belonging
    3. Freedom from decision making
    4. Preservation of dignity and self-worth

Answer: _____   Rationale: _____

_____

_____

Critical Thinking Model for Nursing Care Plan for Compromised Family Coping

45. Imagine that you are the student nurse in the care plan on page 472 of your text. Complete the *Evaluation phase* of the critical thinking model by writing your answers in the appropriate boxes of the model shown. Think about the following.

    • In evaluating Mr. Stevens' plan of care, what knowledge did you apply?

    • In what way might your previous experience influence your evaluation of Mr. Stevens' care?

    • During evaluation, what intellectual and professional standards were applied to Mr. Stevens' care?

    • In what way do critical thinking attitudes play a role in how you approach evaluation of Mr. Stevens' care?

    • How might you adjust Mr. Stevens' care?

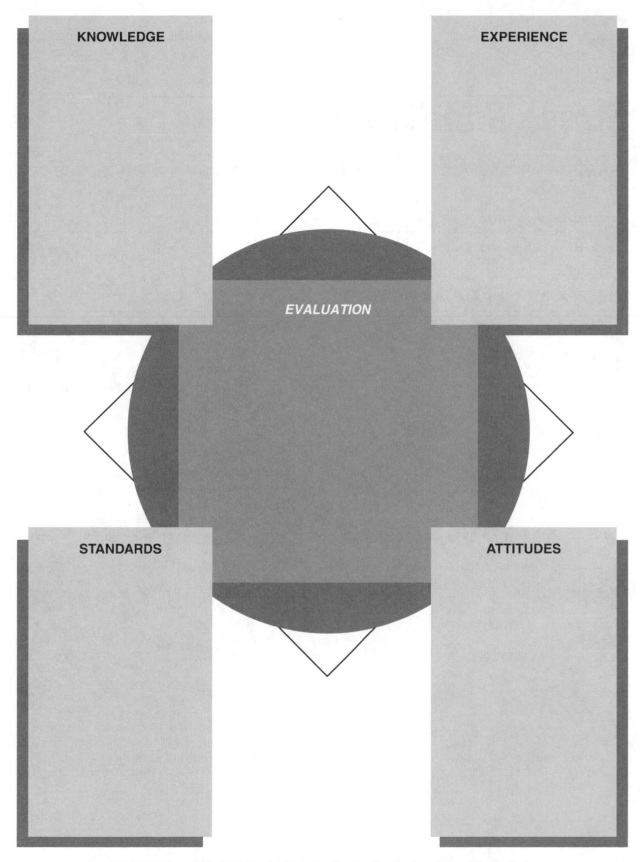

CHAPTER 30   Critical Thinking Model for Nursing Care Plan for *Compromised Family Coping*

31

Stress and Coping

Chapter 31, pp. 485–501

Comprehensive Understanding

Scientific Knowledge Base

Match the following terms.

1. _____ Stress
2. _____ Stressors
3. _____ Appraisal
4. _____ Trauma
5. _____ Fight-or-flight response
6. _____ General adaptation syndrome
7. _____ Endorphins
8. _____ Alarm reaction
9. _____ Resistance stage
10. _____ Exhaustion stage
11. _____ Primary appraisal
12. _____ Secondary appraisal
13. _____ Coping
14. _____ Ego-defense mechanisms
15. _____ Distress
16. _____ Eustress
17. _____ Posttraumatic stress disorder
18. _____ Acute distress disorder
19. _____ Flashbacks
20. _____ Developmental crisis

a. Damaging stress
b. Consists of the person displaying at least three acute dissociative symptoms
c. Disruptive forces operating within or on any system
d. Evaluating an event for its personal meaning
e. Stress that protects health, is motivating
f. A three-stage reaction to stress
g. Arousal of the sympathetic nervous system
h. A trauma occurs and its effects will sometimes last well after the event ends
i. Allow a person to cope with stress indirectly
j. An experience a person is exposed to, through a stimulus or stressor
k. How people interpret the impact of the stressor on themselves
l. Recurrent or intrusive recollections of the event
m. Experienced when symptoms persist beyond the duration of the stressor
n. Act on the mind like morphine and opiates, producing a sense of well-being
o. Rising hormone levels result in increased blood volume, blood glucose levels, epinephrine and norepinephrine amounts, heart rate, blood flow to the muscles, oxygen intake, and mental alertness
p. Occurs when the body is no longer able to resist the effects of the stressor
q. Focuses on possible coping strategies
r. Body stabilizes and responds in the opposite manner to the alarm reaction
s. Person's effort to manage psychological stress
t. Requires new coping skills and occurs as the person moves through life's stages

21. Identify the three structures that control the body's response to a stressor.

    a. _____

    b. _____

    c. _____

Nursing Knowledge Base

Summarize the following models related to stress and coping.

22. Neuman Systems Model:

    _____

    _____

23. Pender's health promotion model:

    _____

    _____

The following factors can potentially be stressors. Give some examples.

24. Situational factors:

    _____

    _____

25. Maturational factors:

    _____

    _____

26. Sociocultural factors:

    _____

    _____

Nursing Process

Assessment

27. Identify three subjective areas that are used to assess a client's level of stress.

    a. _____

    b. _____

    c. _____

28. Identify some objective findings related to stress and coping.

    a. _____

    b. _____

    c. _____

    d. _____

e. _____

f. _____

g. _____

Nursing Diagnosis

29. Identify the defining characteristics of *ineffective coping*.

    _____

    _____

Planning

30. Desirable outcomes for persons experiencing stress are:

    a. _____

    b. _____

    c. _____

    d. _____

Implementation

Health Promotion

31. Identify the primary modes of intervention for stress.

    a. _____

    b. _____

    c. _____

32. Identify the areas about which the nurse can educate clients and their families to reduce stress.

    a. _____

    b. _____

    c. _____

    d. _____

    e. _____

    f. _____

    g. _____

    h. _____

Acute Care

33. Crisis intervention is:

    _____

    _____

Evaluation

34. The desired outcomes for a client recovering from acute stress are:

_____

_____

Review Questions

Select the appropriate answer and cite the rationale for choosing that particular answer.

35. Which definition does not characterize stress?
    1. Efforts to maintain relative constancy within the internal environment
    2. A condition eliciting an intellectual, behavioral, or metabolic response
    3. Any situation in which a nonspecific demand requires an individual to respond or take action
    4. A phenomenon affecting social, psychological, developmental, spiritual, and physiological dimensions

    Answer: _____   Rationale: _____

    _____

    _____

36. Major homeostatic mechanisms are controlled by all of the following except:
    1. Thymus gland
    2. Pituitary gland
    3. Medulla oblongata
    4. Reticular formation

    Answer: _____   Rationale: _____

    _____

    _____

37. Which of the following is an example of the general adaptation syndrome?
    1. Alarm reaction
    2. Inflammatory response
    3. Fight-or-flight response
    4. Ego-defense mechanisms

    Answer: _____   Rationale: _____

    _____

    _____

38. Crisis intervention is a specific measure used for helping a client resolve a particular, immediate stress problem. This approach is based on:
    1. An in-depth analysis of a client's situation
    2. The ability of the nurse to solve the client's problems
    3. Effective communication between the nurse and client
    4. Teaching the client how to use ego-defense mechanisms

    Answer: _____   Rationale: _____

    _____

    _____

Critical Thinking Model for Nursing Care Plan for Caregiver Role Strain

39. Imagine that you are Janet, the nurse in the care plan on page 495 of your text. Complete the *Evaluation phase* of the critical thinking model by writing your answers in the appropriate boxes of the model shown. Think about the following.

    - In evaluating the care of Carl and Evelyn, what knowledge did Janet apply?

    - In what way might Janet's previous experience influence the evaluation of Carl's care?

    - During evaluation, what intellectual and professional standards were applied to Carl's care?

    - In what way do critical thinking attitudes play a role in how Janet approaches the evaluation of Carl's care?

    - How might Janet adjust Carl's care?

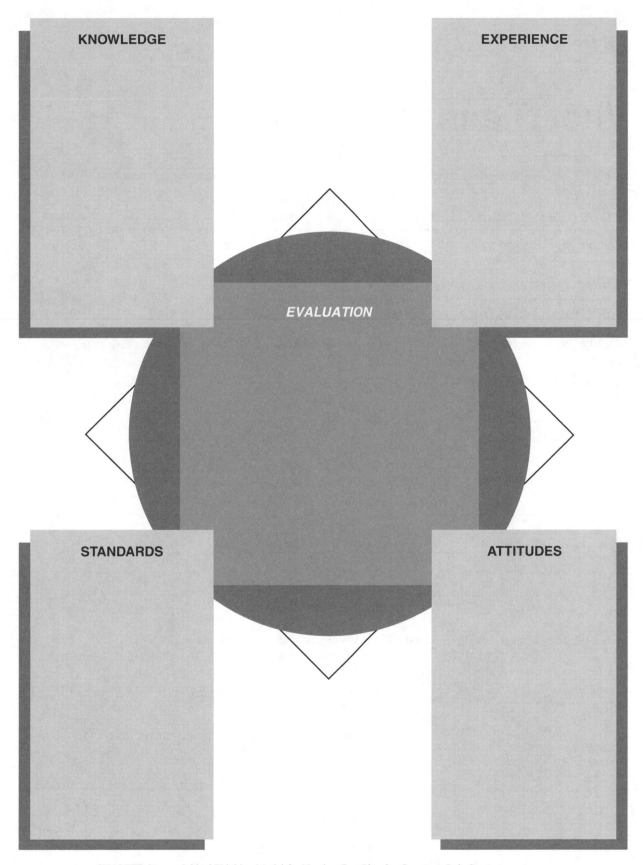

KNOWLEDGE

EXPERIENCE

EVALUATION

STANDARDS

ATTITUDES

CHAPTER 31   Critical Thinking Model for Nursing Care Plan for *Caregiver Role Strain*

32

Vital Signs

Preliminary Reading

Chapter 32, pp. 502–551

Comprehensive Understanding

Guidelines for Taking Vital Signs

Identify the guidelines that assist the nurse with incorporating vital sign measurement into practice.

1. _____
2. _____
3. _____
4. _____
5. _____
6. _____
7. _____
8. _____
9. _____
10. _____
11. _____
12. _____

Body Temperature

Match the following terms that address the physiology of body temperature.

13. _____ Core temperature
14. _____ Thermoregulation
15. _____ Hypothalamus
16. _____ Basal metabolic rate
17. _____ Shivering
18. _____ Nonshivering thermogenesis
19. _____ Radiation
20. _____ Conduction
21. _____ Convection
22. _____ Evaporation

a. Involuntary body response to temperature differences in the body
b. Transfer of heat from the surface of one object to the surface of another without direct contact
c. Transfer of heat away by air movement
d. Transfer of heat energy when a liquid is changed to a gas
e. The heat produced by the body at absolute rest
f. Controls body temperature
g. Vascular brown tissue is metabolized for heat production in the neonate
h. Temperature of the deep tissues
i. Transfer of heat from one object to another with direct contact
j. Mechanisms that regulate the balance between heat lost and heat produced

23. List the six factors that affect body temperature.

    a. _____

    b. _____

    c. _____

    d. _____

    e. _____

    f. _____

Match the following terms that address temperature alterations.

24. _____ Pyrexia
25. _____ Pyrogens
26. _____ Hyperthermia
27. _____ Malignant hyperthermia
28. _____ Heatstroke
29. _____ Heat exhaustion
30. _____ Hypothermia
31. _____ Frostbite

a. Occurs when the body is exposed to subnormal temperatures
b. Body's inability to promote heat loss or reduce heat production
c. A dangerous heat emergency
d. Cold that overwhelms the body's ability to produce heat
e. Fever
f. Hereditary condition of uncontrolled heat production
g. Profuse diaphoresis with excess water and electrolyte loss
h. Bacteria and viruses that elevate body temperature

32. Briefly explain the following patterns of fever.

    a. Sustained: _____

    b. Intermittent: _____

    c. Remittent: _____

    d. Relapsing: _____

Nursing Process and Thermoregulation

Assessment

33. List at least one advantage and one disadvantage of each of the following temperature sites.

    a. oral: _____

    b. tympanic: _____

    c. rectal: _____

    d. axilla: _____

    e. skin: _____

    f. temporal artery: _____

34. State the formulas for the following conversions.

    a. Fahrenheit to Celsius: _____

    b. Celsius to Fahrenheit: _____

Nursing Diagnosis

35. Identify four nursing diagnoses related to thermoregulation.

    a. _____

    b. _____

    c. _____

    d. _____

Planning

36. Identify goals for temperature alterations related to the environment.

    a. Short term: _____

    b. Long term: _____

Implementation

Health Promotion

37. Identify the clients who are at risk for hypothermia.

    _____

Acute Care

38. Explain the differences related to febrile states in each of the following.

    a. Children: _____

    _____

    _____

    b. Hypersensitivities to drugs: _____

    _____

    _____

39. Give an example of each type of fever therapy.

    a. Pharmacological: _____

    _____

    _____

    b. Nonpharmacological: _____

    _____

    _____

40. First aid treatment for heatstroke is:

    _____

    _____

41. Summarize the treatment for hypothermia.

    _____

    _____

Evaluation

42. Identify evaluative measures for temperature alterations.

    _____

    _____

Pulse

43. Identify the two most common pulse rate assessments.

    a. _____

    b. _____

44. Identify the measurement criteria for the following pulse sites.
    a. Temporal:
    b. Carotid:
    c. Apical:
    d. Brachial:
    e. Radial:
    f. Ulnar:
    g. Femoral:
    h. Popliteal:
    i. Posterior tibial:
    j. Dorsalis pedis:

45. List the characteristics to identify when assessing the following.

    a. Radial pulse: _____

    _____

    b. Apical pulse: _____

    _____

46. List the acceptable pulse ranges for the following.
    a. Infant:

    b. Toddler:

    c. Preschooler:

    d. School-age child:

    e. Adolescent:

    f. Adult:

47. Identify seven factors that may increase or decrease the pulse rate.

    a. _____
    b. _____
    c. _____
    d. _____
    e. _____
    f. _____
    g. _____

Define the following terms.

48. *Tachycardia:*

    _____

    _____

49. *Bradycardia:*

    _____

    _____

50. *Pulse deficit:*

    _____

    _____

51. *Dysrhythmia:*

    _____

    _____

Respiration

Define the following terms related to respirations.

52. *Ventilation:* _____

_____

_____

53. *Diffusion:* _____

_____

_____

54. *Perfusion:* _____

_____

_____

55. *Hypoxemia:* _____

_____

_____

Mechanics of Breathing

56. Identify which phase of respirations is active and which is passive.

a. Inspiration: _____

_____

_____

b. Expiration: _____

_____

_____

Assessment of Ventilations

57. Identify factors that influence the character of respirations and the mechanism of each factor.

a. _____
b. _____
c. _____
d. _____
e. _____
f. _____
g. _____
h. _____

58. Identify the acceptable range for respiratory rates for the following age-groups.

a. Newborn: _____
b. Infant: _____
c. Toddler: _____
d. Child: _____
e. Adolescent: _____
f. Adult: _____

Briefly explain the following alterations in breathing patterns.

59. Bradypnea:

_____

60. Tachypnea:

_____

_____

61. Hyperpnea:

_____

_____

62. Apnea:

_____

_____

63. Hyperventilation:

_____

_____

64. Hypoventilation:

_____

_____

65. Cheyne-Stokes:

_____

_____

66. Kussmaul's:

_____

_____

67. Biot's:

_____

_____

68. SaO_2 is:

_____

_____

Blood Pressure

Define the following terms related to blood pressure.

69. *Blood* pressure: _____

_____

_____

70. Systolic: _____

_____

_____

71. Diastolic: _____

_____

_____

72. Pulse *pressure:* _____
_____
_____

Blood pressure is reflected by the following. Briefly explain each.

73. Cardiac output:
_____
_____

74. Peripheral resistance:
_____
_____

75. Blood volume:
_____
_____

76. Viscosity:
_____
_____

77. Elasticity:
_____
_____

78. List eight factors that influence blood pressure.
   a. _____
   b. _____
   c. _____
   d. _____
   e. _____
   f. _____
   g. _____
   h. _____

79. Identify the optimal blood pressure for the following ages.
   a. Newborn: _____
   b. 1 month: _____
   c. 1 year: _____
   d. 6 years: _____
   e. 10 to 13 years: _____
   f. 14 to 17 years: _____
   g. Greater than 18 years: _____

80. Fill in the table below.

Category	Systolic	Diastolic
Normal		
Prehypertension		
Stage 1 hypertension		
Stage 2 hypertension		

81. List the risk factors that are linked to hypertension.
_____
_____

82. Identify the risk factors for orthostatic hypotension.
_____
_____

83. Identify the following Korotkoff sounds.
    First: _____
    Second: _____
    Third: _____
    Fourth: _____
    Fifth: _____

84. Define *auscultatory gap*.
    _____
    _____

Health Promotion and Vital Signs

85. Identify at least one teaching consideration that emphasizes health promotion for the following vital signs.
    a. Temperature: _____
    b. Pulse: _____
    c. Blood pressure: _____
    d. Respirations: _____

86. Identify at least two variations that are unique to the older adult.
    a. Temperature:
       _____
       _____

    b. Pulse rate:
       _____
       _____

    c. Blood pressure:
       _____
       _____

    d. Respirations:
       _____
       _____

Review Questions

Select the appropriate answer and cite the rationale for choosing that particular answer.

87. The skin plays a role in temperature regulation by:
    1. Insulating the body
    2. Constricting blood vessels
    3. Sensing external temperature variations
    4. All of the above

    Answer: _____ Rationale: _____
    _____
    _____

88. The nurse bathes the client who has a fever with cool water. The nurse does this to increase heat loss by means of:
    1. Radiation
    2. Convection
    3. Conduction
    4. Condensation

    Answer: _____ Rationale: _____
    _____
    _____

89. The nurse is assessing a client who she suspects has the nursing diagnosis hyperthermia related to vigorous exercise in hot weather. In reviewing the data the nurse knows that the most important sign of heatstroke is:
    1. Confusion
    2. Excess thirst
    3. Hot, dry skin
    4. Muscle cramps

    Answer: _____ Rationale: _____
    _____
    _____

90. The nurse is auscultating Mrs. McKinnon's blood pressure. The nurse inflates the cuff to 180 mm Hg. At 156 mm Hg, the nurse hears the onset of a tapping sound. At 130 mm Hg the sound changes to a murmur or swishing. At 100 mm Hg the sound momentarily becomes sharper, and at 92 mm Hg it becomes muffled. At 88 mm Hg the sound disappears. Mrs. McKinnon's blood pressure is:
    1. 130/88
    2. 156/88
    3. 180/92
    4. 180/130

    Answer: _____ Rationale: _____
    _____
    _____

33

Health Assessment and Physical Examination

Preliminary Reading

Chapter 33, pp. 552–640

Comprehensive Understanding

Purposes of Physical Examination

1. List the five nursing purposes for performing a physical assessment.

    a. _____

    _____

    b. _____

    _____

    c. _____

    _____

    d. _____

    _____

    e. _____

    _____

Skills of Physical Assessment

2. List six principles to facilitate accurate inspection of body parts.

    a. _____

    _____

    b. _____

    _____

    c. _____

    _____

    d. _____

    _____

    e. _____

    _____

    f. _____

    _____

3. Define *palpation*. _____

_____

_____

4. Identify the information obtained through percussion. _____

_____

_____

5. Define *auscultation*. _____

_____

_____

Preparation for Examination

6. Proper preparation for examination should include:

   a. _____

   b. _____

   c. _____

   d. _____

   e. _____

7. List seven variations in the nurse's individual style that are appropriate when examining children.

   a. _____

   _____

   b. _____

   _____

   c. _____

   _____

   d. _____

   _____

   e. _____

   _____

   f. _____

   _____

   g. _____

   _____

8. List seven variations in the nurse's individual style that are appropriate when examining older adults.

   a. _____

   _____

   b. _____

   _____

   c. _____

   _____

d. _____

e. _____

_____

f. _____

_____

g. _____

_____

General Survey

List at least 12 specific observations of the client's general appearance and behavior that should be reviewed.

9. _____

10. _____

11. _____

12. _____

13. _____

14. _____

15. _____

16. _____

17. _____

18. _____

19. _____

20. _____

21. Identify some signs of client abuse.

   _____

   _____

22. Identify the questions related to the following acronym.

   C _____

   A _____

   G _____

   E _____

23. List three actions that should be taken to ensure accurate weight measurement of a hospitalized client.

   a. _____

   b. _____

   c. _____

Skin, Hair, and Nails

24. List the risks for skin lesions in the hospitalized client.

_____

_____

Define the following terms.

25. *Melanoma:* _____

_____

26. *Pigmentation:* _____

_____

27. For each skin color variation, identify the mechanism that produces color change, common causes of the variation, and the optimal sites for assessment (see Table 1).

_____

_____

_____

_____

28. Identify two conditions that are due to excessive dryness.

    a. _____

    b. _____

Define the following terms.

29. *Indurated:* _____

_____

_____

30. *Turgor:* _____

_____

_____

31. *Edema:* _____

_____

_____

32. *Senile keratosis:* _____

_____

_____

33. *Cherry angiomas:* _____

_____

_____

Briefly describe the following primary skin lesions, and give an example of each.

34. Macule: _____

_____

_____

35. Papule: _____

_____

_____

36. Nodule: _____

_____

_____

37. Tumor: _____

_____

_____

38. Wheal: _____

_____

_____

39. Vesicle: _____

_____

_____

40. Pustule: _____

_____

_____

41. Ulcer: _____

_____

_____

42. Atrophy:_____

_____

_____

43. Name the three types of lice.

  a. _____

  b. _____

  c. _____

Briefly describe the following abnormalities of the nail bed.

44. Clubbing: _____

_____

_____

45. Beau's lines: _____

_____

_____

46. Koilonychia: _____

_____

_____

47. Splinter hemorrhages: _____

_____

_____

48. Paronychia: _____

_____

_____

Head and Neck

Define the following head abnormalities.

49. Hydrocephalus: _____

_____

50. Acromegaly: _____

_____

Define the following common eye and visual abnormalities.

51. Hyperopia: _____

_____

52. Myopia: _____

_____

53. Presbyopia: _____

_____

54. Retinopathy: _____

_____

55. Strabismus: _____

_____

56. Cataracts: _____

_____

57. Glaucoma: _____

_____

58. Macular degeneration: _____

_____

59. Examination of the eye includes assessment of five areas. Name them.

a. _____

b. _____

c. _____

d. _____

e. _____

60. Identify the structures of the external eye that you would inspect.

a. _____

b. _____

c. _____

d. _____

e. _____

f. _____

g. _____

Define the following terms related to the external eye.

61. *Exophthalmos:* _____

_____

_____

62. *Ectropion:* _____

_____

_____

63. *Entropion:* _____

_____

_____

64. *Conjunctivitis:* _____

_____

_____

65. *Arcus senilis:* _____

_____

_____

66. *PERRLA:* _____

_____

_____

67. Identify the internal eye structures that you would examine with an ophthalmoscope.

_____

_____

68. Identify the three parts of the ear canal.

a. _____

b. _____

c. _____

69. List the steps of hearing (sound traveling through the ear by air and bone conduction).

a. _____

b. _____

c. _____

d. _____

e. _____

70. Identify the three types of hearing loss.

a. _____

b. _____

c. _____

Explain the following tuning fork tests.

71. Weber's test: _____

_____

72. Rinne test: _____

_____

Define the following terms that relate to the nose.

73. Excoriation: _____

_____

74. *Polyps:* _____

_____

Define the following terms that relate to the oral cavity.

75. *Leukoplakia:* _____

_____

76. *Varicosities:* _____

_____

77. *Exostosis:* _____

_____

78. Assessment of the neck includes: _____

_____

Thorax and Lungs

79. Define *vocal* or *tactile fremitus.*

_____

_____

Define the following normal breath sounds heard over the posterior thorax.

80. *Vesicular:* _____

_____

81. *Bronchovesicular:* _____

82. *Bronchial:* _____

_____

83. Complete the following table of adventitious breath sounds.

Sound	Site Auscultated	Cause	Character
Crackles			
Rhonchi (sonorous wheeze)			
Wheezes (sibilant wheeze)			
Pleural friction rub			

Heart

Explain the following terms related to assessment of the heart.

84. Point of maximal impulse:

_____
_____

85. S_1: _____
_____
_____

86. S_2: _____
_____
_____

87. S_3: _____
_____
_____

88. S_4: _____
_____
_____

Identify the appropriate sites for inspection and palpation of the following.

89. Angle of Louis: _____

_____

90. Aortic area: _____

_____

91. Pulmonic area: _____

_____

92. Second pulmonic area: _____

_____

93. Tricuspid area: _____

_____

94. Mitral area: _____

_____

95. Epigastric area: _____

_____

96. Define *murmur*. _____

_____

97. List the six factors to assess when a murmur is detected.

  a. _____

  b. _____

  c. _____

  d. _____

  e. _____

  f. _____

Vascular System

Explain the following conditions that are related to the vascular system.

98. Syncope: _____ _____

_____

99. Occlusion: _____

_____

100. Atherosclerosis: _____

_____

101. Bruit: _____

_____

102. Explain the steps the nurse would use to assess venous pressure.

  a. _____

  _____

  _____

  b. _____

  _____

  _____

  c. _____

  _____

  _____

  d. _____

  _____

  e. _____

  _____

103. Complete the following table by listing the signs of venous and arterial insufficiency.

Assessment criterion	Venous	Arterial
Color		
Temperature		
Pulse		
Edema		
Skin changes		

104. Describe how you would assess for phlebitis.

_____
_____
_____
_____

Breasts

105. The American Cancer Society (2006) recommends the following guidelines for early detection of breast cancer.

a. _____
_____

b. _____
_____

c. _____
_____

d. _____
_____

e. _____
_____

f. _____
_____

Define the following terms.

106. *Metastasize:* _____
_____
_____
_____

107. *Benign (fibrocystic) breast disease:* _____
_____
_____
_____

Abdomen

Define the following terms related to the abdomen.

108. *Striae:* _____
_____
_____

109. *Hernias:* _____
_____
_____

110. *Distention:* _____

_____

_____

111. *Peristalsis:* _____

_____

_____

112. *Paralytic ileus:* _____

_____

_____

113. *Borborygmi:* _____

_____

_____

114. *Rebound tenderness:* _____

_____

_____

115. *Aneurysm:* _____

_____

_____

Female Genitalia and Reproductive Tract

Define the following terms related to the female genitourinary tract.

116. *Chancres:* _____

_____

_____

117. *Papanicolaou specimen:* _____

_____

_____

Male Genitalia

118. Identify the common symptoms of testicular cancer.

_____

_____

_____

_____

_____

Rectum and Anus

119. The purpose of digital examination is:

_____

_____

_____

_____

Musculoskeletal System

Define the following terms.

120. *Kyphosis:* _____

_____

121. *Lordosis:* _____

_____

122. *Scoliosis:* _____

_____

123. *Osteoporosis:* _____

_____

124. *Goniometer:* _____

_____

Identify the correct range of motion for the following terms.

125. Flexion: _____

126. Extension: _____

127. Hyperextension: _____

128. Pronation: _____

129. Supination: _____

130. Abduction: _____

131. Adduction: _____

132. Internal rotation: _____

133. External rotation: _____

134. Eversion: _____

135. Inversion: _____

136. Dorsiflexion: _____

137. Plantar flexion: _____

Define the following terms related to muscle tone and strength.

138. *Hypertonicity:* _____

_____

139. *Hypotonicity:* _____

_____

140. *Atrophied:* _____

_____

Neurological System

141. The purpose of the Mini-Mental State Examination is to measure:

_____

_____

_____

142. Delirium is characterized by:

_____

_____

_____

143. The purpose of the Glasgow coma scale is to:

_____

_____

_____

144. Briefly explain the two types of aphasia.

a. Receptive:

_____

_____

_____

b. Expressive:

_____

_____

_____

145. Identify the 12 cranial nerves.

a. _____

b. _____

c. _____

d. _____

e. _____

f. _____

g. _____

h. _____

i. _____

j. _____

k. _____

l. _____

146. The sensory pathways of the central nervous system conduct what type of sensations?

_____

147. Identify the functions of the sensory nerves that you would assess.

_____

_____

148. Identify the functions of the cerebellum.

_____

_____

149. Identify the two types of normal reflexes.

a. _____

b. _____

Review Questions

Select the appropriate answer and cite the rationale for choosing that particular answer.

150. The component that should receive the highest priority before a physical examination is:
    1. Preparation of the equipment
    2. Preparation of the environment
    3. Physical preparation of the client
    4. Psychological preparation of the client

Answer: _____   Rationale: _____

_____

_____

151. The nurse assesses the skin turgor of the client by:
    1. Inspecting the buccal mucosa with a penlight
    2. Palpating the skin with the dorsum of the hand
    3. Grasping a fold of skin on the back of the forearm and releasing
    4. Pressing the skin for 5 seconds, releasing, and noting each centimeter of depth

Answer: _____   Rationale: _____

_____

_____

152. While examining Mr. Parker, the nurse notes a circumscribed elevation of skin filled with serous fluid on his upper lip. The lesion is 0.4 cm in diameter. This type of lesion is called a:
    1. Macule
    2. Nodule
    3. Vesicle
    4. Pustule

Answer: _____   Rationale: _____

_____

_____

153. When assessing the client's thorax, the nurse should:
    1. Complete the left side and then the right side
    2. Compare symmetrical areas from side to side
    3. Begin with the posterior lobes on the right side
    4. Change the position of the stethoscope between inspiration and expiration

Answer: _____ Rationale: _____

_____

_____

154. In a client with pneumonia, the nurse hears high-pitched, continuous musical sounds over the bronchi on expiration. These sounds are called:
    1. Rhonchi
    2. Crackles
    3. Wheezes
    4. Friction rubs

Answer: _____ Rationale: _____

_____

_____

155. The second heart sound (S_2) occurs when:
    1. Systole begins
    2. There is rapid ventricular filling
    3. The mitral and tricuspid valves close
    4. The aortic and pulmonic valves close

Answer: _____ Rationale: _____

_____

_____

34

Infection Prevention and Control

Preliminary Reading

Chapter 34, pp. 641–685

Comprehensive Understanding

Scientific Knowledge Base

Match the following terms that are related to the infectious process.

1. _____ Pathogen
2. _____ Colonization
3. _____ Infectious disease
4. _____ Communicable disease
5. _____ Symptomatic
6. _____ Asymptomatic
7. _____ Dose
8. _____ Virulence
9. _____ Host resistance
10. _____ Immunocompromised
11. _____ Reservoir
12. _____ Carriers
13. _____ Aerobic bacteria
14. _____ Anaerobic bacteria
15. _____ Bacteriostasis
16. _____ Bactericidal

a. Susceptibility of the host
b. Persons who show no symptoms of illness but who have the pathogens that are transferred to others
c. Prevention of the growth and reproduction of bacteria by cold temperatures
d. Infectious agent
e. Bacteria that require oxygen for survival
f. Having an impaired immune system
g. Clinical signs and symptoms of an illness
h. Bacteria that thrive with little or no free oxygen
i. A temperature or chemical that destroys bacteria
j. A place where a pathogen survives
k. Sufficient number of organisms
l. An infectious disease that is transmitted directly from one person to another
m. Organism that multiplies but does not cause an infection
n. An illness with no clinical signs or symptoms
o. Illnesses such as viral meningitis or pneumonia
p. Ability to survive in the host or outside the body

17. Development of an infection occurs in a cycle that depends on the following elements.

a. _____
b. _____
c. _____
d. _____
e. _____
f. _____

Explain the most common modes of transmission.

18. Direct: _____

19. Indirect: _____

20. Droplet: _____

21. Airborne: _____

22. Vehicles: _____

23. Vector: _____

24. Define *susceptibility*. _____

_____

The Infection Process

25. Describe the two types of infections.

    a. Localized: _____

       _____

    b. Systemic: _____

Explain the normal body defenses against infection.

26. Normal flora: _____

_____

_____

27. Body system defenses: _____

_____

_____

28. Inflammation: _____

_____

_____

Acute inflammation is an immediate response to cellular injury. Explain each briefly.

29. Vascular and cellular responses: _____

_____

_____

30. Inflammatory exudate: _____

_____

_____

31. Tissue repair: _____

_____

_____

Define the following types of health care–associated infections (nosocomial).

32. Exogenous: _____

_____

_____

33. Endogenous: _____

_____

_____

34. Identify the sites and causes of health care–associated infections, and give an example of each.

    a. _____

       _____

    b. _____

       _____

    c. _____

       _____

    d. _____

       _____

The Nursing Process in Infection Control Assessment

The following risks need to be assessed in the adult. Give an example of each.

35. Age: _____

_____

_____

36. Lifestyle—high-risk behaviors: _____

_____

_____

37. Occupation: _____

_____

_____

38. Diagnostic procedures: _____

_____

_____

39. Hereditary: _____

_____

_____

40. Travel history: _____

_____

_____

41. Trauma: _____

_____

_____

42. Nutrition: _____

_____

_____

43. Fill in the following table.

Laboratory Value	Normal (Adult) Values	Indication of Infection
WBC count		
Erythrocyte sedimentation rate		
Iron level		
Cultures of urine and blood		
Cultures and Gram stain of wound, sputum, and throat		
Neutrophils		
Lymphocytes		
Monocytes		
Eosinophils		
Basophils		

Nursing Diagnosis

44. Identify some common nursing diagnoses that apply to clients at risk or who have an actual infection.

   a. _____

   b. _____

   c. _____

   d. _____

   e. _____

   f. _____

Planning

45. List four common goals for the client with an actual or potential risk for infection.

   a. _____
   _____

   b. _____
   _____

   c. _____
   _____

   d. _____
   _____

Implementation

Health Promotion

46. List the ways a nurse can teach clients and their families to prevent an infection from developing and/or spreading.

   a. _____
   _____

   b. _____
   _____

   c. _____
   _____

   d. _____
   _____

   e. _____
   _____

   f. _____
   _____

The nurse follows certain principles and procedures to prevent infection and to control its spread. Briefly explain each one.

47. Concept of asepsis:

   _____
   _____

48. Medical asepsis:

   _____
   _____

Explain the following methods of controlling or eliminating infectious agents.

49. Proper cleansing: _____
   _____
   _____

50. Disinfection: _____
   _____
   _____

51. Sterilization of objects: _____
   _____
   _____

52. Control or elimination of reservoirs: _____
   _____
   _____

53. Control of portals of exit: _____
   _____
   _____

54. Control of transmission: _____
   _____
   _____

55. Define *hand hygiene*. _____
   _____
   _____

The isolation guidelines of the Centers for Disease Control and Prevention contain a two-tiered approach. Explain each one.

56. Standard precautions (Tier 1):

   _____
   _____

57. Transmission categories (Tier 2):

   _____
   _____

Identify the rationale for the following personal protective equipment.

58. Gowns: _____

_____

59. Masks: _____

60. Protective eyewear: _____

_____

61. Gloves: _____

_____

62. Identify some common waste materials that are considered infectious or medical waste.

a. _____

b. _____

c. _____

d. _____

e. _____

63. List the nine responsibilities of the infection control professional.

a. _____

_____

b. _____

_____

c. _____

_____

d. _____

_____

e. _____

_____

f. _____

_____

g. _____

_____

h. _____

_____

i. _____

_____

64. Identify clinical situations in which the nurse would use surgical asepsis.

a. _____

_____

b. _____

_____

c. _____

_____

List the seven principles of surgical asepsis.

65. _____

_____

66. _____

_____

67. _____

_____

68. _____

_____

69. _____

_____

70. _____

_____

71. _____

_____

72. List in order the steps for performing a sterile procedure.

a. _____

_____

b. _____

_____

c. _____

_____

d. _____

_____

e. _____

_____

f. _____

_____

g. _____

_____

h. _____

Evaluation

73. The expected outcome is the absence of signs and symptoms of infection. List some ways the nurse can monitor the client.

a. _____

_____

b. _____

_____

c. _____

_____

d. _____

_____

Review Questions

Select the appropriate answer and cite the rationale for choosing that particular answer.

74. Which of the following is not an element in the development or chain of infection?
    1. Means of transmission
    2. Infectious agent or pathogen
    3. Formation of immunoglobulin
    4. Reservoir for pathogen growth

Answer: _____ Rationale: _____
_____
_____

75. The severity of a client's illness will depend on all of the following except:
    1. Incubation period
    2. Extent of infection
    3. Susceptibility of the host
    4. Pathogenicity of the microorganism

Answer: _____ Rationale: _____
_____
_____

76. Which of the following best describes an iatrogenic infection?
    1. It results from a diagnostic or therapeutic procedure.
    2. It results from an extended infection of the urinary tract.
    3. It involves an incubation period of 3 to 4 weeks before it can be detected.
    4. It occurs when clients are infected with their own organisms as a result of immunodeficiency.

Answer: _____ Rationale: _____
_____
_____

77. The nurse sets up a nonbarrier sterile field on the client's over-bed table. In which of the following instances is the field contaminated?
    1. Sterile saline solution is spilled on the field.
    2. The nurse, who has a cold, wears a double mask.
    3. Sterile objects are kept within a 1-inch border of the field.
    4. The nurse keeps the top of the table above his or her waist.

Answer: _____ Rationale: _____
_____
_____

78. When a client on respiratory isolation must be transported to another part of the hospital, the nurse:
    1. Places a mask on the client before leaving the room
    2. Obtains a health care provider's order to prohibit the client from being transported
    3. Instructs the client to cover his or her mouth and nose with a tissue when coughing or sneezing
    4. Advises other health team members to wear masks and gowns when coming in contact with the client

Answer: _____ Rationale: _____
_____
_____

35

Medication Administration

Preliminary Reading

Chapter 35, pp. 686–770

Comprehensive Understanding

Scientific Knowledge Base

1. Briefly summarize the roles of the following in relation to the regulation of medications.

   a. Federal government:

   _____

   b. State government:

   _____

   c. Health care institutions:

   _____

   d. Nurse Practice Act:

   _____

A single medication may have three different names. Define each one.

2. Chemical name: _____

3. Generic name: _____

4. Trade name: _____

5. A medication classification indicates: _____

6. The form of the medication determines its: _____

7. Pharmacokinetics is: _____

8. Absorption is: _____

9. Identify the factors that influence drug absorption.

   a. _____
   b. _____
   c. _____
   d. _____
   e. _____

10. Identify the factors that affect the rate and extent of medication distribution.

    a. _____

    b. _____

    c. _____

11. Explain the role of metabolism.

    _____

    _____

12. Identify the primary organ for drug excretion, and explain what happens if this organ function declines.

    _____

    _____

Define the following predicted or unintended effects of drugs.

13. Therapeutic effects: _____

    _____

14. Side effects: _____

    _____

15. Adverse effects: _____

    _____

16. Toxic effects: _____

    _____

17. Idiosyncratic reactions: _____

    _____

18. Allergic reactions: _____

    _____

19. Anaphylactic reactions: _____

    _____

20. A medication interaction is: _____

    _____

21. A synergistic effect is: _____

    _____

Define the following terms related to medication dose responses.

22. Serum concentration: _____

    _____

23. Peak concentration: _____

    _____

24. Serum half-life: _____

    _____

Explain the following time intervals of medication actions.

25. Onset of drug action:_____

    _____

26. Peak action: _____

    _____

27. Trough: _____

    _____

28. Duration of action:_____

    _____

29. Plateau: _____

    _____

30. Identify the three types of oral routes.

    a. _____

    b. _____

    c. _____

31. List the four major sites for parenteral injections.

    a. _____

    b. _____

    c. _____

    d. _____

Define the following advanced techniques of medication administration.

32. Epidural: _____

    _____

33. Intrathecal: _____

    _____

34. Intraosseous: _____

    _____

35. Intraperitoneal: _____

    _____

36. Intrapleural: _____

    _____

37. Intraarterial: _____

    _____

38. Intracardiac:_____

    _____

39. Intraarticular: _____

    _____

40. Identify five methods for applying medications to mucous membranes.

    a. _____

    b. _____

    c. _____

    d. _____

    e. _____

41. Identify the benefit of the inhalation route.

    _____

42. Identify the three types of measurement used in medication therapy.

    a. _____

    b. _____

    c. _____

43. A solution is: _____

    _____

Nursing Knowledge Base

44. Write out the formula used to determine the correct dose when preparing solid or liquid forms of medications. _____

    _____

    _____

45. Write out the formula applied to accurately calculate pediatric dosages. _____

    _____

    _____

Briefly explain the common types of medication orders.

46. Verbal: _____

47. Standing or routine: _____

48. prn: _____

49. Single (one-time): _____

50. STAT: _____

51. Now: _____

52. List the medication distribution systems.

    a. _____

    b. _____

53. Identify the common medication errors that can cause client harm.

    _____

    _____

54. Identify the process for medication reconciliation.

    a. _____

    b. _____

    c. _____

    d. _____

Critical Thinking

55. List the six rights of medication administration, and briefly explain each one.

    a. _____

    _____

    b. _____

    _____

    _____

    c. _____

    _____

    d. _____

    _____

    _____

    e. _____

    _____

    f. _____

    _____

    _____

56. Briefly summarize *The Patient Care Partnership* related to medication administration.

    a. _____

    _____

    _____

    b. _____

    _____

    _____

    c. _____

    _____

    d. _____

    _____

    _____

    e. _____

    _____

f. _____
   _____
   _____
g. _____
   _____
   _____
h. _____
   _____
   _____

Nursing Process and Medication Administration

Assessment

57. Identify the areas the nurse needs to assess to determine the need for and potential response to medication therapy.
    a. _____
    b. _____
    c. _____
    d. _____
    e. _____
    f. _____
    g. _____
    h. _____
    i. _____

Nursing Diagnosis

Identify potential nursing diagnoses used during the administration of medications.

58. _____
59. _____
60. _____
61. _____
62. _____
63. _____
64. _____
65. _____
66. _____

Planning

67. Identify the outcomes for a client with newly diagnosed type 2 diabetes
    a. _____
    b. _____
    c. _____
    d. _____

Implementation

68. Identify factors that can influence the client's compliance with the medication regimen.
    _____
    _____
    _____

69. Identify the components of medication orders.
    a. _____
    b. _____
    c. _____
    d. _____
    e. _____
    f. _____
    g. _____

70. The recording of medication includes:
    _____
    _____

71. Explain the two types of polypharmacy.
    a. Rational: _____
       _____
       _____
    b. Irrational: _____
       _____
       _____

Evaluation

72. Identify two goals for safe and effective medication administration.
    a. _____
    b. _____

Oral Administration

73. Identify the precautions to take when administering any oral preparation.

    a. _____

    b. _____

    c. _____

    d. _____

    e. _____

    f. _____

    g. _____

    h. _____

    i. _____

    j. _____

    k. _____

    l. _____

74. Identify the guidelines to ensure safe administration of transdermal or topical medications.

    a. _____

    b. _____

    c. _____

    d. _____

    e. _____

    f. _____

75. The most common form of nasal instillation is:_____

76. List four principles for administering eye instillations.

    a. _____

    b. _____

    c. _____

    d. _____

77. Failure to instill ear drops at room temperature causes:

    a. _____

    b. _____

    c. _____

78. Vaginal medications are available as: _____
_____

79. Rectal suppositories are used for: _____

80. Explain the following types of inhalation inhalers:

    a. Metered-dose inhalers (MDIs): _____
    _____

    b. Dry power inhalers (DPIs): _____
    _____

Identify the aseptic techniques to use to prevent an infection during an injection.

81. _____

82. _____

83. _____

84. _____

85. Identify the factors that must be considered when selecting a needle for an injection.

    a. _____
       _____
       _____

    b. _____
       _____
       _____

86. Describe each of the following.

    a. Ampule: _____
       _____
       _____

    b. Vial:_____
       _____
       _____

87. List the three principles to follow when mixing medications from two vials.

    a. _____
       _____
       _____

    b. _____
       _____
       _____
       _____

    c. _____
       _____
       _____

88. Insulin is classified by:

    _____
    _____

89. Identify the principles when mixing two kinds of insulin in the same syringe.

    a. _____
    b. _____
    c. _____
    d. _____
    e. _____
    f. _____

90. List the techniques used to minimize client discomfort that is associated with injections.

    a. _____
    b. _____
    c. _____
    d. _____
    e. _____
    f. _____
    g. _____

91. Identify the best sites for subcutaneous (Sub-Q) injections.

    _____
    _____
    _____

92. What is the maximum amount of water-soluble medication given by the Sub-Q route?

    _____

93. What angles should be utilized when administering a Sub-Q injection?

    _____
    _____

94. What is the angle of insertion for an intramuscular (IM) injection?

    _____

95. Indicate the maximum volume of medication for IM injection in each of the following groups.

    a. Well-developed adult: _____
       _____

    b. Older children, older adults, or thin adults: _____
       _____

    c. Older infants and small children: _____
       _____

Describe the characteristics of the following intramuscular injection sites.

96. Vastus lateralis: _____
    _____
    _____

97. Ventrogluteal: _____
    _____
    _____

98. Deltoid: _____
    _____
    _____

99. Explain the rationale for the Z-track method in IM injections.

    _____
    _____

100. Explain the rationale for intradermal injections.

    _____
    _____

101. List the methods a nurse can use to administer medications intravenously.

    a. _____
    b. _____
    c. _____

102. Identify the advantages of the intravenous (IV) route of administration.

    a. _____
    b. _____
    c. _____

103. The disadvantages of IV bolus medications are:

    a. _____
    b. _____

104. List the advantages of using volume-controlled infusions.

    a. _____
    b. _____
    c. _____

105. What is a piggyback set?

    _____

106. What is a tandem setup?

    _____

107. What is a volume-control administration set?

    _____

108. What is a miniinfusion pump?

    _____

109. List the three advantages of using intermittent venous access devices.

    a. _____
    b. _____
    c. _____

Review Questions

Select the appropriate answer and cite the rationale for choosing that particular answer.

110. The study of how drugs enter the body, reach their sites of action, are metabolized, and exit from the body is called:
    1. Pharmacology
    2. Pharmacopoeia
    3. Pharmacokinetics
    4. Biopharmaceutica

Answer: _____   Rationale: _____

_____

111. Which statement correctly characterizes drug absorption?
    1. Most drugs must enter the systemic circulation to have a therapeutic effect.
    2. Oral medications are absorbed more quickly when administered with meals.
    3. Mucous membranes are relatively impermeable to chemicals, making absorption slow.
    4. Drugs administered subcutaneously are absorbed more quickly than those injected intramuscularly.

Answer: _____   Rationale: _____

_____

112. The onset of drug action is the time it takes for a drug to:
    1. Produce a response
    2. Accelerate the cellular process
    3. Reach its highest effective concentration
    4. Produce blood serum concentration and maintenance

Answer: _____   Rationale: _____

_____

113. Which of the following is not a parenteral route of administration?
    1. Buccal
    2. Intradermal
    3. Intramuscular
    4. Subcutaneous

Answer: _____   Rationale: _____

_____

114. Using the body surface area formula, what dose of drug X should a child who weighs 12 kg (body surface area = 0.54 m^2) receive if the normal adult dose of drug X is 300 mg?
    1. 50 mg
    2. 90 mg
    3. 100 mg
    4. 200 mg

Answer: _____   Rationale: _____

_____

115. The nurse is preparing an insulin injection in which both regular and NPH will be mixed. Into which vial should the nurse inject air first?
    1. The vial of regular insulin
    2. The vial of NPH
    3. Either vial, as long as modified insulin is drawn up first

4. Neither vial; it is not necessary to put air into vials before withdrawing medication

Answer: _____   Rationale: _____

_____

_____

36

Complementary and Alternative Therapies

Preliminary Reading

Chapter 36 pp. 771–785

Comprehensive Understanding

Describe the difference between the following terms.

1. Complementary therapies:

   _____

   _____

2. Alternative therapies:

   _____

   _____

3. Explain the following alternative medical systems.

   a. Acupuncture: _____

   b. Ayurveda: _____

   c. Homeopathic medicine: _____

   d. Latin American practices: _____

   e. Native American practices: _____

   f. Naturopathic medicine: _____

   g. Traditional Chinese medicine (TCM): _____

4. Explain the following biologically based therapies.

   a. The "Zone": _____

   b. Macrobiotic diet: _____

   c. Orthomolecular medicine: _____

   d. European phytomedicines: _____

   e. Traditional Chinese herbal medicines: _____

   f. Ayurvedic herbs: _____

5. Explain the following manipulative and body-based methods.

   a. Acupressure: _____
_____
_____

   b. Chiropractic medicine: _____
_____
_____

   c. Feldenkrais method: _____
_____
_____

   d. Tai chi: _____
_____
_____

   e. Massage therapy: _____
_____
_____

   f. Simple touch: _____
_____
_____
_____

6. Explain the following mind-body interventions.

   a. Art therapy: _____
_____
_____

   b. Biofeedback: _____
_____
_____

   c. Dance therapy: _____
_____
_____

   d. Breathwork: _____
_____
_____

   e. Guided imagery: _____
_____
_____
_____

   f. Meditation: _____
_____
_____
_____

   g. Music therapy: _____
_____
_____

   h. Healing intention: _____
_____
_____

   i. Psychotherapy: _____
_____
_____

   j. Yoga: _____
_____
_____
_____

7. Explain the following energy therapies.

   a. Biofield: _____
_____
_____

   b. Bioelectromagnetic-based therapies:
_____
_____
_____

Nursing-Accessible Therapies

8. Explain the cascade of changes that are associated with the stress response.
_____

9. The relaxation response is:
_____
_____

10. Progressive relaxation training helps to:
_____
_____

11. Passive relaxation involves teaching:
_____
_____

12. The outcome of relaxation therapy is: _____
_____

13. Identify the limitations of relaxation therapy.
_____
_____

14. Meditation is: _____
_____

15. Identify the indications for the use of meditation. _____
_____

16. Identify the limitations of meditation.
_____
_____

17. Imagery is: _____
_____

18. Creative visualization is: _____
_____

19. Identify the clinical applications of imagery.
_____
_____

Training-Specific Therapies

20. Biofeedback is: _____
_____
_____
_____

21. Identify some clinical applications for the use of biofeedback:
_____
_____

22. Identify the limitations of biofeedback.
_____
_____

23. Therapeutic touch is:
_____
_____

24. Therapeutic touch consists of five phases. Explain each one.
a. Centering: _____
_____
_____
_____

b. Assessment: _____
_____
_____
_____

c. Unruffling: _____
_____
_____
_____

d. Treatment: _____
_____
_____
_____

e. Evaluation: _____
_____
_____
_____

25. Identify the clinical applications of therapeutic touch.
_____
_____

26. Identify the limitations of therapeutic touch.
_____
_____

27. Chiropractic therapy is:
_____
_____

28. Identify the clinical applications of chiropractic therapy.
_____
_____

29. Identify the limitations of chiropractic therapy.
_____
_____

30. Traditional Chinese medicine is:
_____
_____

31. Explain the following terms related to TCM:
a. Yin and yang: _____
b. *Qi:* _____
c. Meridians: _____
d. Acupoints: _____
e. Acupuncture: _____

32. Describe the clinical applications of acupuncture.

_____

_____

33. Identify the limitations of acupuncture.

_____

_____

34. Herbal therapy is:

_____

_____

35. Identify the clinical applications of herbal therapy.

_____

_____

36. Identify the limitations of herbal therapy.

_____

_____

Nursing Role in Complementary and Alternative Therapies

37. Explain what the integrative medicine approach is.

_____

_____

Review Questions

Select the appropriate answer and cite the rationale for choosing that particular answer.

38. Clients choose to use unconventional therapy because:
    1. They are willing to pay more to feel better
    2. They are dissatisfied with conventional medicine
    3. They want religious approval for the remedies they use
    4. It is now widely accepted by the Food and Drug Administration

Answer: _____   Rationale: _____

_____

_____

39. The Dietary Supplement and Health Education Act states that:
    1. The Food and Drug Administration must evaluate all herbal therapies
    2. Herbs, vitamins, and minerals may be sold with their therapeutic advantages listed on the label
    3. Herbs, vitamins, and minerals may be sold as long as no therapeutic claims are made on the label
    4. In conjunction with the Food and Drug Administration, all supplements are considered safe for use

Answer: _____   Rationale: _____

_____

_____

40. Which of the following steps should nurses take to be better informed about alternative therapies?
    1. Review herb manufacturers' literature on specific herbs
    2. Read current books and magazines on alternative therapies
    3. Familiarize themselves with general principles of phytotherapy
    4. Familiarize themselves with recent case studies on alternative therapies

Answer: _____   Rationale: _____

_____

_____

37

Activity and Exercise

Preliminary Reading

Chapter 37, pp. 786–810

Comprehensive Understanding

Scientific Knowledge Base

Match the following terms.

1. _____ Posture
2. _____ Activities of daily living
3. _____ Body alignment
4. _____ Body balance
5. _____ Coordinated body movement
6. _____ Friction
7. _____ Activity tolerance
8. _____ Isotonic contractions
9. _____ Isometric contractions
10. _____ Resistive isometric exercises
11. _____ Fibrous joints
12. _____ Cartilaginous joints
13. _____ Synovial joints
14. _____ Ligaments
15. _____ Tendons
16. _____ Cartilage
17. _____ Antagonistic muscles
18. _____ Synergistic muscles
19. _____ Antigravity muscles
20. _____ Proprioception

a. The awareness of the position of the body and its parts
b. Bands of tissue that connect muscle to bone
c. Muscles that are involved with joint stabilization
d. ADLs
e. The amount of exercise or activity that the person is able to perform
f. Have little movement but are elastic and use cartilage to separate body surfaces
g. Freely movable joints
h. Nonvascular supporting tissue
i. Muscles that bring about movement of a joint
j. Muscles that contract to accomplish movement
k. Maintained by the coordinated movements of the musculoskeletal and nervous systems
l. Movement that is the result of weight, center of gravity, and balance
m. The force that occurs in a direction to oppose movement
n. Occurs with a low center of gravity and a wide, stable base of support
o. Exercises that involve tightening or tensing of muscles without moving body parts
p. Refers to the relationship of one body part to another body part
q. Exercises that cause muscle contraction and change in muscle length
r. Bands of fibrous tissue that bind joints and connect bones and cartilage
s. Contraction of muscles while pushing against a stationary object or resisting the movement of the object
t. Joints that fit closely together and are fixed

Identify the principles for safe client transfer and positioning.

21. _____

22. _____

144

23. _____

24. _____

25. _____

26. _____

27. _____

28. Identify the pathological conditions that influence body alignment and mobility.

    a. _____

    b. _____

    c. _____

    d. _____

Nursing Knowledge Base

Identify the descriptive characteristics of body alignment and mobility related to the following developmental changes.

29. Infants: _____

    _____

30. Toddlers: _____

    _____

31. Adolescence: _____

    _____

32. Young to middle adults: _____

    _____

33. Older adults: _____

    _____

Nursing Process

Assessment

Briefly explain how assessment of body alignment and posture is carried out.

34. Standing: _____

    _____

35. Sitting: _____

    _____

36 Recumbent: _____

    _____

There are three components to assess in regard to mobility. Explain each.

37. Range of motion (ROM):

    _____

    _____

38. Gait: _____

    _____

    _____

39. Exercise: _____

    _____

    _____

40. Identify some factors that affect activity tolerance.

    _____

    _____

Nursing Diagnosis

41. Identify the nursing diagnoses that are related to activity and exercise.

    a. _____

    b. _____

    c. _____

    d. _____

    e. _____

    f. _____

    g. _____

Planning

42. List three outcomes for a client with deficits in activity and exercise.

    a. _____

    b. _____

    c. _____

Implementation

Health Promotion Activities

43. Explain how to calculate the client's maximum heart rate (MHR).

    _____

    _____

44. An exercise program can consist of the following. Explain each one.

    a. Aerobic exercise:

    _____
    _____

    b. Stretching and flexibility exercises:

    _____
    _____

    c. Resistance training:

    _____
    _____

Acute Care

Briefly explain how the following maintain joint mobility and prevent contractures.

45. Stretching and isometric exercises:

    _____
    _____

46. ROM:

    _____
    _____

47. Walking:

    _____
    _____

48. Identify the two types of canes that are available and their use.

    a. _____
    b. _____

49. Explain the four standard crutch gaits.

    a. Four-point: _____
    b. Three-point:_____
    c. Two-point: _____
    d. Swing-through: _____

Explain how the nurse would implement a plan of care to increase activity and exercise in the following specific disease conditions.

50. Coronary heart disease (CHD):

    _____
    _____

51. Hypertension:

    _____
    _____

52. Chronic obstructive pulmonary disease:

    _____
    _____

53. Diabetes mellitus:

    _____
    _____

Evaluation

54. Identify the areas to evaluate to determine the effectiveness of the nursing interventions to enhance activity and exercise.

    a. _____
    b. _____
    c. _____
    d. _____
    e. _____

Review Questions

Select the appropriate answer and cite the rationale for choosing that particular answer.

55. White, shiny, flexible bands of fibrous tissue binding joints together and connecting various bones and cartilage types are known as:
    1. Joints
    2. Muscles
    3. Tendons
    4. Ligaments

Answer: _____ Rationale: _____

_____
_____

56. The nurse would expect all of the following physiological effects of exercise on the body systems except:
    1. Change in metabolic rate
    2. Decreased cardiac output
    3. Increased respiratory rate and depth
    4. Increased muscle tone, size, and strength

Answer: _____ Rationale: _____

_____
_____

Critical Thinking Model for Nursing Care Plan for Activity Intolerance

57. Imagine that you are the nurse in the care plan on page 798 of your text. Complete the *Planning phase* of the critical thinking model by writing your answers in the appropriate boxes of the model shown. Think about the following.

- In developing Mrs. Smith's plan of care, what knowledge did the nurse apply?

- In what way might the nurse's previous experience assist in developing a plan of care for Mrs. Smith?

- When developing a plan of care, what intellectual or professional standards were applied to Mrs. Smith?

- What critical thinking attitudes might have been applied in developing Mrs. Smith's plan?

- How will the nurse accomplish the goals of the plan of care?

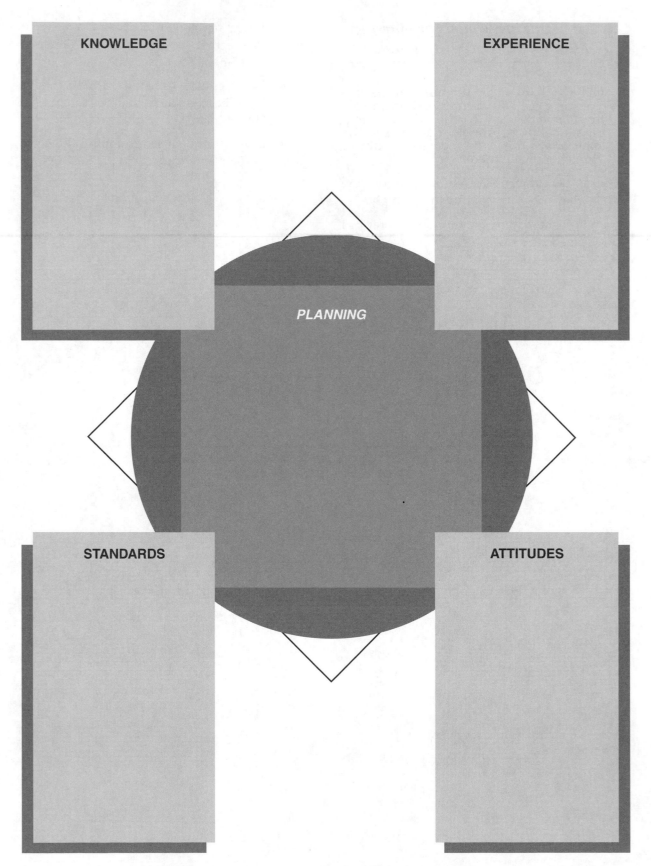

CHAPTER 37   Critical Thinking Model for Nursing Care Plan for *Activity Intolerance*

38

Client Safety

Preliminary Reading

Chapter 38, pp. 811–848

Comprehensive Understanding

Scientific Knowledge Base

Match the following terms to the scientific knowledge.

1. _____ Environment
2. _____ Carbon monoxide
3. _____ Food poisoning
4. _____ Food and Drug Administration (FDA)
5. _____ Hypothermia
6. _____ Relative humidity
7. _____ Immunization
8. _____ Air pollution
9. _____ Land pollution
10. _____ Water pollution
11. _____ Noise pollution
12. _____ Bioterrorism

a. Core temperature is 35° C or below
b. Staphylococcal and clostridial bacteria are the most common types
c. Contamination of lakes, rivers, and streams by industrial pollutants
d. Includes all of the physical and psychosocial factors that influence the life and the survival of the client
e. Uncomfortable noise levels
f. Contamination of the atmosphere with a harmful chemical
g. Federal agency responsible for regulating the manufacture, processing, and distribution of foods, drugs, and cosmetics
h. Process by which resistance to an infectious disease is produced
i. Caused by improper disposal of radioactive waste products
j. The use of anthrax, smallpox, pneumonic plague, and botulism
k. Colorless, odorless, poisonous gas
l. Amount of water vapor in the air compared with the maximum amount of water vapor that the air could contain

Nursing Knowledge Base

13. In addition to being knowledgeable about the environment, nurses must be familiar with:

    a. _____

    b. _____

    c. _____

    d. _____

14. Identify the individual risk factors that can pose a threat to safety.

    a. _____
    b. _____
    c. _____
    d. _____

15. List the four major risks to client safety in the health care environment.

    a. _____
    b. _____
    c. _____
    d. _____

Safety and the Nursing Process

Assessment

16. Identify the specific client assessments to perform when considering possible threats to the client's safety.

    a. _____
    b. _____
    c. _____
    d. _____
    e. _____

Identify the features that should alert nurses to the possibility of a bioterrorism-related outbreak.

17. _____
18. _____
19. _____
20. _____
21. _____
22. _____
23. _____
24. _____

Nursing Diagnosis

Identify actual or potential nursing diagnoses that apply to clients whose safety is threatened.

25. _____
26. _____
27. _____
28. _____

29. _____
30. _____
31. _____
32. _____
33. _____

Planning

34. Identify the expected outcomes that focus on the client's need for safety.

    a. _____
    b. _____
    c. _____

Implementation

Health Promotion

35. Identify general preventive measures to ensure a safer environment.

    a. _____
    b. _____
    c. _____
    d. _____

Acute Care

36. List eight measures to prevent falls in the health care setting.

    a. _____
    b. _____
    c. _____
    d. _____
    e. _____
    f. _____
    g. _____
    h. _____

37. A physical restraint is:

    _____
    _____

38. Use of restraints must meet the following objectives.

    a. _____
    b. _____
    c. _____
    d. _____

39. Explain why an Ambularm is used.

_____

40. Explain the mnemonic RACE to set priorities in case of fire.

R _____

A _____

C _____

E _____

41. A poison is:

_____

42. Explain seizure precautions to take.

_____

_____

43. Identify the measures with which the nurse must be familiar to reduce exposure to radiation.

_____

_____

Briefly explain the four phases of the emergency management plan.

44. Mitigation: _____

_____

45. Preparedness: _____

_____

46. Response: _____

_____

47. Recovery: _____

_____

Review Questions

Select the appropriate answer and cite the rationale for choosing that particular answer.

48. Which of the following would most threaten an individual's safety?
    1. 70% humidity
    2. Carbon dioxide
    3. Lack of water supply
    4. Unrefrigerated fresh vegetables

Answer: _____ Rationale: _____

_____

_____

49. The developmental stage that carries the highest risk of an injury from a fall is:
    1. Preschool
    2. Adulthood
    3. School-age
    4. Older adulthood

Answer: _____ Rationale: _____

_____

_____

50. Mrs. Field falls asleep while smoking in bed and drops the burning cigarette on her blanket. When she awakens, her bed is on fire, and she quickly calls the nurse. On observing the fire, the nurse should immediately:
    1. Report the fire
    2. Attempt to extinguish the fire
    3. Assist Mrs. Fields to a safe place
    4. Close all windows and doors to contain the fire

Answer: _____ Rationale: _____

_____

_____

51. Sixteen-year-old Jimmy is admitted to an adolescent unit with a diagnosis of substance abuse. The nurse examines Jimmy and finds that he has bloodshot eyes, slurred speech, and an unstable gait. He smells of alcohol and is unable to answer questions appropriately. The appropriate nursing diagnosis would be:
    1. Self-care deficit related to alcohol abuse
    2. Deficient knowledge related to alcohol abuse
    3. Disturbed thought processes related to sensory overload
    4. High risk for injury related to impaired sensory perception

Answer: _____ Rationale: _____

_____

_____

Critical Thinking Model for Nursing Care Plan for Risk for Injury

52. Imagine that you are Mr. Key, the nurse in the care plan on page 825 of your text. Complete the *Assessment phase* of the critical thinking model by writing your answers in the appropriate boxes of the model shown. Think about the following.

- In developing Ms. Cohen's plan of care, what knowledge did Mr. Key apply?

- In what way might Mr. Key's previous experience assist in this case?

- What intellectual or professional standards were applied to Ms. Cohen?

- What critical thinking attitudes might have been applied in this case?

- As you review your assessment, what key areas did you cover?

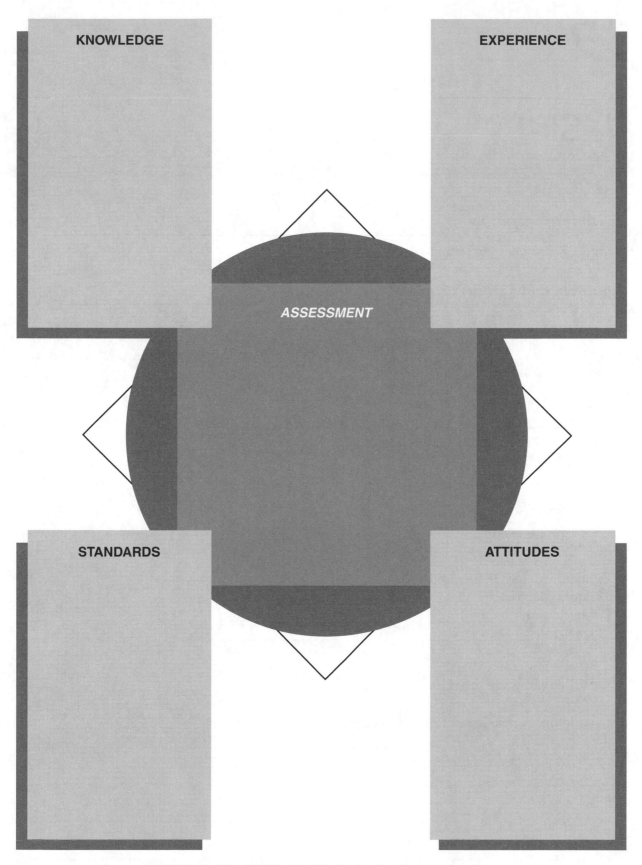

KNOWLEDGE

EXPERIENCE

ASSESSMENT

STANDARDS

ATTITUDES

CHAPTER 38   Critical Thinking Model for Nursing Care Plan for *Risk for Injury*

39

Hygiene

Preliminary Reading

Chapter 39, pp. 849–906

Comprehensive Understanding

1. Explain the three primary layers of the skin.
   a. Epidermis: _____
   b. Dermis: _____
   c. Subcutaneous: _____

2. Identify the functions of the skin.
   a. _____
   b. _____
   c. _____
   d. _____

3. Define the following terms related to feet, hands, and nails.
   a. Cuticle: _____
   b. Lunula: _____

4. Define the following terms related to the oral cavity.
   a. Buccal glands: _____
   b. Mastication: _____
   c. Gingivitis: _____

Nursing Knowledge Base

5. Identify the factors that influence a personal preference for hygiene.
   a. _____
   b. _____
   c. _____
   d. _____
   e. _____
   f. _____
   g. _____

The Nursing Process

Assessment

6. Assessment of the skin includes:

_____

_____

7. Common skin problems can affect how hygiene is administered. Describe the hygiene provided for the following.

    a. Dry skin: _____

    _____

    _____

    b. Acne: _____

    _____

    _____

    c. Skin rashes: _____

    _____

    _____

    d. Contact dermatitis: _____

    _____

    _____

    e. Abrasion: _____

    _____

    _____

8. Briefly explain the risk factors for skin impairment.

    a. Immobilization: _____

    _____

    _____

    b. Reduced sensation: _____

    _____

    _____

    c. Nutrition and hydration: _____

    _____

    _____

    d. Secretions and excretions: _____

    _____

    _____

    e. Vascular insufficiency: _____

    _____

    _____

    f. External devices: _____

    _____

    _____

9. Identify the characteristics of the following foot and nail problems.

    a. Calluses: _____

    _____

    _____

    b. Corns: _____

    _____

    _____

    c. Plantar warts: _____

    _____

    _____

    d. Tinea pedis: _____

    _____

    _____

    e. Ingrown nails: _____

    _____

    _____

    f. Foot odors: _____

    _____

    _____

10. Halitosis is: _____

    _____

    _____

11. Identify the characteristics of the following hair and scalp conditions.

    a. Dandruff: _____

    _____

    _____

    b. Ticks: _____

    _____

    _____

    c. Pediculosis: _____

    _____

    _____

    d. Pediculosis capitis: _____

    _____

    _____

    e. Pediculosis corporis: _____

    _____

    _____

    f. Pediculosis pubis: _____

    _____

    _____

g. Alopecia:

_____

_____

12. Give examples of clients at risk for hygiene problems.

a. Oral problems:

_____

_____

b. Skin problems:

_____

_____

c. Foot problems:

_____

_____

d. Eye care problems:

_____

_____

Nursing Diagnosis

List 10 possible nursing diagnoses that apply to clients in need of hygienic care.

13. _____

_____

14. _____

_____

15. _____

_____

16. _____

_____

17. _____

_____

18. _____

_____

19. _____

_____

20. _____

_____

21. _____

_____

22. _____

_____

Planning

23. Identify three expected outcomes for "client's musculoskeletal system remains free of breakdown or contractures."

a. _____

b. _____

c. _____

Implementation

24. List the educational tips for clients about hygiene practices.

a. _____

b. _____

c. _____

d. _____

Acute and Restorative Care

25. Briefly explain the following types of baths.

a. Complete bed bath:

_____

_____

b. Partial bed bath:

_____

_____

c. Sponge bath:

_____

_____

d. Tub bath:

_____

_____

e. Bed bath/travel bath:

_____

_____

26. State guidelines that the nurse needs to follow regardless of the type of bath.

a. _____

b. _____

c. _____

d. _____

e. _____

27. Identify the clients at risk for skin break-down in the perineal area.

_____

_____

28. Identify the benefits of a back rub.

_____

_____

List the guidelines to include when advising clients with peripheral neuropathy or vascular insufficiency about foot care.

29. _____

_____

30. _____

_____

31. _____

_____

32. _____

_____

33. _____

_____

34. _____

_____

35. _____

_____

36. _____

_____

37. _____

_____

38. _____

_____

39. _____

_____

40. _____

_____

41. _____

_____

Briefly explain the benefits of the following in relation to oral hygiene.

42. Brushing:

_____

_____

43. Flossing:

_____

_____

44. Denture care:

_____

_____

Briefly describe the rationale for the following interventions.

45. Brushing and combing:

_____

_____

46. Shampooing:

_____

_____

47. Shaving:

_____

_____

48. Mustache and beard care:

_____

_____

49. Describe basic eye care for a client.

_____

_____

50. The three types of contact lenses that are available are:
    a. _____
    b. _____
    c. _____

51. Describe each of the following techniques necessary in caring for an artificial eye.
    a. Removal:

    _____

    _____

    b. Cleansing:

    _____

    _____

    c. Reinsertion:

    _____

    _____

    d. Storage:

    _____

    _____

52. Describe the procedure for removal of impacted cerumen.

_____

_____

53. Describe the following types of hearing aids.
    a. In-the-canal (ITC):

    _____

    _____

    b. In-the-ear (ITE):

    _____

    _____

    c. Behind-the-ear (BTE):

    _____

    _____

54. Describe the following common bed positions.
    a. Fowler's:

    _____

    _____

    b. Semi-Fowler's:

    _____

    _____

    c. Trendelenburg's:

    _____

    _____

    d. Reverse Trendelenburg's:

    _____

    _____

    e. Flat:

    _____

    _____

Review Questions

Select the appropriate answer and cite the rationale for choosing that particular answer.

55. Mr. Gray is a 19-year-old client in the rehabilitation unit. He is completely paralyzed below the neck. The most appropriate bath for Mr. Gray is a:
    1. Partial bed bath
    2. Complete bed bath
    3. Sitz bath
    4. Tepid bath

    Answer: _____   Rationale: _____

    _____

    _____

56. All of the following will help maintain skin integrity in the older adult except:
    1. Environmental air that is cold and dry
    2. Use of warm water and mild cleansing agents for bathing
    3. Bathing every other day
    4. Drinking 8 to 10 glasses of water a day

    Answer: _____   Rationale: _____

    _____

    _____

57. When preparing to give complete AM care to a client, what would the nurse do first?
    1. Gather the necessary equipment and supplies.
    2. Remove the client's gown or pajamas while maintaining privacy.
    3. Assess the client's preferences for bathing practices.
    4. Lower the side rails, and assist the client with assuming a comfortable position.

    Answer: _____   Rationale: _____

    _____

    _____

58. Mrs. Veech is a diabetic. Which intervention should be included in her teaching plan regarding foot care?
    1. Use a pumice stone to smooth corns and calluses.
    2. File toenails straight across and square.
    3. Apply powder to dry areas along the feet and between the toes.
    4. Wear elastic stockings to improve circulation.

Answer: _____ Rationale: _____
_____
_____

59. Assessment of the hair and scalp reveals that John has head lice. An appropriate intervention would be:
    1. Shave hair off the affected area
    2. Place oil on the hair and scalp until all of the lice are dead
    3. Shampoo with medicated shampoo and repeat 12 to 24 hours later
    4. Shampoo with regular shampoo and dry with hairdryer set at the hottest setting

Answer: _____ Rationale: _____
_____
_____

Critical Thinking Model for Nursing Care Plan for Bathing/Hygiene Self-Care Deficit

60. Imagine that you are Jeannette, the nurse in the care plan on page 865 of your text. Complete the *Planning phase* of the critical thinking model by writing your answers in the appropriate boxes of the model shown. Think about the following.

    - In developing Mrs. Wyatt's plan of care, what knowledge did Jeannette apply?

    - In what way might Jeannette's previous experience assist in developing a plan of care for Mrs. Wyatt?

    - When developing a plan of care, what intellectual and professional standards were applied?

    - What critical thinking attitudes might have been applied in developing Mrs. Wyatt's plan of care?

    - How will Jeannette accomplish the goals?

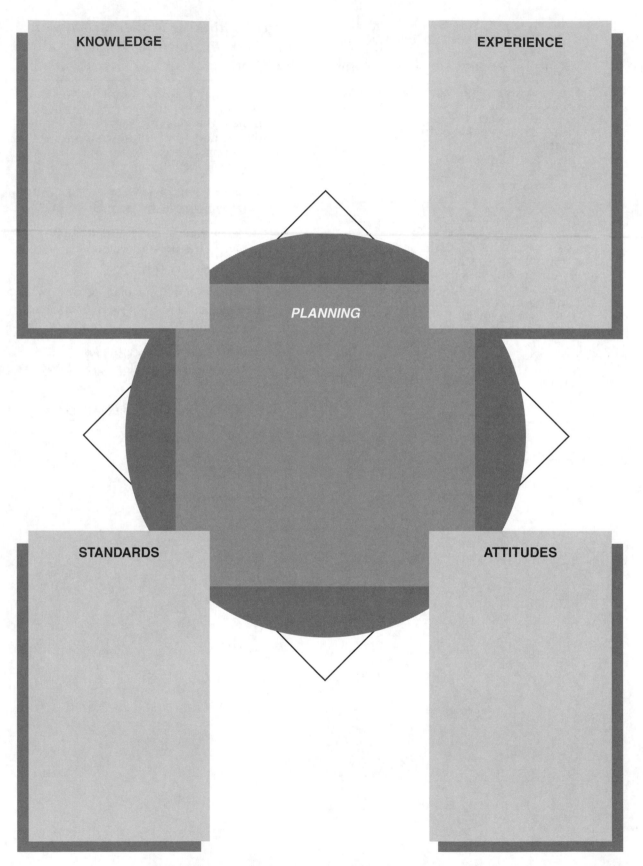

KNOWLEDGE

EXPERIENCE

PLANNING

STANDARDS

ATTITUDES

CHAPTER 39   Critical Thinking Model for *Bathing/Hygiene Self-Care Deficit*

40

Oxygenation

Preliminary Reading

Chapter 40, pp. 907–965

Comprehensive Understanding

Match the following cardiopulmonary physiology terms.

1. _____ Frank-Starling law
2. _____ Cardiac output
3. _____ Cardiac index
4. _____ Stroke volume
5. _____ Preload
6. _____ Afterload
7. _____ ECG
8. _____ Normal sinus rhythm (NSR)

a. Reflects the electrical activity of the conduction system
b. End-diastolic volume
c. As the myocardium stretches, the strength of the contraction increases
d. Normal sequence on the electrocardiogram (ECG)
e. Amount of blood ejected from the left ventricle each minute
f. Amount of blood ejected from the ventricle with each contraction
g. The resistance to left ventricular ejection
h. Is determined by dividing the cardiac output by the body surface area (BSA)

Explain what the following waves in the conduction system represent and the normal values for each.

9. P wave:

_____

_____

10. PR interval:

_____

_____

11. QRS complex:

_____

_____

12. QT interval:

_____

_____

Match the following key terms that relate to respiratory physiology.

13. _____ Ventilation
14. _____ Work of breathing
15. _____ Inspiration
16. _____ Expiration
17. _____ Compliance
18. _____ Airway resistance
19. _____ Diffusion
20. _____ Deoxyhemoglobin
21. _____ Neural regulation
22. _____ Chemical regulation

a. Central nervous system (CNS) control of respiratory rate, depth, and rhythm
b. Reduced hemoglobin
c. Influence of carbon dioxide and hydrogen ions on the rate and depth of respirations
d. Pressure difference between the mouth and the alveoli in relation to the rate of flow of inspired gas
e. Process of moving gases into and out of the lungs
f. Process for the exchange of respiratory gases in the alveoli and the capillaries of the body tissues
g. Effort required to expand and contract the lungs
h. Ability of the lungs to distend or to expand in response to increased intraalveolar pressure
i. Active process stimulated by chemical receptors in the aorta
j. Passive process dependent on the elastic recoil properties of the lungs

23. Identify the factors that affect oxygenation.

a. _____
b. _____
c. _____
d. _____

24. Identify conditions that affect chest wall movement.

a. _____
b. _____
c. _____
d. _____
e. _____
f. _____
g. _____

25. Briefly describe the following dysrhythmias.

a. Sinus tachycardia:

_____
_____

b. Sinus bradycardia:

_____
_____

c. Atrial fibrillation:

_____
_____

d. Ventricular tachycardia:

_____
_____

e. Ventricular fibrillation:

_____
_____

26. Explain the difference between the following types of heart failure.

a. Left-sided:

_____
_____

b. Right-sided:

_____
_____

27. Explain the difference between the following impaired valvular functions.

a. Stenosis:

_____
_____

b. Regurgitation:

_____
_____

Describe the following disorders.

28. Myocardial ischemia:

_____
_____

29. Angina pectoris:

_____
_____

30. Myocardial infarction:

_____

_____

31. Acute coronary syndrome:

_____

_____

Explain the following alterations in respiratory functioning.

32. Hyperventilation:

_____

_____

33. Hypoventilation:

_____

_____

34. Atelectasis:

_____

_____

35. Hypoxia:

_____

_____

36. Cyanosis:

_____

_____

Nursing Knowledge Base

Identify the cardiopulmonary risk factors for the following developmental levels.

37. Infants and toddlers:

_____

_____

38. School-age children and adolescents:

_____

_____

39. Young and middle-age adults:

_____

_____

40. Older adults:

_____

_____

41. List the lifestyle modifications to decrease cardiopulmonary risks.

a. _____

b. _____

c. _____

d. _____

e. _____

42. List four occupational pollutants.

a. _____

b. _____

c. _____

d. _____

Nursing Process

Assessment

43. Explain the focus of the nursing history to meet oxygen needs for the following.

a. Cardiac function:

_____

_____

b. Respiratory function:

_____

_____

44. Explain the differences between the following types of chest pain.

a. Cardiac pain:

_____

_____

b. Pleuritic chest pain:

_____

_____

c. Musculoskeletal pain:

_____

_____

Explain how the following affect oxygenation.

45. Fatigue:

_____

_____

46. Dyspnea: _____

_____

_____

47. Orthopnea: _____

_____

_____

48. Cough: _____

_____

_____

49. Wheezing: _____

_____

_____

Briefly explain the following techniques used during the physical examination to assess tissue oxygenation.

50. Inspection: _____

_____

_____

51. Palpation: _____

_____

_____

52. Percussion: _____

_____

_____

53. Auscultation: _____

_____

_____

54. Describe the following diagnostic tests used to determine the adequacy of the cardiac conduction system.

   a. Holter monitor:

   _____

   _____

   b. Exercise stress test:

   _____

   _____

   c. Thallium stress test:

   _____

   _____

   d. Electrophysiological study (EPS):

   _____

   _____

   e. Echocardiography:

   _____

   _____

   f. Scintigraphy:

   _____

   _____

   g. Cardiac catheterization and angiography:

   _____

   _____

55. Describe the following tests used to measure the adequacy of ventilation and oxygenation.

   a. Pulmonary function tests:

   _____

   _____

   b. Peak expiratory flow rate (PEFR):

   _____

   _____

   c. Bronchoscopy:

   _____

   _____

   d. Lung scan:

   _____

   _____

   e. Thoracentesis:

   _____

   _____

Nursing Diagnosis

List the nursing diagnoses that are appropriate for the client with alterations in oxygenation.

56. _____

_____

57. _____

_____

58. _____

_____

59. _____

_____

60. _____

_____

61. _____

_____

62. _____

_____

63. _____

_____

64. _____

_____

65. _____

_____

66. _____

_____

67. _____

_____

Planning

68. List the specific outcomes for maintaining a patent airway.

    a. _____
    b. _____
    c. _____
    d. _____

Implementation

69. List the modalities appropriate for a client with dyspnea.

    a. _____
    b. _____
    c. _____
    d. _____
    e. _____
    f. _____

70. List the interventions that promote mobilization of pulmonary secretions.

    a. _____
    b. _____
    c. _____
    d. _____

71. List the common suctioning techniques.

    a. _____
    b. _____
    c. _____

Nursing interventions that maintain or promote lung expansion include the following noninvasive techniques. Briefly explain each one.

72. Positioning:

    _____
    _____

73. Incentive spirometry:

    _____
    _____

74. Identify the three reasons for inserting chest tubes.

    a. _____
    b. _____
    c. _____

75. Define the following.

    a. Hemothorax:

    _____
    _____

    b. Pneumothorax:

    _____
    _____

76. The goal of oxygen therapy is:

    _____
    _____

77. Describe the following methods of oxygen delivery, and identify the advantages and disadvantages of each.

    a. Nasal cannula: _____
    _____
    _____

    b. Face mask: _____
    _____
    _____

    c. Venturi mask: _____
    _____
    _____

78. Identify the indications for a client to receive home oxygen therapy.

    _____
    _____

79. The "ABCs" of cardiopulmonary resuscitation are:

A _____

B _____

C _____

80. The goal of cardiopulmonary rehabilitation for the client to maintain an optimal level of health focuses on:

a. _____

b. _____

c. _____

d. _____

e. _____

Briefly explain the following techniques used to improve ventilation and oxygenation.

81. Coughing techniques:

_____

_____

82. Respiratory muscle training:

_____

_____

83. Pursed-lip breathing:

_____

_____

84. Diaphragmatic breathing:

_____

_____

Evaluation

85. List the evaluative criteria for a client with alterations in oxygenation.

a. _____

b. _____

c. _____

d. _____

e. _____

Review Questions

Select the appropriate answer and cite the rationale for choosing that particular answer.

86. Ventilation, perfusion, and exchange of gases are the major purposes of:
1. Respiration
2. Circulation
3. Aerobic metabolism
4. Anaerobic metabolism

Answer: _____ Rationale: _____

_____

_____

87. Afterload refers to:
1. The resistance to left ventricular ejection
2. The amount of blood in the left ventricle at the end of diastole
3. The amount of blood ejected from the left ventricle each minute
4. The amount of blood ejected from the left ventricle with each contraction

Answer: _____ Rationale: _____

_____

_____

88. The movement of gases into and out of the lungs depends on:
1. 50% oxygen content in the atmospheric air
2. The pressure gradient between the atmosphere and the alveoli
3. The use of accessory muscles of respiration during expiration
4. The amount of carbon dioxide dissolved in the fluid of the alveoli

Answer: _____ Rationale: _____

_____

_____

89. Mr. Isaac comes to the emergency depart-
    ment complaining of difficulty breathing.
    An objective finding associated with his
    dyspnea might include:
    1. Feelings of heaviness in the chest
    2. Complaints of shortness of breath
    3. Use of accessory muscles of respiration
    4. Statements about a sense of impending
       doom

Answer: _____ Rationale: _____
_____
_____

90. The use of chest physiotherapy to mobi-
    lize pulmonary secretions involves the
    use of:
    1. Hydration
    2. Percussion
    3. Nebulization
    4. Humidification

Answer: _____ Rationale: _____
_____
_____

Critical Thinking Model for Nursing Care Plan for Ineffective Airway Clearance

91. Imagine that you are the student nurse
    in the care plan on page 928 of your text.
    Complete the *Assessment phase* of the
    critical thinking model by writing your
    answers in the appropriate boxes of the
    model shown. Think about the following.

- What knowledge base was applied to Mr.
  Edwards?

- In what way might your previous experience apply in this case?

- What intellectual or professional standards were applied to Mr. Edwards?

- What critical thinking attitudes did you
  use in assessing Mr. Edwards?

- As you review your assessment, what key
  areas did you cover?

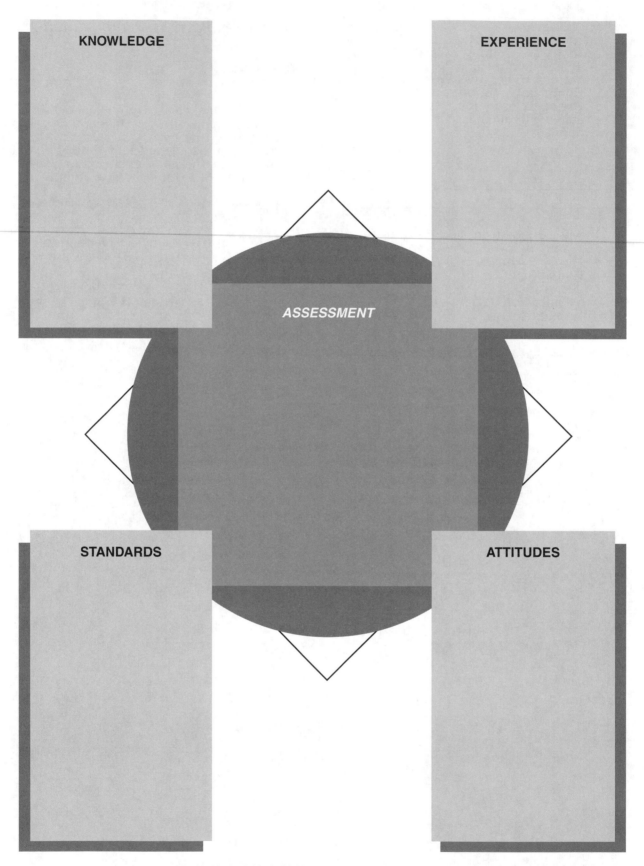

KNOWLEDGE

EXPERIENCE

ASSESSMENT

STANDARDS

ATTITUDES

CHAPTER 40   Critical Thinking Model for *Ineffective Airway Clearance*

41

Fluid, Electrolyte, and Acid-Base Balance

Preliminary Reading

Chapter 41, pp. 966–1027

Comprehensive Understanding

Scientific Knowledge Base

1. Body fluids are distributed in two distinct compartments. Briefly explain each one.
   a. Extracellular: _____
   b. Intracellular: _____

Define the following terms related to the composition of body fluids.

2. *Cations:* _____

3. *Anions:* _____

4. *mEq/L:* _____

5. *Solute:* _____

Define the following terms related to the movement of body fluids.

6. *Osmosis:* _____

7. *Osmols:* _____

8. *Osmotic pressure:* _____

9. *Osmolality:* _____

10. *Osmolarity:* _____

11. *Isotonic solution:* _____

12. *Hypertonic solution:* _____

13. *Hypotonic solution:* _____

14. *Diffusion:* _____

15. *Concentration gradient:* _____

16. *Filtration:* _____

17. *Active transport:* _____

18. List the three ways that body fluids are regulated.

    a. _____

    b. _____

    c. _____

Define the following terms related to the regulation of body fluids.

19. *Osmoreceptors:* _____

    _____

20. *Hypovolemia:* _____

    _____

21. *Dehydration:* _____

    _____

22. *Antidiuretic hormone:* _____

    _____

23. Changes in renal perfusion initiate the renin-angiotension-aldosterone mechanism. Explain the mechanism.

    a. Angiotension I: _____

    _____

    _____

    _____

b. Angiotension II: _____

    _____

    _____

    _____

c. Aldosterone: _____

    _____

    _____

    _____

24. What is atrial natriuretic peptide?

    _____

    _____

25. List the four organs of water loss.

    a. _____

    b. _____

    c. _____

    d. _____

26. Explain the difference between the following water losses.

    a. Insensible water loss:

    _____

    _____

Electrolyte	Values	Function	Regulatory Mechanism
Sodium			
Potassium			
Calcium			
Magnesium			
Chloride			
Bicarbonate			
Phosphate			

b. Sensible water loss:

_____

_____

27. Give the normal values, function, and regulatory mechanisms for the major body electrolytes in the following table.

28. Identify the three types of acid-base regulators in the body.

a. _____

b. _____

c. _____

Imbalance	Laboratory Finding	Signs and Symptoms
Hyponatremia		
Hypernatremia		
Hypokalemia		
Hyperkalemia		
Hypocalcemia		
Hypercalcemia		
Hypomagnesemia		
Hypermagnesemia		

29. For each electrolyte disturbance, identify the diagnostic laboratory finding and list at least four characteristic signs and symptoms in the following table.

30. Briefly explain the following components of acid-base balance.

a. pH: _____

_____

_____

b. $PaCO_2$: _____

_____

_____

c. PaO_2: _____

_____

_____

d. Oxygen saturation: _____

_____

_____

e. Base excess: _____

_____

_____

f. Bicarbonate: _____

_____

_____

31. The four primary types of acid-base imbalances are listed in the following table. For each acid-base imbalance, identify the diagnostic laboratory finding and list the characteristic signs and symptoms.

Acid-Base Imbalance	Laboratory Findings	Signs and Symptoms
Respiratory acidosis		
Respiratory alkalosis		
Metabolic acidosis		
Metabolic alkalosis		

32. Identify the risk factors for fluid, electrolyte, and acid-base imbalances, and give an example of each.

a. _____
_____
_____
_____

b. _____
_____
_____
_____

c. _____
_____
_____

d. _____
_____
_____

e. _____
_____
_____

f. _____
_____
_____

g. _____
_____
_____
_____

Nursing Process

Assessment

Explain how the following can affect fluid, electrolyte, and acid-base balances.

33. Age: _____
_____
_____

34. Acute illness: _____
_____
_____

35. Surgery: _____
_____
_____

36. Burns: _____
_____

37. Respiratory disorders: _____
_____
_____

38. Head injury: _____

39. Chronic illness: _____

40. Cancer: _____

41. Cardiovascular disease: _____

42. Renal disorders: _____

43. Gastrointestinal disturbances: _____

44. Environmental factors: _____

45. Diet: _____

46. Lifestyle: _____

47. Medication: _____

48. Indicate the possible fluid, electrolyte, or acid-base imbalances associated with each physical finding.

    a. Weight loss of 5% to 8%: _____

    b. Irritability: _____

    c. Lethargy: _____

d. Periorbital edema: _____

e. Sticky, dry mucous membranes: _____

f. Chvostek's sign: _____

g. Distended neck veins: _____

h. Dysrhythmias: _____

i. Weak pulse: _____

j. Low blood pressure: _____

k. Third heart sound: _____

l. Increased respiratory rate: _ _____

m. Crackles: _____

n. Anorexia: _____

o. Abdominal cramps:_ _____

p. Poor skin turgor: _____

q. Oliguria or anuria: _____

r. Increased urine specific gravity: _____

_____

_____

s. Muscle cramps, tetany: _____

_____

_____

t. Hypertonicity of muscles on palpation:

_____

_____

u. Decreased or absent deep tendon reflexes:

_____

_____

v. Increased temperature: _____

_____

_____

w. Distended abdomen: _____

_____

_____

x. Cold, clammy skin: _____

_____

_____

y. 2+ edema: _____

_____

_____

Nursing Diagnosis

List potential or actual nursing diagnoses for a client with fluid, electrolyte, or acid-base imbalances.

49. _____

_____

50. _____

_____

51. _____

_____

52. _____

_____

53. _____

_____

54. _____

_____

55. _____

_____

56. _____

_____

57. _____

_____

58. _____

_____

Planning

59. List three goals that are appropriate for a client with altered fluid status.

a. _____

b. _____

c. _____

Implementation

Briefly describe the rationale for the following interventions.

60. Enteral replacement of fluids:

_____

_____

61. Restriction of fluids:

_____

_____

62. Parenteral replacement of fluids and electrolytes:

_____

_____

63. Total parenteral nutrition:

_____

_____

64. Intravenous (IV) therapy:

_____

_____

65. Vascular access devices:

_____

_____

66. Give an example of the following types of electrolyte solutions.

a. Isotonic:

_____

_____

b. Hypotonic:

_____

_____

c. Hypertonic:

_____

_____

67. Complete the grid below describing complications of IV therapy.

_____

_____

Complication	Assessment Finding	Nursing Action
Infiltration		
Phlebitis		
Fluid overload		
Bleeding		

68. A venipuncture is:

_____

_____

69. Electronic infusion pumps are necessary for:

_____

_____

70. Line maintenance involves:

a. _____

b. _____

c. _____

71. The objectives for blood transfusions are:

a. _____

b. _____

c. _____

72. The ABO system includes:

_____

_____

73. The universal blood donor is:

_____

_____

74. The universal blood recipient is:

_____

_____

75. A transfusion reaction is:

_____

_____

76. Define *autotransfusion*.

_____

_____

77. Identify the nursing interventions associated with blood transfusions.

a. _____

b. _____

c. _____

d. _____

e. _____

f. _____

g. _____

h. _____

78. Briefly describe the following acute transfusion reactions and their causes:

a. Acute hemolytic:

_____

_____

b. Febrile, nonhemolytic:

_____

_____

c. Mild allergic:

_____

_____

d. Anaphylactic:

_____

_____

e. Circulatory overload:

_____

_____

f. Sepsis:

_____

_____

79. List the five signs and symptoms most commonly associated with transfusion reactions.

a. _____
b. _____
c. _____
d. _____
e. _____

List the steps the nurse should follow if a transfusion reaction is suspected.

80. _____
81. _____
82. _____
83. _____
84. _____
85. _____
86. _____
87. _____

Review Questions

Select the appropriate answer and cite the rationale for choosing that particular answer.

88. The body fluids constituting the interstitial fluid and blood plasma are:
1. Hypotonic
2. Hypertonic
3. Intracellular
4. Extracellular

Answer: _____ Rationale: _____

_____

_____

89. Mrs. Green's arterial blood gas results are as follows: pH, 7.32; $PaCO_2$, 52 mm Hg; PaO_2, 78 mm Hg; HCO_3^-, 24 mEq/L. Mrs. Green has:
1. Metabolic acidosis
2. Metabolic alkalosis
3. Respiratory acidosis
4. Respiratory alkalosis

Answer: _____ Rationale: _____

_____

_____

90. Mr. Frank is an 82-year-old client who has had a 3-day history of vomiting and diarrhea. Which symptom would you expect to find on a physical examination?
1. Tachycardia
2. Hypertension
3. Neck vein distention
4. Crackles in the lungs

Answer: _____ Rationale: _____

_____

_____

91. Which of the following is most likely to result in respiratory alkalosis?
1. Steroid use
2. Fad dieting
3. Hyperventilation
4. Chronic alcoholism

Answer: _____ Rationale: _____

_____

_____

Critical Thinking Model for Ineffective Airway Clearance/Risk for Deficient Fluid Volume

92. Imagine that you are the student nurse in the care plan on page 988 of your text. Complete the *Planning phase* of the critical thinking model by writing your answers in the appropriate boxes of the model shown. Think about the following.

- In developing Mrs. Bottomley's plan of care, what knowledge did you apply?

- In what way might your previous experience assist you in developing a plan of care for Mrs. Bottomley?

- When developing a plan of care, what intellectual and professional standards were applied?

- What critical thinking attitudes might have been applied to developing Mrs. Bottomley's care?

- How will you accomplish the goals of the plan of care?

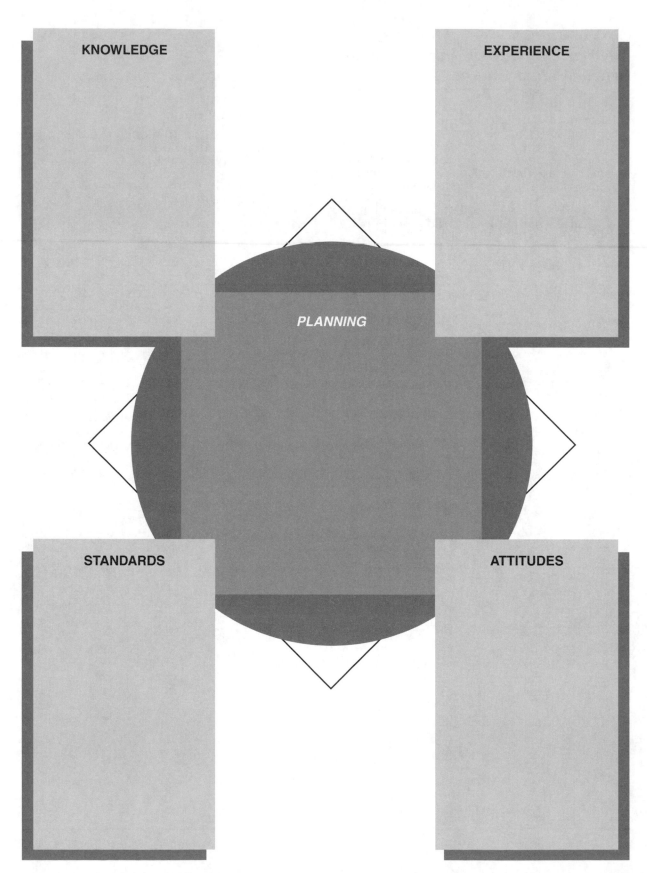

CHAPTER 41   Critical Thinking Model for *Ineffective Airway Clearance/Risk for Deficient Fluid Volume*

42

Sleep

Preliminary Reading

Chapter 42, pp. 1028–1050

Comprehensive Understanding

Scientific Knowledge Base

Match the following terms related to sleep.

1. _____ Sleep
2. _____ Circadian rhythm
3. _____ Biological clock
4. _____ NREM
5. _____ REM
6. _____ Dreams
7. _____ Nocturia
8. _____ Hypersomnolence
9. _____ Polysomnogram
10. _____ Insomnia
11. _____ Sleep hygiene
12. _____ Sleep apnea
13. _____ Excessive daytime sleepiness (EDS)
14. _____ Narcolepsy
15. _____ Cataplexy
16. _____ Sleep deprivation
17. _____ Parasomnias

a. Urination during the night, which disrupts the sleep cycle
b. Involves the use of electroencephalogram (EEG), electromyogram (EMG), and electrooculogram (EOG) to monitor stages of sleep
c. Results in impaired waking function, poor work performance, accidents, and emotional problems
d. Most common sleep complaint, signaling an underlying physical or psychological disorder
e. More common in children, an example is sudden infant death syndrome (SIDS)
f. Cyclical process that alternates with longer periods of wakefulness
g. Rapid eye movement phase at the end of each sleep cycle
h. Synchronizes sleep cycles
i. Influences the pattern of major biological and behavioral functions
j. Sleep that progresses through four stages (light to deep)
k. More vivid and elaborate during REM sleep and are functionally important to learning
l. Characterized by the lack of airflow through the nose and mouth for 10 seconds or longer during sleep
m. Practices that the client associates with sleep
n. Inadequacies in either the quantity or quality of nighttime sleep
o. Problem clients experience as a result of dyssomnia
p. Sudden muscle weakness during intense emotions at any time during the day
q. Dysfunction of mechanisms that regulate the sleep and wake states (excessive daytime sleepiness)

Nursing Knowledge Base

18. Complete the following table listing the normal sleep patterns and rituals for the following developmental stages.

Developmental Stage	Sleep Patterns	Usual Rituals
Neonates		
Infants		
Toddlers		
Preschoolers		
School-age children		
Adolescents		
Young adults		
Middle adults		
Older adults		

Describe how each of the following affects sleep, and give an example of each.

19. Drugs and substances: _____
_____
_____

20. Lifestyle: _____
_____
_____

21. Usual sleep patterns: _____
_____
_____

22. Emotional stress: _____
_____
_____

23. Environment: _____
_____
_____

24. Exercise and fatigue: _____
_____
_____

25. Food and caloric intake: _____
_____
_____

Nursing Process

Assessment

26. Identify sources for sleep assessment.

_____

_____

27. List the components of a sleep history.

   a. _____

   b. _____

   c. _____

   d. _____

   e. _____

   f. _____

   g. _____

   h. _____

Nursing Diagnosis

List the common nursing diagnoses related to sleep problems.

28. _____

29. _____

30. _____

31. _____

32. _____

33. _____

34. _____

35. _____

36. _____

37. _____

Planning

List four goals appropriate for a client needing rest or sleep.

38. _____

39. _____

40. _____

41. _____

Implementation

Many factors affect the ability to gain adequate rest and sleep. Briefly give examples of each of the following in relation to health promotion.

42. Environmental controls:

_____

_____

43. Promoting bedtime routines:

_____

_____

44. Promoting safety:

_____

45. Promoting comfort:

_____

_____

46. Establishing periods of rest and sleep:

_____

_____

47. Stress reduction:

_____

_____

48. Bedtime snacks:

_____

_____

49. Pharmacological approaches:

_____

_____

Acute Care

For each of the following situations, give two examples of nursing measures that will promote sleep.

50. Environmental controls:

   a. _____

   b. _____

51. Promoting comfort:

   a. _____

   b. _____

52. Establishing periods of rest and sleep:

   a. _____

   b. _____

53. Promoting safety:

   a. _____

   b. _____

54. Stress reduction:

    a. _____

    b. _____

Evaluation

55. With regard to sleep disturbances, the client is the source for outcomes evaluation. List three outcomes for a client with a sleep disturbance.

    a. _____

    b. _____

    c. _____

Review Questions

Select the appropriate answer and cite the rationale for choosing that particular answer.

56. The 24-hour day-night cycle is known as:
    1. Ultradian rhythm
    2. Circadian rhythm
    3. Infradium rhythm
    4. Non-REM rhythm

Answer: _____   Rationale: _____

_____

_____

57. Which of the following substances will promote normal sleep patterns?
    1. Alcohol
    2. Narcotics
    3. L-tryptophan
    4. Beta-blockers

Answer: _____   Rationale: _____

_____

_____

58. All of the following are symptoms of sleep deprivation except:
    1. Irritability
    2. Hyperactivity
    3. Decreased motivation
    4. Rise in body temperature

Answer: _____   Rationale: _____

_____

_____

59. Mrs. Peterson complains of difficulty falling asleep, awakening earlier than desired, and not feeling rested. She attributes these problems to leg pain that is secondary to her arthritis. What would be the appropriate nursing diagnosis for her?
    1. Fatigue related to leg pain
    2. Insomnia related to arthritis
    3. Deficient knowledge related to sleep hygiene measures
    4. Insomnia related to chronic leg pain

Answer: _____   Rationale: _____

_____

_____

60. A nursing care plan for a client with sleep problems has been implemented. All of the following would be expected outcomes except:
    1. Client reports satisfaction with amount of sleep
    2. Client falls asleep within 1 hour of going to bed
    3. Client reports no episodes of awakening during the night
    4. Client rates sleep as an 8 or above on the visual analog scale

Answer: _____   Rationale: _____

_____

_____

Critical Thinking Model for Nursing Care Plan for Insomnia

61. Imagine that you are the nurse in the care plan on page 1042 of your text. Complete the *Evaluation phase* of the critical thinking model by writing your answers in the appropriate boxes of the model shown. Think about the following.

    - What knowledge did you apply in evaluating Julie's care?

    - In what way might your previous experience influence your evaluation of Julie's care?

    - During evaluation, what intellectual and professional standards were applied to Julie's care?

    - In what way do critical thinking attitudes play a role in how you approach the evaluation of Julie's plan?

    - How might you evaluate Julie's plan of care?

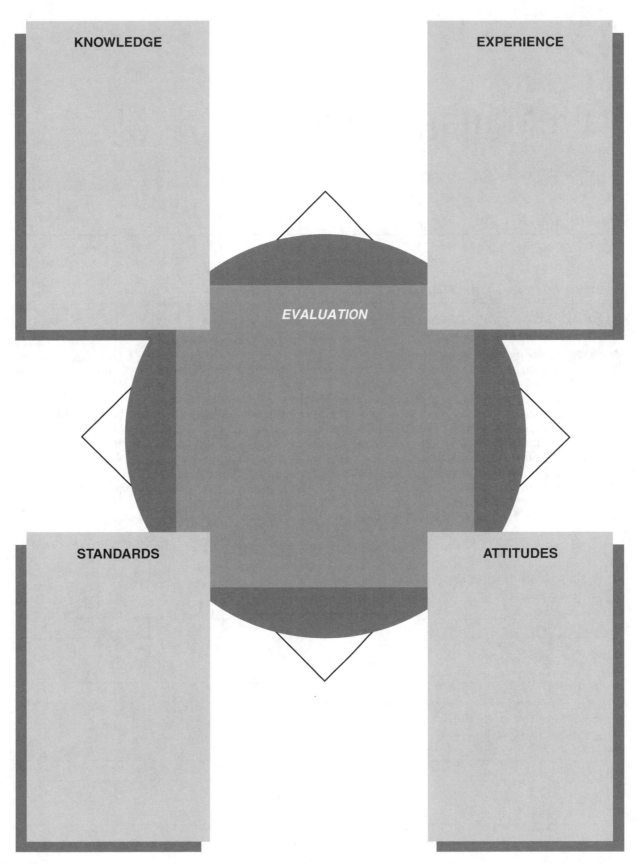

KNOWLEDGE

EXPERIENCE

EVALUATION

STANDARDS

ATTITUDES

CHAPTER 42   Critical Thinking Model for *Insomnia*

43

Pain Management

Preliminary Reading

Chapter 43, pp. 1051–1084

Comprehensive Understanding

Scientific Knowledge Base

Match the following terms related to pain.

1. _____ Transduction
2. _____ Nociceptor
3. _____ Substance P
4. _____ Serotonin
5. _____ Prostaglandins
6. _____ Bradykinin
7. _____ Neuromodulators
8. _____ Perception
9. _____ Modulation
10. _____ Pain threshold
11. _____ Pain tolerance

a. Binds to receptors on peripheral nerves, increasing pain stimuli
b. Causes vasodilation and edema
c. The energy of thermal, chemical, or mechanical stimuli is converted to electrical energy
d. Level of pain a person is willing to put up with
e. The point at which a person is aware of pain
f. Sensory peripheral pain nerve fiber
g. Inhibition of the pain impulse of the nociceptive process
h. Increase sensitivity to pain
i. Body's natural supply of morphinelike substances
j. Inhibits pain transmission
k. The point at which a person feels pain

12. Explain the difference between the following.
    a. Acute pain:

    _____

    _____

    b. Chronic pain:

    _____

    _____

13. Define the following terms related to pain.
    a. *Chronic episodic pain:*

    _____

    _____

    b. *Idiopathic pain:*

    _____

    _____

Nursing Knowledge Base

14. Pain is classified by inferred pathology. Describe the following.

    a. Nociceptive pain: _____
    _____
    _____

    b. Somatic pain: _____
    _____
    _____

    c. Visceral pain: _____
    _____
    _____

    d. Neuropathic pain: _____
    _____
    _____

    e. Deafferentation pain: _____
    _____
    _____

    f. Sympathetically maintained pain: _____
    _____
    _____

    g. Polyneuropathies: _____
    _____
    _____

    h. Mononeuropathies: _____
    _____
    _____

15. Identify the physiological factors that influence pain.
    a. _____
    b. _____
    c. _____
    d. _____

16. Identify the social factors that can influence pain.
    a. _____
    b. _____
    c. _____

17. Identify the spiritual factors that can influence pain.
    _____
    _____
    _____
    _____

18. Identify the psychological factors that can influence pain.
    a. _____
    b. _____ .

19. Identify the cultural factors that can influence pain.
    a. _____
    b. _____

Nursing Process
Assessment

20. Identify the ABCDE clinical approach to pain assessment and management.
    A: _____
    B: _____
    C: _____
    D: _____
    E: _____

21. Identify the common characteristics of pain that the nurse would assess.
    a. _____
    b. _____
    c. _____
    d. _____
    e. _____
    f. _____
    g. _____
    h. _____
    i. _____
    j. _____

Nursing Diagnosis

List potential or actual nursing diagnoses related to a client in pain.

22. _____
    _____

23. _____
    _____

24. _____
    _____

25. _____
    _____

26. _____

_____

27. _____

_____

28. _____

_____

29. _____

_____

30. _____

_____

31. _____

_____

Planning

List the client outcomes appropriate for the client experiencing pain.

32. _____

_____

33. _____

_____

34. _____

_____

Implementation

35. The Agency for Healthcare Research and Quality (AHRQ) guidelines for acute pain management cite nonpharmacological interventions appropriate for clients who meet certain criteria. List those criteria.

a. _____

b. _____

c. _____

d. _____

e. _____

Nonpharmacological interventions such as the following lessen pain. Briefly explain each one.

36. Relaxation: _____

_____

_____

37. Distraction: _____

_____

_____

38. Music: _____

_____

39. Cutaneous stimulation: _____

_____

_____

40. Herbals: _____

_____

41. Reducing pain perception: _____

_____

_____

42. Identify the three types of analgesics used for pain relief.

a. _____

b. _____

c. _____

43. Adjuvants/coanalgesics are:

_____

_____

44. Explain the benefits of patient-controlled analgesia (PCA).

_____

_____

45. Explain the purpose of perineural local anesthetic infusion.

_____

_____

46. Explain the purpose of topical analgesics.

_____

_____

Explain the differences between the following.

47. Local anesthesia:

_____

_____

48. Regional anesthesia:

_____

_____

49. Epidural analgesia:

_____

_____

50. Complications of opioid epidural analgesia are:

_____

_____

51. List the goals for the care of a client with epidural infusions. Describe one action for each goal.

a. _____

b. _____

c. _____

d. _____

e. _____

f. _____

52. Explain the difference between the following.

a. Transdermal fentanyl.

_____

_____

b. Transmucosal fentanyl.

_____

_____

53. Identify the following types of breakthrough pain.

a. Incident pain: _____

_____

_____

b. End-of-dose pain: _____

_____

_____

c. Spontaneous pain: _____

_____

_____

54. Give some examples of barriers to effective pain management.

a. Client: _____

_____

_____

b. Health care provider: _____

_____

_____

c. Health care system: _____

_____

_____

55. Explain the difference between the following types of dependence.

a. Physical dependence: _____

_____

_____

b. Drug tolerance: _____

_____

_____

c. Addiction: _____

_____

_____

d. Pseudoaddiction: _____

_____

_____

e. Pseudotolerance: _____

_____

56. Define *placebo*._____

_____

Explain the purpose of the following.

57. Pain clinics: _____

_____

_____

58. Palliative care: _____

_____

59. Hospice: _____

_____

_____

Evaluation

60. Identify some principles to evaluate related to pain management.

_____

_____

Review Questions

Select the appropriate answer and cite the rationale for choosing that particular answer.

61. Pain is a protective mechanism warning of tissue injury and is largely a (an):
    1. Objective experience
    2. Subjective experience
    3. Acute symptom of short duration
    4. Symptom of a severe illness or disease

    Answer: _____ Rationale: _____
    _____
    _____

62. A substance that can cause analgesia when it attaches to opiate receptors in the brain is:
    1. Endorphin
    2. Bradykinin
    3. Substance P
    4. Prostaglandin

    Answer: _____ Rationale: _____
    _____
    _____

63. To adequately assess the quality of a client's pain, which question would be appropriate?
    1. "Is it a sharp pain or a dull pain?"
    2. "Tell me what your pain feels like."
    3. "Is your pain a crushing sensation?"
    4. "How long have you had this pain?"

    Answer: _____ Rationale: _____
    _____
    _____

64. The use of client distraction in pain control is based on the principle that:
    1. Small C fibers transmit impulses via the spinothalamic tract
    2. The reticular formation can send inhibitory signals to gating mechanisms
    3. Large A fibers compete with pain impulses to close gates to painful stimuli
    4. Transmission of pain impulses from the spinal cord to the cerebral cortex can be inhibited

    Answer: _____ Rationale: _____
    _____
    _____

65. Teaching a child about painful procedures is best achieved by:
    1. Early warnings of the anticipated pain
    2. Storytelling about the upcoming procedure
    3. Relevant play directed toward procedure activities
    4. Avoiding explanations until the pain is experienced

    Answer: _____ Rationale: _____
    _____
    _____

Critical Thinking Model for Nursing Care Plan for Insomnia

66. Imagine that you are the student nurse in the care plan on page 1069 of your text. Complete the *Assessment phase* of the critical thinking model by writing your answers in the appropriate boxes of the model shown. Think about the following.

    - What knowledge base was applied to Mrs. Mays?

    - In what way might previous experience assist you in this case?

    - What intellectual or professional standards were applied to the care of Mrs. Mays?

    - What critical thinking attitudes did you use in assessing Mrs. Mays?

    - As you review your assessment, what key areas did you cover?

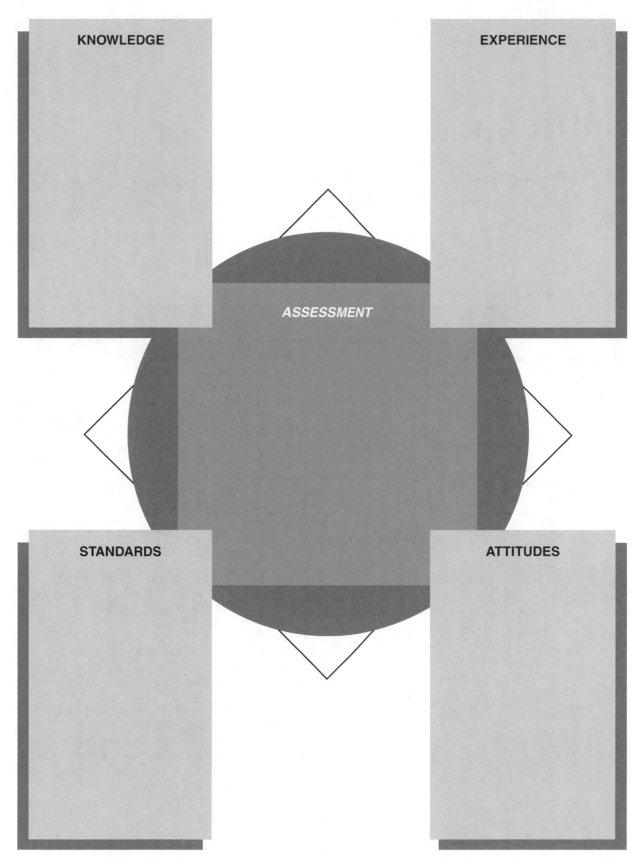

KNOWLEDGE

EXPERIENCE

ASSESSMENT

STANDARDS

ATTITUDES

CHAPTER 43   Critical Thinking Model for Nursing Care Plan for *Acute Pain*

44

Nutrition

Preliminary Reading

Chapter 44, pp. 1085–1128

Comprehensive Understanding

Match the following biochemical units of nutrition.

1. _____ Basal metabolic rate (BMR)
2. _____ Resting energy expenditure (REE)
3. _____ kcal
4. _____ Nutrient density
5. _____ Saccharides
6. _____ Simple carbohydrates
7. _____ Fiber
8. _____ Proteins
9. _____ Amino acid
10. _____ Indispensable amino acids
11. _____ Dispensable amino acids
12. _____ Nitrogen balance
13. _____ Lipids
14. _____ Triglycerides
15. _____ Saturated fatty acids
16. _____ Unsaturated fatty acids
17. _____ Monounsaturated fatty acids
18. _____ Polyunsaturated fatty acids
19. _____ Water
20. _____ Fat-soluble vitamins
21. _____ Hypervitaminosis
22. _____ Water-soluble vitamins
23. _____ Trace elements

a. Vitamin C and B complex
b. Inorganic elements that act as catalysts in biochemical reactions
c. Energy needed to maintain life-sustaining activities for a specific period of time at rest
e. Made up of three fatty acids attached to a glycerol
d. Simplest form of protein
f. The intake and output of nitrogen are equal
g. Have two or more double carbon bonds
h. Resting metabolic rate over a 24-hour period
i. Kilocalorie
j. Are found primarily in sugars
k. Includes soluble (pectin) and insoluble (cellulose)
l. Makes up 60% to 70% of total body weight
m. Most calorie-dense nutrient, provides 9 kcal/g
n. The proportion of essential nutrients to the number of kilocalories
o. Carbohydrate units
p. Alanine, asparagine, and glutamic acid
q. Unequal number of hydrogen atoms are attached and the carbon atoms attach to each other with a double bond
r. Each carbon has two attached hydrogen atoms
s. Histidine, lysine, and phenylalanine
t. Results from megadoses of supplemental vitamins, fortified food, and large intake of fish oils
u. Vitamins A, D, E, K
v. A source of energy (4 kcal/g)
w. Fatty acids with one double bond

Match the following key terms related to the digestive system.

24. _____ Enzymes
25. _____ Peristalsis
26. _____ Chyme
27. _____ Active transport
28. _____ Passive diffusion
29. _____ Osmosis
30. _____ Phagocytosis
31. _____ Metabolism
32. _____ Anabolism
33. _____ Catabolism
34. _____ Glycogenolysis
35. _____ Glycogenesis
36. _____ Gluconeogenesis

a. Anabolism of glucose into glycogen for storage
b. Acidic, liquefied mass
c. Catabolism of glycogen into glucose, carbon dioxide, and water
d. Building of more complex biochemical substances by synthesis of nutrients
e. Breakdown of biochemical substances into simpler substances, occurring during a negative nitrogen balance
f. Proteinlike substances that act as catalysts to speed up chemical reactions
g. Particles move from an area of greater concentration to an area of lesser concentration
h. Wavelike muscular contractions
i. Catabolism of amino acids and glycerol into glucose for energy
j. Engulfing of large molecules of nutrients by the absorbing cell
k. Movement of water through a membrane that separates solutions of different concentrations, do not need a special "carrier"
l. Force by which particles move outward from an area of greater concentration to lesser concentration
m. All biochemical reactions within the cells of the body

37. Explain the four components of the dietary reference intake (DRI).

   a. Estimated average requirement (EAR):

   _____
   _____

   b. Recommended dietary allowance (RDA):

   _____
   _____

   c. Adequate intake (AI):

   _____
   _____

   d. Upper intake level (UL):

   _____
   _____

38. List the key dietary recommendations for the general population.

   a. _____
   b. _____
   c. _____
   d. _____
   e. _____
   f. _____
   g. _____
   h. _____
   i. _____

Nursing Knowledge Base

39. List the benefits of breast-feeding an infant.

   a. _____
   b. _____
   c. _____
   d. _____
   e. _____
   f. _____

Explain why the following should not be used in infant formula.

40. Cow's milk:

   _____
   _____

41. Honey and corn syrup:

   _____
   _____

42. List the indications of an infant's readiness to begin solid foods.

   a. _____
   b. _____
   c. _____

43. Identify the factors that contribute to child-hood obesity.

a. _____

b. _____

c. _____

d. _____

e. _____

44. Identify the factors that influence the adolescent's diet.

a. _____

b. _____

c. _____

d. _____

e. _____

45. Identify the diagnostic criteria for the following eating disorders.

a. Anorexia nervosa:

_____

_____

b. Bulimia nervosa:

_____

_____

46. Explain the importance of folic acid intake in the pregnant woman:

_____

_____

47. List the factors that influence the nutritional status of the older adult.

a. _____

b. _____

c. _____

d. _____

e. _____

f. _____

Explain the following types of vegetarian diets:

48. Ovolactovegetarian:

_____

_____

49. Lactovegetarian:

_____

_____

50. Vegan:

_____

_____

51. Fruitarian:

_____

_____

Nursing Process

Assessment

52. List the five components of a nutritional assessment, and briefly explain.

a. _____

b. _____

c. _____

d. _____

e. _____

53. Dysphagia is:

_____

_____

54. For each assessment area, list at least two signs of poor nutrition.

a. General appearance:

_____

_____

b. Weight:

_____

_____

c. Posture:

_____

_____

d. Muscles:

_____

_____

e. Nervous system:

_____

_____

f. Gastrointestinal function:

_____

_____

g. Cardiovascular function:

_____

_____

h. General vitality:

_____

_____

i. Hair:

_____

_____

j. Skin:

_____

_____

k. Face and neck:

_____

_____

l. Lips:

_____

_____

m. Mouth, oral membranes:

_____

_____

n. Gums:

_____

_____

o. Tongue:

_____

_____

P. Teeth:

_____

_____

q. Eyes:

_____

_____

r. Neck:

_____

_____

s. Nails:

_____

_____

t. Legs, feet:

_____

_____

u. Skeleton:

_____

_____

Nursing Diagnosis

List the potential or actual nursing diagnoses for altered nutritional status.

55. _____

56. _____

57. _____

58. _____

59. _____

60. _____

61. _____

62. _____

63. _____

64. _____

Planning

65. List the goals for a client with nutritional problems.

a. _____

b. _____

c. _____

d. _____

e. _____

Implementation

66. Identify the food source for the following food-borne diseases.

a. Botulism: _____

_____

_____

b. Escherichia coli: _____

_____

_____

c. Listeriosis: _____

_____

_____

d. Perfringens enteritis: _____

_____

e. Salmonellosis: _____

_____

_____

f. Shigellosis: _____

_____

g. Staphylococcus: _____

_____

_____

67. Identify the clients who are at risk for aspiration.

_____

_____

68. Identify the four levels of the dysphagia diet.

a. _____

b. _____

c. _____

d. _____

69. Identify the four levels of liquid.

a. _____

b. _____

c. _____

d. _____

70. Identify the following types of enteral formulas.

a. Polymeric:

_____

_____

b. Modular:

_____

_____

c. Elemental:

_____

_____

d. Specialty:

_____

_____

71. List the benefits of enteral feedings compared to parenteral nutrition (PN).

a. _____

b. _____

c. _____

72. List the three factors on which safe administration of parenteral nutrition depends.

a. _____

b. _____

c. _____

73. Lipid emulsions are:

_____

_____

74. Identify the complications of enteral tube feedings and possible cause.

a. _____

b. _____

c. _____

d. _____

e. _____

f. _____

g. _____

h. _____

i. _____

j. _____

75. List the potential complications of parenteral nutrition, and identify the symptoms of each.

a. _____

b. _____

c. _____

d. _____

e. _____

76. Explain the goal of transition from PN to enteral nutrition (EN) and/or oral feeding.

_____

_____

77. Medical nutrition therapy is:

_____

_____

Identify the nutritional interventions for the following common disease states.

78. *Helicobacter pylori:* _____

_____

_____

79. Inflammatory bowel disease:

_____

_____

80. Malabsorption syndromes:

_____

_____

81. Diverticulitis: _____

_____

_____

82. Diabetes mellitus (DM): _____

_____

_____

83. Cardiovascular disease: _____

_____

_____

84. Cancer: _____

_____

_____

85. Human immunodeficiency virus (HIV):

_____

_____

Evaluation

86. Identify the ongoing evaluative measures.

_____

_____

Review Questions

Select the appropriate answer and cite the rationale for choosing that particular answer.

87. Which nutrient is the body's most preferred energy source?
    1. Fat
    2. Protein
    3. Vitamin
    4. Carbohydrate

    Answer: _____   Rationale: _____

    _____

    _____

88. Positive nitrogen balance would occur in which condition?
    1. Infection
    2. Starvation
    3. Pregnancy
    4. Burn injury

    Answer: _____   Rationale: _____

    _____

    _____

89. Mrs. Nelson is talking with the nurse about the dietary needs of her 23-month-old daughter, Laura. Which of the following responses by the nurse would be appropriate?
    1. "Use skim milk to cut down on the fat in Laura's diet."
    2. "Laura should be drinking at least 1 quart of milk per day."
    3. "Laura needs less protein in her diet now because she isn't growing as fast."
    4. "Laura needs fewer calories in relation to her body weight now than she did as an infant."

    Answer: _____   Rationale: _____

    _____

    _____

90. All of the following clients are at risk for alteration in nutrition except:
    1. Client L, whose weight is 10% above his ideal body weight
    2. Client J, who is 86 years old, lives alone, and has poorly fitting dentures
    3. Client M, a 17-year-old girl who weighs 90 pounds and frequently complains about her baby fat
    4. Client K, who has been allowed nothing by mouth (NPO) for 7 days following bowel surgery and is receiving 3000 mL of 10% dextrose per day

    Answer: _____   Rationale: _____

    _____

    _____

91. Which of the following is the most accurate method of bedside confirmation of placement of a small-bore nasogastric tube?
    1. Assess the client's ability to speak.
    2. Test the pH of withdrawn gastric contents.
    3. Auscultate the epigastrium for gurgling or bubbling.
    4. Assess the length of the tube that is outside the client's nose.

    Answer: _____   Rationale: _____

    _____

    _____

92. A client who has been hospitalized after experiencing a heart attack will most likely receive a diet consisting of:
    1. Low fat, low sodium, and low carbohydrates
    2. Low fat, low sodium, and high carbohydrates
    3. Low fat, high protein, and high carbohydrates
    4. Liquids for several days, progressing to a soft and then a regular diet

    Answer: _____   Rationale: _____

    _____

    _____

Critical Thinking Model for Nursing Care Plan for Imbalanced Nutrition: Less Than Body Requirement

93. Imagine that you are the nurse practitioner in the care plan on page 1107 of your text. Complete the *Assessment phase* of the critical thinking model by writing your answers in the appropriate boxes of the model shown. Think about the following:

- In developing Mrs. Cooper's plan of care, what knowledge did Maria apply?

- In what ways might the nurse practitioner's previous experience assist in developing Mrs. Cooper's plan of care?

- When developing a plan of care for Mrs. Cooper, what intellectual and professional standards were applied?

- What critical thinking attitudes might have been applied in developing Mrs. Cooper's plan of care?

- How will the nurse practitioner accomplish these goals?

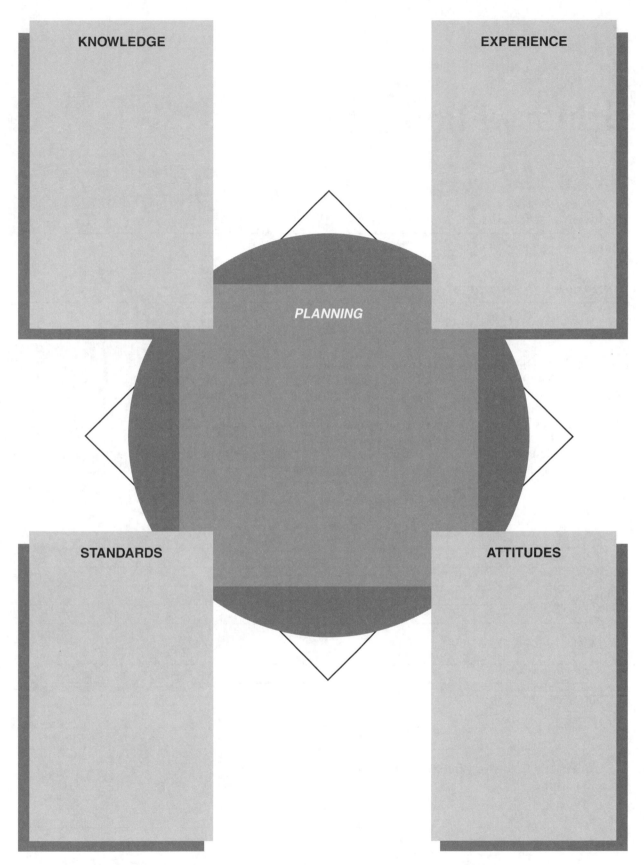

KNOWLEDGE

EXPERIENCE

PLANNING

STANDARDS

ATTITUDES

CHAPTER 44   Critical Thinking Model for *Imbalanced Nutrition: Less Than Body Requirements*

45

Urinary Elimination

Preliminary Reading

Chapter 45, pp. 1129–1173

Comprehensive Understanding

Scientific Knowledge Base

Match the following terms related to urinary elimination.

1. _____ Nephron
2. _____ Proteinuria
3. _____ Erythropoietin
4. _____ Renin
5. _____ Micturition
6. _____ Renal calculus
7. _____ Reflex incontinence

a. Loss of voluntary control, micturition reflex pathway is intact
b. Reflux of urine from the bladder into the ureters
c. Presence of large proteins in the urine
d. Functional unit of the kidneys that forms the urine
e. Kidney stone
f. Enzyme that coverts angiotensinogen into angiotensin I
g. Functions within the bone marrow to stimulate red blood cell (RBC) production

8. List source of the factors that influence urination.
   a. _____
   b. _____
   c. _____
   d. _____
   e. _____

9. Explain uremic syndrome.
   _____
   _____

10. Identify some indications for dialysis.
    _____
    _____

11. Explain the following alterations in fluid balance.
    a. Nocturia:
    _____
    _____

    b. Polyuria:
    _____
    _____

c. Oliguria:

_____

_____

d. Anuria:

_____

_____

Explain the following alterations in urinary elimination.

12. Urinary diversion:

_____

_____

13. Urinary retention:

_____

_____

14. Urinary tract infection (UTI):

_____

_____

15. Urinary incontinence:

_____

_____

16. List the signs or symptoms of UTIs.

a. _____

b. _____

c. _____

d. _____

e. _____

f. _____

g. _____

17. Identify some indications for urinary diversions.

_____

_____

Briefly describe the following urinary diversions.

18. Ileal loop or conduit: _____

_____

_____

19. Nephrostomy: _____

_____

_____

Nursing Process

Assessment

Nursing History

20. List the three major factors to be explored during a nursing history in regard to urinary elimination.

a. _____

b. _____

c. _____

Match the following common types of urinary alterations.

21. _____ Urgency
22. _____ Dysuria
23. _____ Frequency
24. _____ Hesitancy
25. _____ Polyuria
26. _____ Oliguria
27. _____ Nocturia
28. _____ Dribbling
29. _____ Incontinence
30. _____ Hematuria
31. _____ Retention
32. _____ Residual urine

a. Accumulation of urine in the bladder, with the inability to empty fully
b. May be due to stress incontinence
c. Greater than 100 mL of urine remaining after voiding
d. Due to loss of pelvic muscle tone, fecal impaction, overactive bladder
e. Painful or difficult urination
f. Blood in the urine
g. Due to increased fluid intake, pregnancy, and diuretics
h. Large amounts of urine voided
i. Due to prostate enlargement, anxiety, or urethral edema
j. Feeling of the need to void immediately
k. Diminished urinary output relative to intake
l. Nighttime voiding often due to coffee or alcohol

33. Identify the primary structures that the nurse would assess.

_____

_____

Describe the following characteristics of urine.

34. Color:

_____

_____

35. Clarity:

_____

_____

36. Odor:

_____

_____

37. Describe the following types of urine specimens collected for testing.

  a. Random: _____

_____

_____

  b. Clean-voided or midstream:_____

_____

_____

  c. Sterile:_____

_____

_____

  d. Timed urine:_____

_____

_____

Common urine tests include the following. Briefly explain each.

38. Urinalysis: _____

_____

_____

39. Specific gravity: _____

_____

_____

40. Urine culture: _____

_____

_____

41. Briefly explain the purpose of each of the following noninvasive diagnostic examinations.

  a. Abdominal roentgenogram: _____

_____

_____

  b. Intravenous pyelogram (IVP): _____

_____

_____

  c. Urodynamic testing:_____

_____

_____

  d. Computerized axial tomography (CT) scan:

_____

_____

  e. Ultrasound: _____

_____

_____

42. Explain the purpose of the following invasive procedures.

  a. Endoscopy: _____

_____

_____

  b. Arteriogram: _____

_____

_____

Nursing Diagnosis

List the potential or actual nursing diagnoses related to urinary elimination.

43. _____

44. _____

45. _____

46. _____

47. _____

48. _____

49. _____

50. _____

Planning

51. List the goals appropriate for a client with a urinary elimination problem.

  a. _____

  b. _____

  c. _____

Implementation

Health Promotion

52. List the techniques that may be used to stimulate the micturition reflex.

    a. _____

    b. _____

    c. _____

    d. _____

53. List two interventions for each of the following types of urinary incontinence.

    a. Functional: _____

    _____

    _____

    b. Stress: _____

    _____

    _____

    c. Urge: _____

    _____

    _____

    d. Mixed: _____

    _____

    _____

    e. Reflex: _____

    _____

    _____

54. Identify substances that can increase urine acidity.

    _____

    _____

55. State the indications for the following types of catheterizations.

    a. Intermittent:

    _____

    _____

    b. Short-term indwelling:

    _____

    _____

    c. Long-term indwelling:

    _____

    _____

Acute Care

Explain the nursing measures taken to prevent infection and maintain an unobstructed flow of urine in catheterized clients.

56. Perineal hygiene: _____

    _____

    _____

57. Catheter care: _____

    _____

    _____

58. Fluid intake: _____

    _____

    _____

59. Irrigations and instillations: _____

    _____

    _____

Briefly explain the two alternatives to urinary catheterization.

60. Suprapubic catheter: _____

    _____

    _____

61. Condom catheter: _____

    _____

    _____

Explain the purpose of the following.

62. Pelvic floor exercises (PFEs/Kegel exercises):

    _____

    _____

63. Bladder retraining: _____

    _____

    _____

64. Habit training: _____

    _____

    _____

65. Self-catheterization: _____

    _____

    _____

Evaluation

66. Identify how the nurse would evaluate the effectiveness of the interventions utilized.

_____

_____

Review Questions

Select the appropriate answer and cite the rationale for choosing that particular answer.

67. Mrs. Rantz complains of leaking urine when she coughs or laughs. This is known as:
    1. Urge incontinence
    2. Stress incontinence
    3. Reflex incontinence
    4. Functional incontinence

Answer: _____ Rationale: _____

_____

_____

68. Ms. Hathaway has a urinary tract infection. Which of the following symptoms would you expect her to exhibit?
    1. Dysuria
    2. Oliguria
    3. Polyuria
    4. Proteinuria

Answer: _____ Rationale: _____

_____

_____

69. The nurse is working in the radiology department with a client who is having an intravenous pyelogram. Which of the following complaints by the client is an abnormal response?
    1. Frequent, loose stools
    2. Thirst and feeling "worn out"
    3. Shortness of breath and audible wheezing
    4. Feeling dizzy and warm with obvious facial flushing

Answer: _____ Rationale: _____

_____

_____

70. The urinalysis of Ms. Hathaway reveals a high bacteria count. Ampicillin is prescribed for her urinary tract infection. The teaching plan for the prevention of a UTI should include all of the following except:
    1. Drink at least 2000 mL of fluid daily
    2. Always wipe perineum from front to back
    3. Drink plenty of orange and grapefruit juices
    4. Explain the possible side effects of medication

Answer: _____ Rationale: _____

_____

_____

Critical Thinking Model for Nursing Care Plan for Stress Urinary Incontinence

71. Imagine that you are Mrs. Kay, the nurse in the care plan on page 1147 of your text. Complete the *Assessment phase* of the critical thinking model by writing your answers in the appropriate boxes of the model shown. Think about the following.

    • What knowledge base was applied to the care of Mrs. Grayson?

    • In what way might Mrs. Kay's previous experience assist in this case?

    • What intellectual or professional standards were applied to the care of Mrs. Grayson?

    • What critical thinking attitudes did you utilize in assessing Mrs. Grayson?

    • As you review the assessment, what key areas did Mrs. Kay cover?

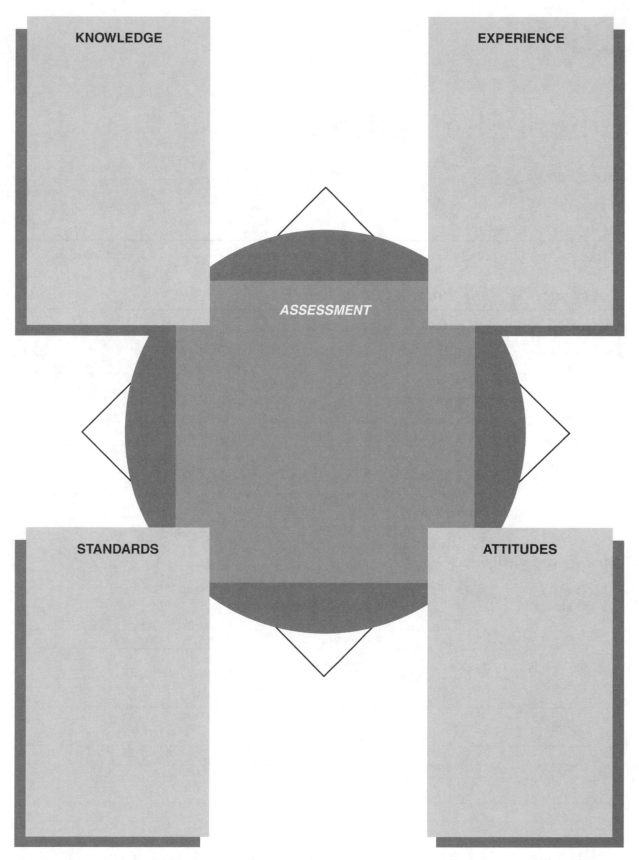

KNOWLEDGE

EXPERIENCE

ASSESSMENT

STANDARDS

ATTITUDES

CHAPTER 45   Critical Thinking Model for *Stress Urinary Incontinence*

46

Bowel Elimination

Preliminary Reading

Chapter 46, pp. 1174–1218

Comprehensive Understanding

Scientific Knowledge Base

Summarize the functions of the following.
1. Mouth: _____

2. Esophagus: _____

3. Stomach: _____

4. Small intestine: _____

5. Large intestine: _____

6. Anus: _____

7. Explain the Valsalva maneuver. _____

Nursing Knowledge Base

8. Explain the normal age-related changes that occur in the gastrointestinal (GI) tract.
   a. Mouth:

   _____

   _____

   b. Esophagus:

   _____

   _____

   c. Stomach:

   _____

   _____

   d. Small intestine:

   _____

   _____

   e. Large intestine:

   _____

   _____

f. Liver:

_____

_____

9. Explain how fiber affects the diet, and give some examples of good fiber sources.

_____

_____

10. Define *lactose intolerance.*

_____

_____

11. Summarize how fluids can affect the character of feces.

_____

_____

12. Summarize the benefits of physical activity:

_____

_____

13. List the diseases of the GI tract that may be associated with stress.

_____

_____

14. List four personal elimination habits that influence bowel function.
    a. _____
    b. _____
    c. _____
    d. _____

15. List conditions that may result in painful defecation.
    a. _____
    b. _____
    c. _____
    d. _____

16. Summarize the effects of anesthetic agents and peristalsis on defecation.

_____

_____

17. Describe the effect of each medication on elimination.

    a. Dicyclomine HCl (Bentyl): _____

    _____

    _____

    b. Narcotics: _____

    _____

    _____

c. Anticholinergics: _____

_____

_____

d. Antibiotics: _____

_____

e. Nonsteroidal antiinflammatory drugs (NSAIDs): _____

_____

f. Aspirin: _____

_____

g. Histamine antagonists: _____

_____

_____

h. Iron: _____

_____

_____

18. List types of diagnostic tests for visualization of GI structures.
    a. _____
    b. _____

19. List four factors that place a client at risk for elimination problems.
    a. _____
    b. _____
    c. _____
    d. _____

20. List the signs of constipation.
    a. _____
    b. _____
    c. _____
    d. _____
    e. _____

21. List common causes of constipation.
    a. _____
    b. _____
    c. _____
    d. _____
    e. _____
    f. _____
    g. _____
    h. _____
    i. _____
    j. _____

22. List the groups of clients in whom constipation could pose a significant health hazard.
    a. _____
    b. _____
    c. _____
    d. _____

23. Define *fecal impaction*.
    _____
    _____

24. List signs and symptoms of fecal impaction.
    a. _____
    b. _____
    c. _____
    d. _____
    e. _____

25. Define *diarrhea*.
    _____
    _____

26. Name the two complications associated with diarrhea.
    a. _____
       _____
       _____
    b. _____
       _____
       _____

27. Explain *Clostridium difficile* infection:
    _____
    _____

28. Explain the following.
    a. Fecal incontinence: _____
       _____
       _____
       _____
    b. Flatulence: _____
       _____
       _____
       _____

29. List four conditions that cause hemorrhoids.
    a. _____
    b. _____
    c. _____
    d. _____

Define the following bowel diversions.

30. *Stoma:* _____
    _____
    _____
    _____

31. *Ileostomy:* _____
    _____
    _____
    _____

32. *Colostomy:* _____
    _____
    _____
    _____

33. Identify the three types of colostomy constructions available.
    a. _____
    b. _____
    c. _____

Nursing Process

Assessment

34. List 15 factors that affect elimination that need to be included in a nursing history for clients with altered elimination status.
    a. _____
    b. _____
    c. _____
    d. _____
    e. _____
    f. _____
    g. _____
    h. _____
    i. _____
    j. _____
    k. _____
    l. _____
    m. _____
    n. _____
    o. _____

Summarize the following steps for assessing the abdomen.

35. Inspection: _____
    _____

36. Auscultation: _____
    _____

37. Palpation: _____

_____

38. Percussion: _____

_____

39. Define *fecal occult blood testing (FOBT)*. _____

_____

40. Describe the normal fecal characteristics.

a. Color: _____

b. Odor: _____

c. Consistency: _____

d. Frequency: _____

e. Amount: _____

f. Shape: _____

g. Constituents: _____

41. List the common radiological and diagnostic tests used with the client with altered bowel elimination.

a. _____

b. _____

c. _____

d. _____

e. _____

f. _____

g. _____

h. _____

j. _____

k. _____

l. _____

Nursing Diagnosis

List the potential or actual nursing diagnoses for a client with alteration in bowel elimination.

42. _____

43. _____

44. _____

45. _____

46. _____

47. _____

Planning

List the overall goals appropriate for clients with elimination problems.

48. _____

49. _____

50. _____

51. _____

52. _____

Implementation

53. List the factors to consider to promote normal defecation.

a. _____

b. _____

c. _____

Acute Care

Identify the primary action of the following.

54. Cathartics and laxatives: _____

_____

55. Antidiarrheals: _____

_____

56. Enemas: _____

_____

Briefly describe the following types of enemas.

57. Cleansing enema: _____

_____

58. Tap water enema: _____

_____

59. Normal saline: _____

_____

60. Hypertonic solution: _____

_____

61. Soapsuds: _____

_____

62. Oil retention: _____

_____

63. Explain the purpose of a carminative enema. _____

_____

64. Explain the physician's or health care provider's order, "Give enemas till clear."

_____

65. List the complications of excessive rectal manipulation.

a. _____

b. _____

c. _____

66. List the purposes of nasogastric (NG) intubation.
    a. _____
    b. _____
    c. _____
    d. _____

67. Explain how the nurse would provide comfort to a client with an NG tube.

    _____
    _____

List the measures included for a successful bowel training program.

68. _____

69. _____

70. _____

71. _____

72. _____

73. _____

74. _____

75. _____

76. _____

Evaluation

77. Identify some positive outcomes for a client with alterations in bowel elimination.

    _____
    _____

Review Questions

Select the appropriate answer and cite the rationale for choosing that particular answer.

78. Most nutrients and electrolytes are absorbed in the:
    1. Colon
    2. Stomach
    3. Esophagus
    4. Small intestine

    Answer: _____   Rationale: _____
    _____
    _____

79. Which of the following should be included in the teaching plan for the client who is scheduled for an upper GI series?
    1. The client will be allowed nothing by mouth (NPO) after midnight.
    2. General anesthetic is usually used for the procedure.
    3. Moderate abdominal pain is common after the procedure.
    4. A cleansing enema will be given the evening before the procedure.

    Answer: _____   Rationale: _____
    _____
    _____

80. Mrs. Anthony is concerned about her breast-fed infant's stool, stating that it is yellow instead of brown. The nurse explains to Mrs. Anthony that:
    1. The stool is normal for an infant
    2. A change to formula may be necessary
    3. It will be necessary to send a stool specimen to the laboratory
    4. Her infant is dehydrated and she should increase his fluid intake

    Answer: _____   Rationale: _____
    _____
    _____

81. After positioning a client on the bedpan, the nurse should:
    1. Leave the head of the bed flat
    2. Raise the head of the bed 30 degrees
    3. Raise the bed to the highest working level
    4. Raise the head of the bed to a 90-degree angle

    Answer: _____   Rationale: _____
    _____
    _____

82. The physician has ordered a cleansing enema for 7-year-old Michael. The nurse realizes the maximum volume to be given would be:
    1. 100 to 150 mL
    2. 150 to 250 mL
    3. 300 to 500 mL
    4. 600 to 700 mL

    Answer: _____   Rationale: _____
    _____
    _____

Critical Thinking Model for Nursing Care Plan for Constipation

83. Imagine that you are Javier, the home care nurse in the care plan on page 1193 of your text. Complete the *Planning phase* of the critical thinking model by writing your answers in the appropriate boxes of the model shown. Think about the following.

- In developing Larry's plan of care, what knowledge did Javier apply?

- In what way might Javier's previous experience assist in developing a plan of care for Larry?

- When developing a plan of care, what intellectual and professional standards were applied?

- What critical thinking attitudes might have been applied in developing a plan for Larry?

- How will Javier accomplish the goals?

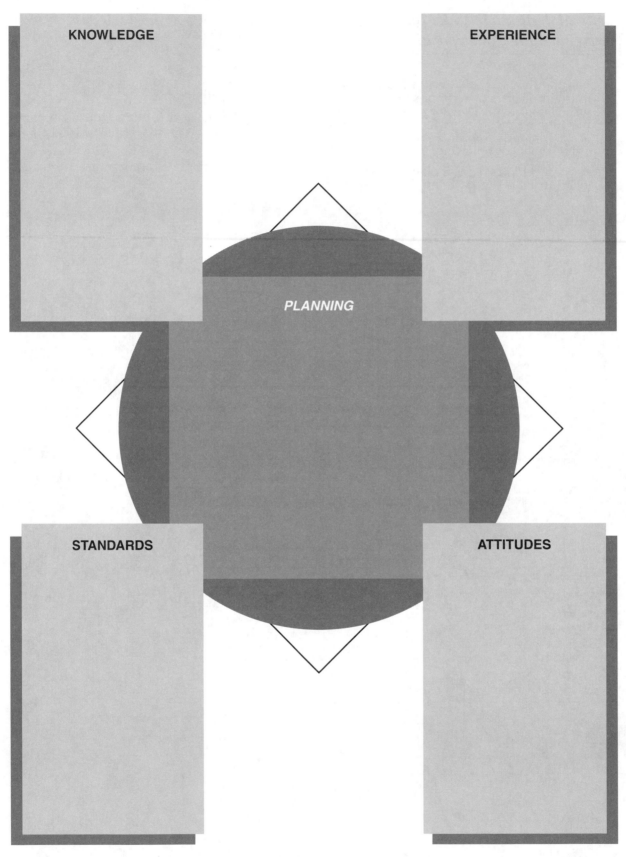

KNOWLEDGE

EXPERIENCE

PLANNING

STANDARDS

ATTITUDES

CHAPTER 46   Critical Thinking Model for *Constipation*

47

Mobility and Immobility

Preliminary Reading

Chapter 47, pp. 1219–1277

Comprehensive Understanding

Scientific Knowledge Base

Match the following terms related to the nature of movement.

1. _____ Movement
2. _____ Mobility
3. _____ Body mechanics
4. _____ Body alignment
5. _____ Balance
6. _____ Friction

a. Force that occurs in a direction to oppose movement
b. Required to maintain a static position
c. Visible aspect and contributes to self-worth and well-being
d. Coordinated efforts of the musculoskeletal and nervous system
e. Used to show self-defense, perform activities of daily living (ADLs) and recreational activities
f. Reduces strain, maintains muscle tone, comfort, conserves energy

Match the following terms related to the physiology and regulation of movement.

7. _____ Long bones
8. _____ Short bones
9. _____ Flat bones
10. _____ Irregular bones
11. _____ Pathological fractures
12. _____ Synostosis joint
13. _____ Cartilaginous joint
14. _____ Fibrous joint
15. _____ Synovial joint
16. _____ Ligaments
17. _____ Tendons
18. _____ Cartilage
19. _____ Concentric tension
20. _____ Eccentric tension
21. _____ Isotonic contraction
22. _____ Isometric contraction
23. _____ Leverage
24. _____ Posture
25. _____ Muscle tone

a. Inducing or compelling force
b. Increased muscle contraction causes muscle shortening resulting in movement
c. Connect muscle to bone
d. Normal state of balanced muscle tension
e. Make up the vertebral column and some bones of the skull
f. Bones jointed by bones with no movement
g. Occur in clusters (carpal bones in the foot)
h. Provide structural contour (skull)
i. Position of the body in relation to the surrounding space
j. Helps control the speed and direction of movement
k. Joint in which a ligament unites two bony surfaces (paired bones of the lower leg)
l. Unites bony components
m. Active movement between concentric and eccentric muscle actions
n. Ball-and-socket joints (hip joint)
o. Nonvascular, supporting tissue (joints and thorax)
p. Causes an increase in muscle tension or muscle work but no shortening or active movement
q. Fibrous tissue that connect bones and cartilages
r. Contribute to height
s. Caused by weakened bone tissue

26. Define the following pathological abnormalities that influence mobility.

    a. *Torticollis:* _____

    b. *Lordosis:* _____

    c. *Kyphosis:* _____

    d. *Scoliosis:* _____

    e. *Congential hip dysplasia:* _____

    f. *Knock-knee:* _____

    g. *Bowlegs:* _____

    h. *Clubfoot:* _____

    i. *Footdrop:* _____

    j. *Pigeon toes:* _____

27. Damage to a component of the central nervous system that regulates voluntary movement results in: _____

    _____

28. Direct trauma to the musculoskeletal system results in: _____

    _____

Nursing Knowledge Base

Define the following terms.

29. *Mobility:* _____

    _____

    _____

    _____

30. *Immobility:* _____

    _____

    _____

    _____

31. Identify the objectives of bed rest.

    a. _____

    b. _____

    c. _____

    d. _____

32. Identify the complications of immobility in relation to the metabolic functioning of the body.

    a. _____

    b. _____

    c. _____

33. Explain the following respiratory changes that occur with immobility.

    a. Atelectasis: _____

    _____

    _____

    _____

    b. Hydrostatic pneumonia: _____

    _____

    _____

    _____

34. Explain the following cardiovascular changes that occur with immobility.

    a. Orthostatic hypotension: _____

    _____

    _____

    _____

    b. Thrombus: _____

    _____

    _____

    _____

35. Identify the complications of immobility in relation to the musculoskeletal system.

    a. _____

    b. _____

    c. _____

    d. _____

    e. _____

    f. _____

36. Identify the complications of immobility in relation to the urinary system.

    a. _____

    b. _____

37. Identify the complication of immobility in relation to the integumentary system.

    _____

38. Identify the psychosocial effects that occur with immobilization.

    a. _____

    b. _____

    c. _____

Nursing Process

Assessment

Briefly describe the four major areas for assessment of client mobility.

39. Range of motion: _____

40. Gait: _____

41. Exercise and activity tolerance: _____

42. Body alignment: _____

Nursing Diagnosis

List the actual or potential nursing diagnoses related to an immobilized or partially immobilized client.

43. _____

44. _____

45. _____

46. _____

47. _____

48. _____

49. _____

Planning

50. List the expected outcomes for the goal "client skin remains intact".
    a. _____
    b. _____

Implementation

51. Identify some examples of health promotion activities that address mobility and immobility.
    a. _____
    b. _____
    c. _____
    d. _____

Identify the nursing interventions that will reduce the impact of immobility on the following body systems:

52. Metabolic system:
    a. _____
    b. _____

53. Respiratory system:
    a. _____
    b. _____
    c. _____

54. Cardiovascular system:
    a. _____
    b. _____
    c. _____

55. Musculoskeletal system:
    a. _____
    b. _____

56. Integumentary system:
    a. _____
    b. _____

57. Elimination system:
    a. _____
    b. _____

58. Psychosocial system:
    a. _____
    b. _____

59. Explain the use for the following.
    a. Trochanter roll: _____
    b. Hand rolls: _____
    c. Trapeze bar: _____

Give a description of the following positions.

60. Fowler's: _____

61. Supine: _____

62. Prone: _____

63. Side-lying: _____

64. Sims': _____

65. Instrumental activities of daily living (IADL) are: _____

66. Describe how you would assist clients with hemiplegia or hemiparesis: _____

Evaluation

67. Identify the evaluative measures.

_____

_____

_____

_____

Review Questions

Select the appropriate answer and cite the rationale for choosing that particular answer.

68. Which of the following is a potential hazard that you should assess when the client is in the prone position?
    1. Plantar flexion
    2. Increased cervical flexion
    3. Internal rotation of the shoulder
    4. Unprotected pressure points at the sacrum and heels

Answer: _____   Rationale: _____

_____

_____

69. Which of the following is a physiological effect of prolonged bed rest?
    1. An increase in cardiac output
    2. A decrease in lean body mass
    3. A decrease in lung expansion
    4. A decrease in urinary excretion of nitrogen

Answer: _____   Rationale: _____

_____

_____

70. All of the following measures are used to assess for deep vein thrombosis except:
    1. Checking for a positive Homans' sign
    2. Asking the client about the presence of calf pain
    3. Observing the dorsal aspect of lower extremities for redness, warmth, and tenderness
    4. Measuring the circumference of each leg daily, placing the tape measure at the midpoint of the knee

Answer: _____   Rationale: _____

_____

_____

71. Which of the following is an appropriate intervention to maintain the respiratory system of the immobilized client?
    1. Turn the client every 4 hours.
    2. Maintain a maximum fluid intake of 1500 mL per day.
    3. Apply an abdominal binder continuously while in bed.
    4. Encourage the client to deep breathe and cough every 1 to 2 hours.

Answer: _____   Rationale: _____

_____

_____

Critical Thinking Model for Nursing Care Plan for Impaired Mobility

72. Imagine that you are the student nurse in the care plan on page 1242 of your text. Complete the *Evaluation phase* of the critical thinking model by writing your answers in the appropriate boxes of the model shown. Think about the following:

   • What knowledge did you apply in evaluating Ms. Adams' care?

   • In what way might your previous experience influence your evaluation of Ms. Adams?

   • During evaluation, what intellectual and professional standards were applied to Ms. Adams' care?

   • In what ways do critical thinking attitudes play a role in how you approach evaluation of Ms. Adams' care?

   • How might you adjust Ms. Adams' care?

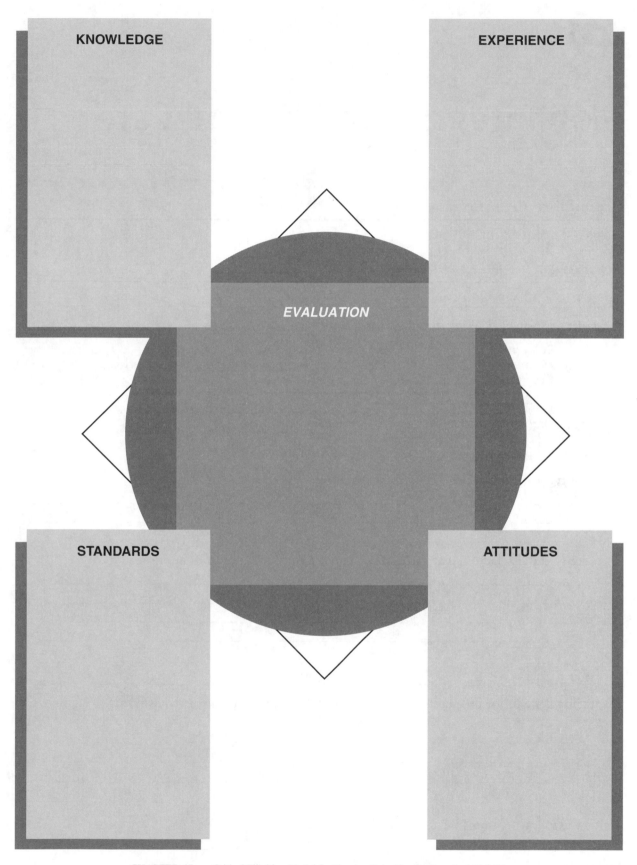

KNOWLEDGE

EXPERIENCE

EVALUATION

STANDARDS

ATTITUDES

CHAPTER 47   Critical Thinking Model for Nursing Care Plan for *Impaired Mobility*

48

Skin Integrity and Wound Care

Preliminary Reading

Chapter 48, pp.1278–1341

Comprehensive Understanding

Scientific Knowledge Base

Match the following key terms related to skin integrity.

1. _____ Epidermis
2. _____ Dermis
3. _____ Collagen
4. _____ Pressure ulcer
5. _____ Blanching
6. _____ Darkly pigmented skin

a. Tough, fibrous protein
b. Localized injury to the skin and underlying tissue over a body prominence
c. Does not blanch
d. Normal red tones of light-skinned clients are absent
e. Top layer of the skin
f. Inner layer of the skin that provides tensile strength and mechanical support

7. Identify the pressure factors that contribute to pressure ulcer development.
   a. _____
   b. _____
   c. _____

8. Identify the risk factors that predispose a client to pressure ulcer formation.
   a. _____
   b. _____
   c. _____
   d. _____
   e. _____
   f. _____

9. Staging systems for pressure ulcers are based on the depth of tissue destroyed. Briefly describe each stage.
   I: _____
   II: _____
   III: _____
   IV: _____

Define the following terms related to wound healing.

10. *Granulation tissue:* _____

11. *Slough:* _____

12. *Eschar:* _____

13. *Exudate:* _____

216

Describe the physiological process involved with wound healing.

14. Primary intention: _____

_____

_____

15. Secondary intention: _____

_____

_____

16. Tertiary intention: _____

_____

_____

_____

17. Identify the three components involved in the healing process of a partial-thickness wound.

  a. _____

  b. _____

  c. _____

Explain the three phases involved in the healing process of a full-thickness wound.

18. Inflammatory phase: _____

_____

19. Proliferative phase: _____

_____

20. Remodeling: _____

_____

Briefly explain the following complications of wound healing.

21. Hemorrhage: _____

_____

_____

22. Health-care associated infection: _____

_____

_____

23. Dehiscence:_____

_____

_____

24. Evisceration:_____

_____

_____

25. Fistulas: _____

_____

_____

Nursing Knowledge Base

26. Identify two types of scales utilized to systematically assess risk for pressure ulcers.

  a. _____

  b. _____

27. List the factors that influence pressure ulcer formation.

  a. _____

  b. _____

  c. _____

  d. _____

  e. _____

Nursing Process

Assessment

Explain the following factors that place a client at risk for a pressure ulcer:

28. Mobility: _____

_____

_____

29. Nutritional status:_____

_____

_____

_____

30. Body fluids:_____

_____

_____

_____

31. Pain: _____

_____

_____

_____

32. Identify the following types of emergency setting wounds.

  a. Abrasion: _____

_____

_____

_____

b. Laceration: _____

_____

_____

c. Puncture: _____

_____

_____

_____

Explain how the nurse assesses the following.

33. Wound appearance: _____

_____

34. Character of wound drainage: _____

_____

_____

35. Drains: _____

_____

_____

36. Wound closures: _____

_____

_____

Nursing Diagnosis

List the potential or actual nursing diagnoses related to impaired skin integrity.

37. _____

38. _____

39. _____

40. _____

41. _____

42. _____

43. _____

44. _____

Planning

45. List possible goals to achieve wound improvement.

a. _____

b. _____

c. _____

Implementation

46. Identify the nursing interventions to perform to prevent pressure ulcer for the following risk factors:

a. Decreased sensory perception:

_____

_____

b. Moisture:

_____

_____

c. Friction and shear:

_____

_____

d. Decreased activity/mobility:

_____

_____

e. Poor nutrition:

_____

_____

Acute Care

47. Explain the rationale for debriding a wound.

_____

48. Identify the four methods of debridement.

a. _____

b. _____

c. _____

d. _____

First aid for wounds includes the following. Briefly explain each one.

49. Hemostasis:

_____

_____

50. Cleansing:

_____

_____

51. Protection:

_____

_____

52. List the purposes of dressings.

a. _____

b. _____

c. _____

d. _____

e. _____

f. _____

g. _____

53. List the clinical guidelines to use when selecting the appropriate dressing.

a. _____

b. _____

c. _____

d. _____

e. _____

f. _____

54. List the advantages of a transparent film dressing.

a. _____

b. _____

c. _____

d. _____

e. _____

f. _____

55. List the functions of hydrocolloid dressings.

a. _____

b. _____

c. _____

d. _____

e. _____

f. _____

g. _____

56. List the advantages of the hydrogel dressing.

a. _____

b. _____

c. _____

d. _____

57. List the Centers for Disease Control and Prevention (CDC) recommendations to follow when changing dressings.

a. _____

b. _____

c. _____

d. _____

58. Summarize the principles of packing a wound.

_____

_____

59. Briefly describe how the Wound Vacuum Assisted Closure (Wound V.A.C.) device works.

_____

_____

60. Identify three principles that are important when cleaning an incision.

a. _____

b. _____

c. _____

61. Summarize the principles of wound irrigation.

_____

_____

62. Explain the purpose for drainage evacuation.

_____

_____

63. Explain the benefits of binders and bandages.

a. _____

b. _____

c. _____

d. _____

e. _____

f. _____

64. List the nursing responsibilities when applying a bandage or binder.

a. _____

b. _____

c. _____

d. _____

65. Describe the physiological responses to the following.

a. Heat applications:

_____

_____

b. Cold applications:

_____

_____

List the factors that influence heat and cold tolerance.

66. _____

67. _____

68. _____

69. _____

70. _____

71. _____

72. _____

73. _____

74. Explain the risk factors for injury from heat and cold applications.

    a. Very young or older clients:

    _____

    _____

    b. Open wounds:

    _____

    _____

    c. Areas of edema:

    _____

    _____

    d. Peripheral vascular disease:

    _____

    _____

    e. Confusion:

    _____

    _____

    f. Spinal cord injury:

    _____

    _____

    g. Abscessed tooth:

    _____

    _____

Explain the rationale for the following types of applications.

75. Warm, moist compresses: _____

    _____

76. Warm soaks: _____

    _____

77. Sitz baths: _____

    _____

78. Aquathermia pads: _____

    _____

79. Commercial hot packs: _____

    _____

80. Cold, moist, and dry compresses:

    _____

81. Cold soaks: _____

    _____

82. Ice bags or collars: _____

    _____

Evaluation

83. List the questions to ask if the identified outcomes were not met.

    a. _____

    b. _____

    c. _____

Review Questions

Select the appropriate answer and cite the rationale for choosing that particular answer.

84. Mr. Post is in a Fowler's position to improve his oxygenation status. The nurse notes that he frequently slides down in the bed and needs to be repositioned. Mr. Post is at risk for developing a pressure ulcer on his coccyx because of:
    1. Friction
    2. Maceration
    3. Shearing force
    4. Impaired peripheral circulation

    Answer: _____ Rationale: _____

    _____

    _____

85. Which of the following is not a subscale on the Braden scale for predicting pressure ulcer risk?
    1. Age
    2. Activity
    3. Moisture
    4. Sensory perception

    Answer: _____ Rationale: _____

    _____

    _____

86. Which of these clients has a nutritional risk for pressure ulcer development?
    1. Client A has an albumin level of 3.5.
    2. Client B has a hemoglobin level within normal limits.
    3. Client C has a protein intake of 0.5 g/kg/day.
    4. Client D has a body weight that is 5% greater than his ideal weight.

Answer: _____ Rationale: _____

_____

_____

87. Mr. Perkins has a stage II ulcer of his right heel. What would be the most appropriate treatment for this ulcer?
    1. Apply a heat lamp to the area for 20 minutes twice daily.
    2. Apply a hydrocolloid dressing, and change it as necessary.
    3. Apply a calcium alginate dressing, and change when strike-through is noted.
    4. Apply a thick layer of enzymatic ointment to the ulcer and the surrounding skin.

Answer: _____ Rationale: _____

_____

_____

Critical Thinking Model for Nursing Care Plan for Impaired Skin Integrity

88. Imagine that you are the nurse in the care plan on page 1302 of your text. Complete the *Assessment phase* of the critical thinking model by writing your answers in the appropriate boxes of the model shown. Think about the following.

- What knowledge base was applied to Mrs. Stein?

- In what way might your previous experience assist you in this case?

- What intellectual or professional standards were applied to Mrs. Stein?

- What critical thinking attitudes did you use in assessing Mrs. Stein?

- As you review your assessment, what key areas did you cover?

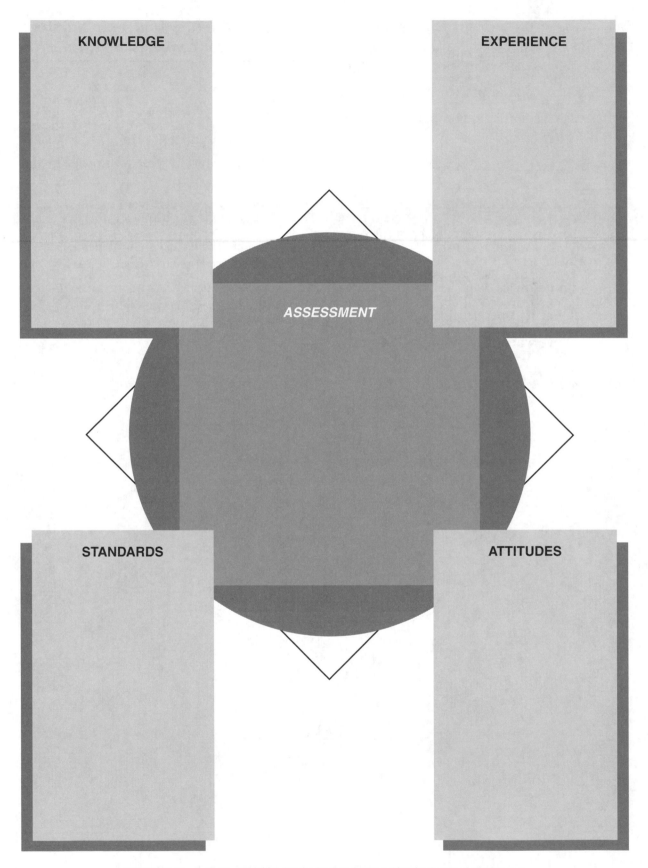

KNOWLEDGE

EXPERIENCE

ASSESSMENT

STANDARDS

ATTITUDES

CHAPTER 48   Critical Thinking Model for Nursing Care Plan for *Impaired Skin Integrity*

49

Sensory Alterations

Preliminary Reading

Chapter 49, pp. 1342–1364

Comprehensive Understanding

Scientific Knowledge Base

Match the following key terms related to sensations.

1. _____ Auditory
2. _____ Tactile
3. _____ Olfactory
4. _____ Gustatory
5. _____ Kinesthetic
6. _____ Stereognosis

a. Enables a person to be aware of position and movement of body parts
b. Taste
c. Hearing
d. Smell
e. Recognition of an object's size, shape, and texture
f. Touch

Match the following terms related to the common sensory deficits.

7. _____ Presbyopia
8. _____ Cataract
9. _____ Dry eyes
10. _____ Glaucoma
11. _____ Diabetic retinopathy
12. _____ Macular degeneration
13. _____ Presbycusis
14. _____ Cerumen
15. _____ Disequilibrium
16. _____ Xerostomia
17. _____ Peripheral neuropathy
18. _____ Stroke

a. Numbness and tingling of the affected area, stumbling gait
b. Results from vestibular dysfunction, vertigo
c. Decreased accommodation of the lens to see near objects clearly
d. Blurring of reading matter, distortion or loss of central vision and vertical lines
e. Caused by clot, hemorrhage, or emboli to the brain
f. Opaque areas of the lens that cause glaring and blurred vision
g. Decrease in salivary production, leading to thicker mucus and dry mouth
h. Decreased tear production that results in itching and burning
i. Progressive hearing disorder in older adults
j. Increase in intraocular pressure resulting in peripheral visual loss, halo effect around lights
k. Earwax, causes a conduction deafness
l. Blood vessel changes of the retina, decreased vision, and macular edema

19. List the three major types of sensory deprivation, and give an example of each.

a. _____

b. _____

c. _____

20. Give an example of the following effects of sensory deprivation.

    a. Cognitive:

    _____

    _____

    b. Affective:

    _____

    _____

    c. Perceptual:

    _____

    _____

21. Define *sensory overload*.

    _____

    _____

Nursing Knowledge Base

22. Identify the factors that influence the capacity to receive or perceive stimuli.

    a. _____

    b. _____

    c. _____

    d. _____

    e. _____

    f. _____

Nursing Process

Assessment

23. Identify the groups that are at high risk for sensory alterations.

    _____

    _____

24. When assessing the client's mental status, the nurse needs to evaluate each of the following. Give an example of each.

    a. Physical appearance and behavior:

    _____

    _____

    b. Cognitive ability:

    _____

    _____

    c. Emotional stability:

    _____

    _____

25. Complete the following table by describing at least one assessment technique for the identified sensory function and the behaviors for an adult and child that would indicate a sensory deficit.

Sense	Assessment Technique	Child Behavior	Adult Behavior
Vision			
Hearing			
Touch			
Smell			
Taste			

26. Identify some common home hazards.

a. _____

b. _____

c. _____

d. _____

e. _____

f. _____

g. _____

h. _____

i. _____

j. _____

k. _____

27. Explain the following types of aphasia.

a. Expressive:

_____

_____

b. Receptive:

_____

_____

Nursing Diagnosis

List the actual or potential nursing diagnoses for a client with sensory alterations.

28. _____

29. _____

30. _____

31. _____

32. _____

33. _____

34. _____

35. _____

36. _____

Planning

37. List goals that would be appropriate for clients with alteration in hearing acuity.

a. _____

b. _____

c. _____

d. _____

Implementation

38. List the three recommended screening interventions for visual impairment.

a. _____

b. _____

c. _____

39. The most common visual problem is:

_____

_____

40. Children at risk for hearing impairment are:

a. _____

b. _____

c. _____

d. _____

e. _____

41. Complete the following table by filling in the normal physiological changes that occur and explaining how the nurse can minimize the loss.

Senses	Physiological Change	Interventions
Vision		
Hearing		
Taste and smell		
Touch		

42. Identify methods to promote communication in the following.

   a. Clients with aphasia:

   _____
   _____
   _____
   _____

   b. Clients with an artifical airway:

   _____
   _____
   _____
   _____

   c. Clients with a hearing impairment:

   _____
   _____
   _____
   _____

Acute Care

43. Identify the approaches to maximize sensory function, and give an example of each.
   a. _____
   b. _____
   c. _____
   d. _____

44. List the principles for reducing loneliness.
   a. _____
   b. _____
   c. _____
   d. _____
   e. _____
   f. _____
   g. _____
   h. _____

Evaluation

45. Explain how the nurse would evaluate whether the measures improved the client's ability to interact within the environment.

   _____
   _____

Review Questions

Select the appropriate answer and cite the rationale for choosing that particular answer.

46. Mr. Green, a 62-year-old farmer, has been hospitalized for 2 weeks for thrombophlebitis. He has no visitors, and the nurse notices that he appears bored, restless, and anxious. The type of alteration occurring because of sensory deprivation is:
   1. Affective
   2. Cognitive
   3. Receptual
   4. Perceptual

Answer: _____   Rationale: _____
_____
_____

47. Which of the following would not provide meaningful stimuli for a client?
   1. Interesting magazines and books
   2. A clock or calendar with large numbers
   3. Family pictures and personal possessions
   4. A television that is kept on all day at a low volume

Answer: _____   Rationale: _____
_____
_____

48. Clients with existing sensory loss must be protected from injury. What determines the safety precautions taken?
    1. The existing dangers in the environment
    2. The financial means to make needed safety changes
    3. The nature of the client's actual or potential sensory loss
    4. The availability of a support system to enable the client to exist in his or her present environment

Answer: _____ Rationale: _____

_____

_____

49. A client who is unable to name common objects or express simple ideas in words or writing suffers from:
    1. Global aphasia
    2. Receptive aphasia
    3. Mental retardation
    4. Expressive aphasia

Answer: _____ Rationale: _____

_____

_____

Critical Thinking Model for Nursing Care Plan for Disturbed Sensory Perception

50. Imagine that you are the community health nurse in the care plan on page 1354 of your text. Complete the *Planning phase* of the critical thinking model by writing your answers in the appropriate boxes of the model shown. Think about the following.

- In developing Judy's plan of care, what knowledge did you apply?

- In what way might your previous experience assist in developing a plan of care for Judy?

- When developing a plan of care, what intellectual and professional standards were applied?

- What critical thinking attitudes might have been applied in developing Judy's plan?

- How will you accomplish the goals?

KNOWLEDGE

EXPERIENCE

PLANNING

STANDARDS

ATTITUDES

CHAPTER 49   Critical Thinking Model for Nursing Care Plan for *Disturbed Sensory Perception*

50

Care of Surgical Clients

Preliminary Reading

Chapter 50, pp. 1365–1408

Comprehensive Understanding

Scientific Knowledge Base

1. List the types of care that perioperative nursing includes.

   a. _____

   b. _____

   c. _____

2. List the benefits of ambulatory surgery.

   a. _____

   b. _____

   c. _____

Match the following descriptions to the surgical procedure classifications.

3. _____ Major

4. _____ Minor

5. _____ Elective

6. _____ Urgent

7. _____ Emergency

8. _____ Diagnostic

9. _____ Ablative

10. _____ Palliative

11. _____ Restorative

12. _____ Procurement

13. _____ Constructive

14. _____ Cosmetic

a. Restores function lost or reduced as result of congenital anomalies

b. Excision or removal of diseased body part

c. Not necessarily emergency

d. Extensive reconstruction, poses great risks to well-being

e. Performed to improve personal appearance

f. Restores function or appearance to traumatized tissues

g. Must be done immediately to save life or preserve function of body part

h. Involves minimal risks compared with major procedures

i. Exploration that allows diagnosis to be confirmed

j. Is not essential and is not always necessary for health

k. Removal of organs/tissues from the dead for transplantation into another

l. Relieves or reduces intensity of disease symptoms, will not produce cure

Nursing Knowledge Base

The Nursing Process in the Preoperative Surgical Phase

Assessment

15. Give an example of the following medical conditions that increase the risks of surgery.

   a. Thrombocytopenia: _____

   b. Diabetes mellitus: _____

   c. Heart disease: _____

d. Obstructive sleep apnea: _____
_____

e. Upper respiratory infection: _____
_____

f. Liver disease: _____
_____

g. Fever: _____
_____

h. Emphysema: _____
_____

i. Acquired immunodeficiency syndrome (AIDS): _____
_____

j. Abuse of street drugs: _____
_____

k. Chronic pain: _____
_____

16. Explain the risk factors for a malnourished client.
   a. _____
   b. _____
   c. _____
   d. _____
   e. _____
   f. _____

17. Explain the risks for the client who is obese.
   a. _____
   b. _____
   c. _____
   d. _____

18. Identify the physiological factors that place the older adult at risk during surgery, and give an example of each.
   a. Cardiovascular system: _____
   _____

   b. Integumentary system: _____
   _____

   c. Pulmonary system: _____
   _____

   d. Renal system: _____
   _____

e. Neurological system: _____
_____

f. Metabolic system: _____
_____

19. Explain how the following drug classes affect the client during surgery.
   a. Antibiotics: _____
   _____
   _____

   b. Antidysrhythmics: _____
   _____
   _____
   _____

   c. Anticoagulants: _____
   _____
   _____
   _____

   d. Anticonvulsants: _____
   _____
   _____
   _____
   _____

   e. Antihypertensives: _____
   _____
   _____
   _____

   f. Corticosteroids: _____
   _____
   _____
   _____

   g. Insulin: _____
   _____
   _____
   _____
   _____

   h. Diuretics: _____
   _____
   _____
   _____

   i. Nonsteroidal antiinflammatory drugs (NSAIDs): _____
   _____
   _____
   _____

   j. Herbal therapies: _____
   _____
   _____
   _____

20. Explain how the following habits affect the client.

    a. Smoking: _____

    _____

    _____

    _____

    b. Alcohol and substance use:_____

    _____

    _____

    _____

21. A comprehensive pain assessment includes:

    a. _____

    b. _____

    c. _____

Briefly explain each of the following factors that need to be assessed in order to understand the impact of surgery on a client's and family's emotional health.

22. Self-concept:_____

    _____

23. Body image: _____

    _____

24. Coping resources: _____

    _____

25. The physical examination of the client before surgery includes:

    a. _____

    b. _____

    c. _____

    d. _____

    e. _____

    f. _____

    g. _____

26. Describe the interpretation of the following diagnostic screening tests for surgical clients.

    a. Complete blood count (CBC): _____

    _____

    _____

    _____

    _____

    b. Serum electrolytes: _____

    _____

    _____

    _____

    _____

    c. Coagulation studies: _____

    _____

    _____

    _____

    _____

    d. Serum creatinine:_____

    _____

    _____

    _____

    _____

    e. Blood urea nitrogen (BUN): _____

    _____

    _____

    _____

    _____

    f. Glucose: _____

    _____

    _____

    _____

    _____

Nursing Diagnosis

List the potential or actual nursing diagnoses appropriate for the preoperative client.

27. _____

28. _____

29. _____

30. _____

31. _____

32. _____

33. _____

34. _____

35. _____

36. _____

37. _____

38. _____

39. _____

40. _____

41. _____

42. _____

43. _____

44. _____

45. _____

Planning

46. Identify the expected outcomes for a client to verbalize the significance of postoperative exercises.

    a. _____
    _____
    _____
    _____

    b. _____
    _____
    _____
    _____

    c. _____
    _____
    _____
    _____

Implementation

47. Identify what the informed consent for surgery involves. _____
    _____
    _____
    _____

48. Describe the criteria developed by the Association of periOperative Registered Nurses (AORN) that may be used in determining the client's understanding of the surgical procedure.

    a. _____
    b. _____
    c. _____
    d. _____
    e. _____
    f. _____
    g. _____
    h. _____

Acute Care

49. Identify the interventions to physically prepare the client for surgery.

    a. _____
    b. _____
    c. _____
    d. _____

50. List the responsibilities of a nurse caring for a client the day of surgery.

    a. _____

    b. _____
    c. _____
    d. _____
    e. _____
    f. _____
    g. _____
    h. _____
    i. _____
    j. _____
    k. _____

51. The signs and symptoms of a latex reaction are: _____
    _____

Transport to the Operating Room

52. List 10 pieces of equipment that should be present in the postoperative bedside unit.

    a. _____
    b. _____
    c. _____
    d. _____
    e. _____
    f. _____
    g. _____
    h. _____
    i. _____
    j. _____

Intraoperative Surgical Phase

53. Explain the responsibilities for the following operating room nurses.

    a. Circulating nurse: _____
    b. Scrub nurse: _____

54. Identify the goals and outcomes for the client goal "maintain skin integrity."

    a. _____
    b. _____

55. The primary focus of intraoperative care is to prevent injury and complications related to:

    a. _____
    b. _____
    c. _____
    d. _____

Explain the following four types of anesthesia.

56. General:_____
_____
_____

57. Regional: _____
_____
_____

58. Local: _____
_____
_____

59. Conscious sedation: _____
_____
_____

Postoperative Surgical Phase

60. Identify the two phases of the postoperative course.
   a. _____
   _____
   _____
   b. _____
   _____
   _____
   _____

61. Identify the responsibilities of the nurse in the postanesthesia care unit (PACU).
_____
_____
_____

62. Identify the outcomes for discharge from the PACU.
_____
_____
_____

The Nursing Process in Postoperative Care

Assessment

63. Describe the frequency of vital sign assessment in the immediate postoperative period. _____
_____
_____

64. List the factors that contribute to airway obstruction in the postoperative client.
   a. _____
   b. _____
   c. _____
   d. _____

65. List the areas the nurse would assess in order to determine a postoperative client's circulatory status.
_____
_____
_____

66. List the complications of malignant hyperthermia._____
_____
_____
_____

67. List the areas the nurse assesses to determine fluid and electrolyte alterations.
   a. _____
   b. _____
   c. _____
   d. _____
   e. _____

68. List the areas of assessment that help to determine a postoperative client's neurological status.
   a. _____
   _____
   _____
   b. _____
   _____
   _____
   c. _____
   _____
   _____
   d. _____
   _____
   _____

69. Explain the following complications related to the skin postoperatively.
   a. Rash: _____
   _____
   b. Abrasions/petechiae:_____
   _____

c. Burns: _____

_____

_____

70. Explain the reasons why distention may occur.

a. _____

_____

_____

b. _____

_____

_____

c. _____

_____

_____

Planning

71. List the typical postoperative orders prescribed by surgeons.

a. _____

_____

_____

b. _____

_____

_____

c. _____

_____

_____

d. _____

_____

_____

e. _____

_____

_____

f. _____

_____

_____

g. _____

_____

_____

h. _____

_____

_____

i. _____

_____

_____

j. _____

_____

_____

72. Identify the expected outcomes for the postoperative client.

a. _____

_____

_____

b. _____

_____

_____

c. _____

_____

_____

d. _____

_____

_____

e. _____

_____

_____

Implementation

List the measures that the nurse would use to promote expansion of the lungs.

73. _____

_____

_____

74. _____

_____

75. _____

_____

76. _____

_____

77. _____

_____

_____

78. _____

_____

79. _____

_____

_____

80. _____

_____

81. _____

_____

_____

82. _____
_____
_____

83. Define the following complications, and give the cause of each.
   a. Atelectasis: _____
   _____
   _____
   _____

   b. Pneumonia: _____
   _____
   _____
   _____

   c. Hypoxemia: _____
   _____
   _____
   _____

   d. Pulmonary embolism: _____
   _____
   _____
   _____

   e. Hemorrhage: _____
   _____
   _____
   _____

   f. Hypovolemic shock: _____
   _____
   _____
   _____

   g. Thrombophlebitis:_____
   _____
   _____
   _____

   h. Thrombus: _____
   _____
   _____
   _____

   i. Embolus: _____
   _____
   _____
   _____

   j. Paralytic ileus:_____
   _____
   _____
   _____

   k. Abdominal distention:_____
   _____
   _____
   _____

   l. Nausea and vomiting: _____
   _____
   _____
   _____

   m. Urinary retention: _____
   _____
   _____
   _____

   n. Urinary tract infection: _____
   _____
   _____
   _____

   o. Wound infection: _____
   _____
   _____
   _____

   p. Wound dehiscence: _____
   _____
   _____
   _____

   q. Wound evisceration: _____
   _____
   _____
   _____

   r. Skin breakdown:_____
   _____
   _____
   _____

   s. Intractable pain:_____
   _____
   _____

List the measures the nurse would utilize to prevent circulatory complications.
84. _____
_____
_____

85. _____
_____
_____

86. _____
_____
_____

87. _____
_____
_____

88. _____
_____
_____

89. _____
_____
_____

90. Identify the sources of a surgical client's pain.
_____
_____
_____

91. List the measures the nurse would provide to promote the return of normal elimination.

    a. _____
    _____
    _____

    b. _____
    _____
    _____

    c. _____
    _____
    _____

    d. _____
    _____
    _____

    e. _____
    _____
    _____

    f. _____
    _____
    _____

92. Identify the measures the nurse would provide to promote normal urinary elimination.

    a. _____
    _____
    _____

    b. _____
    _____
    _____

c. _____
_____
_____

d. _____
_____
_____

93. Identify the measures the nurse would utilize to promote the client's self-concept.

    a. _____
    _____
    _____

    b. _____
    _____
    _____

    c. _____
    _____
    _____

    d. _____
    _____
    _____

    e. _____
    _____
    _____

    f. _____
    _____
    _____

Review Questions

Select the appropriate answer and cite the rationale for choosing that particular answer.

94. Mrs. Young, a 45-year-old diabetic client, is having a hysterectomy in the morning. Because of her history, the nurse would expect:
    1. Impaired wound healing
    2. Fluid and electrolyte imbalances
    3. An increased risk of hemorrhaging
    4. Altered elimination of anesthetic agents

Answer: _____ Rationale: _____
_____
_____

95. The purposes of the nursing history for the client who is to have surgery include all of the following except:
    1. Deciding whether surgery is indicated
    2. Identifying the client's perception and expectations about surgery
    3. Obtaining information about the client's past experience with surgery
    4. Understanding the impact surgery has on the client's and family's emotional health

Answer: _____   Rationale: _____
_____
_____

96. All of the following clients are at risk for developing serious fluid and electrolyte imbalances during and after surgery except:
    1. Client F, who is 1 year old and having a cleft palate repair
    2. Client H, who is 79 years old and has a history of congestive heart failure
    3. Client G, who is 55 years old and has a history of chronic respiratory disease
    4. Client E, who is 81 years old and having emergency surgery for a bowel obstruction following 4 days of vomiting and diarrhea

Answer: _____   Rationale: _____
_____
_____

97. The purpose of postoperative leg exercises is to:
    1. Maintain muscle tone
    2. Promote venous return
    3. Assess range of motion
    4. Exercise fatigued muscles

Answer: _____   Rationale: _____
_____
_____

98. The PACU nurse notices that the client is shivering. This is most commonly caused by:
    1. Cold irrigations used during surgery
    2. Side effects of certain anesthetic agents
    3. Malignant hypothermia, a serious condition
    4. The use of a reflective blanket on the operating room table

Answer: _____   Rationale: _____
_____
_____

Critical Thinking Model for Nursing Care Plan for Deficient Knowledge Regarding Preoperative and Postoperative Care Requirements

99. Imagine that you are the nurse in the care plan on page 1379 of your text. Complete the *Evaluation phase* of the critical thinking model by writing your answers in the appropriate boxes of the model shown. Think about the following.

    • What knowledge did you apply in evaluating Mrs. Campana's care?

    • In what way might your previous experience influence your evaluation of Mrs. Campana's care?

    • During evaluation, what intellectual and professional standards were applied to Mrs. Campana's care?

    • In what way do critical thinking attitudes play a role in how you approach evaluation of Mrs. Campana's care?

    • How might you adjust Mrs. Campana's care?

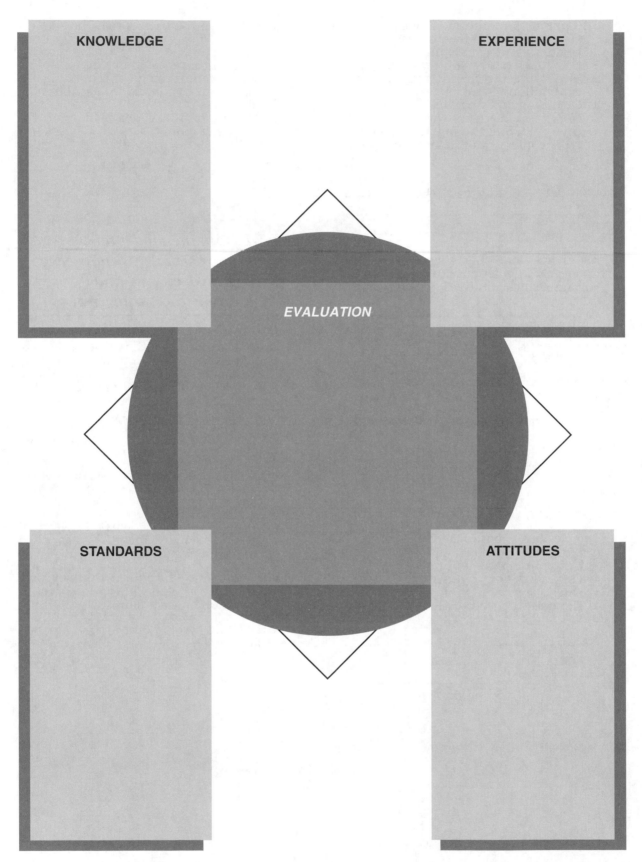

KNOWLEDGE

EXPERIENCE

EVALUATION

STANDARDS

ATTITUDES

CHAPTER 50   Critical Thinking Model for Nursing Care Plan for *Deficient Knowledge Regarding*
Preoperative and Postoperative Care Requirements

STUDENT: _____ DATE: _____

INSTRUCTOR: _____ DATE: _____

CHECKLIST
Skill 32-1 Measuring Body Temperature

	S	U	NP	Comments
1. Assess for temperature alterations and factors that influence body temperature.	____	____	____	_____
2. Determine any previous activity that interferes with accuracy of temperature measurement. When taking oral temperature, wait 20 to 30 minutes before measuring temperature if client has smoked or ingested hot or cold liquids or foods.	____	____	____	_____
3. Determine appropriate temperature site and device for client.	____	____	____	_____
4. Explain route by which temperature will be taken and importance of maintaining proper position until reading is complete.	____	____	____	_____
5. Perform hand hygiene.				
6. Assist client in assuming comfortable position that provides easy access to temperature measurement site.	____	____	____	_____
7. Obtain temperature reading:				
A. Oral temperature measurement with electronic thermometer				
(1) Apply disposable gloves (optional).	____	____	____	_____
(2) Remove thermometer pack from charging unit. Attach oral probe (blue tip) to thermometer unit. Grasp top of probe stem, being careful not to apply pressure on the ejection button.	____	____	____	_____
(3) Slide disposable plastic probe cover over thermometer probe stem until cover locks in place.	____	____	____	_____
(4) Ask client to open mouth; then gently place thermometer probe under tongue in posterior sublingual pocket lateral to center of lower jaw.	____	____	____	_____
(5) Ask client to hold thermometer probe with lips closed.	____	____	____	_____
(6) Leave thermometer probe in place until audible signal occurs and temperature appears on digital display. Remove thermometer probe from under client's tongue.	____	____	____	_____
(7) Push ejection button on thermometer stem to discard plastic probe cover into appropriate receptacle.	____	____	____	_____
(8) Return thermometer stem to storage position of recording unit.	____	____	____	_____
(9) If gloves were worn, remove and dispose of them in appropriate receptacle. Perform hand hygiene.	____	____	____	_____
(10) Return thermometer to charger.	____	____	____	_____
B. Rectal temperature measurement with electronic thermometer				
(1) Draw curtain around bed and/or close room door. Assist client to Sims' position with upper leg flexed. Move aside bed linen to expose only anal area. Keep client's upper body and lower extremities covered with sheet or blanket.	____	____	____	_____
(2) Apply clean gloves.	____	____	____	_____
(3) Remove thermometer pack from charging unit. Attach rectal probe stem (red tip) to thermometer unit. Grasp top of probe stem, being careful not to apply pressure on the ejection button.				

Continued

239

	S	U	NP	Comments

(4) Slide disposable plastic probe cover over thermometer probe until cover locks in place.   ____ ____ ____ _____

(5) Squeeze liberal portion of lubricant on tissue. Dip probe cover's end into lubricant, covering 2.5 to 3.5 cm (1 to 1 ½ inches) for adult.   ____ ____ ____ _____

(6) With nondominant hand, separate buttocks to expose anus. Ask client to breathe slowly and relax.   ____ ____ ____ _____

(7) Gently insert thermometer probe into anus in direction of umbilicus 2.5 to 3.5 cm (1 to 1 ½ inches) for adult. Do not force thermometer. If resistance is felt, withdraw thermometer immediately. Never force thermometer.   ____ ____ ____ _____

(8) Once positioned, hold thermometer probe in place until audible signal indicates completion and client's temperature appears on digital display; remove thermometer probe from anus.   ____ ____ ____ _____

(9) Push ejection button on thermometer stem to discard plastic probe cover into an appropriate receptacle. Wipe probe stem with alcohol swab, paying particular attention to ridges where probe stem cover connects to probe.   ____ ____ ____ _____

(10) Return thermometer probe stem to storage position of recording unit.

(11) Wipe client's anal area with soft tissue to remove lubricant or feces, and discard tissue. Assist client in assuming a comfortable position.   ____ ____ ____ _____

(12) Remove and dispose of gloves in appropriate receptacle. Perform hand hygiene.   ____ ____ ____ _____

(13) Return thermometer to charger. Verify that charger and probes are wiped with alcohol daily.   ____ ____ ____ _____

C. Axillary temperature measurement with electronic thermometer

(1) Draw curtain around bed and/or close door. Assist client to a supine or sitting position. Move clothing or gown away from shoulder and arm.   ____ ____ ____ _____

(2) Remove thermometer pack from charging unit. Be sure oral probe stem (blue tip) is attached to thermometer unit. Grasp top of thermometer probe stem, being careful not to apply pressure on the ejection button.   ____ ____ ____ _____

(3) Slide disposable plastic probe cover over thermometer stem until cover locks in place.   ____ ____ ____ _____

(4) Raise client's arm away from torso; inspect for skin lesion and excessive perspiration. Insert thermometer probe into center of axilla, lower arm over probe, and place arm across client's chest.   ____ ____ ____ _____

(5) Once positioned, hold thermometer probe in place until audible signal occurs and temperature appears on digital display. Remove thermometer probe from axilla.   ____ ____ ____ _____

(6) Push ejection button on thermometer stem to discard plastic probe cover into appropriate receptacle.   ____ ____ ____ _____

(7) Return thermometer stem to storage position of recording unit.   ____ ____ ____ _____

(8) Assist client in assuming a comfortable position, replacing linen or gown.   ____ ____ ____ _____

(9) Perform hand hygiene.   ____ ____ ____ _____

(10) Return thermometer to charger.   ____ ____ ____ _____

Continued

	S	U	NP	Comments

D. Tympanic membrane temperature with electronic thermometer

    (1) Assist client in assuming comfortable position with head turned toward side, away from nurse. If client has been lying on one side, use upper ear. Right-handed persons need to obtain temperature from client's right ear. Left-handed people need to obtain temperature from client's left ear.

    (2) Note if there is obvious earwax in the ear canal.

    (3) Remove handheld thermometer unit from charging base, being careful not to apply pressure on the ejection button.

    (4) Slide clean disposable speculum cover over otoscope-like lens tip until it locks into place, being careful not to touch lens cover.

    (5) If holding handheld unit with right hand, obtain temperature from client's right ear; left-handed persons obtain temperature from client's left ear.

    (6) Insert speculum into ear canal following manufacturer's instructions for tympanic probe positioning:

       a. Pull ear pinna backward, up, and out for an adult. For children under 2 years of age, point covered speculum tip toward midpoint between eyebrow and sideburns.

       b. Move thermometer in a figure-eight pattern.

       c. Fit speculum tip snugly into canal, and do not move, pointing speculum tip toward nose.

    (7) Once positioned, press scan button on handheld unit. Leave speculum in place until audible signal indicates completion and client's temperature appears on digital display.

    (8) Carefully remove speculum from auditory meatus.

    (9) Push ejection button on handheld unit to discard speculum cover into appropriate receptacle.

    (10) If temperature is abnormal or a second reading is necessary, replace speculum cover and wait 2 to 3 minutes before repeating the measurement in the same ear. Repeat measurement in other ear, or try an alternative temperature site or instrument.

    (11) Return handheld unit to charging base.

    (12) Assist client to a comfortable position.

    (13) Perform hand hygiene.

8. Discuss findings with client as needed.

9. If temperature is being assessed for the first time, establish temperature as baseline if within normal range.

10. Compare temperature reading with previous baseline and normal temperature range for client's age-group.

STUDENT: _____ DATE: _____

INSTRUCTOR: _____ DATE: _____

Skill 32-2 Assessing the Radial and Apical Pulses

	S	U	NP	Comments
1. Determine need to assess radial or apical pulse.				
A. Assess for any risk factors for pulse alterations.	____	____	____	_____
B. Assess for signs and symptoms of altered stroke volume and cardiac output, such as dyspnea, fatigue, chest pain, orthopnea, syncope, palpitations (person's unpleasant awareness of heartbeat), jugular venous distention, edema of dependent body parts, cyanosis, or pallor of skin.	____	____	____	_____
C. Assess for signs and symptoms of peripheral vascular disease such as pale, cool extremities; thin, shiny skin with decreased hair growth; thickened nails.	____	____	____	_____
2. Assess for factors that influence pulse rate and rhythm: age, exercise, position changes, fluid balance, medications, temperature, and sympathetic stimulation.	____	____	____	_____
3. Determine previous baseline apical rate (if available) from client's record. Otherwise note baseline radial rate.	____	____	____	_____
4. Explain that you will assess pulse or heart rate. Encourage client to relax and not speak. If client was active, wait 5 to 10 minutes before assessing pulse.	____	____	____	_____
5. Perform hand hygiene.				
6. If necessary, draw curtain around bed and/or close door.	____	____	____	_____
7. Obtain pulse measurement:	____	____	____	_____
A. Radial pulse				
(1) Assist client to supine or sitting position.	____	____	____	_____
(2) If supine, place client's forearm straight alongside body or across lower chest or upper abdomen with wrist extended straight. If sitting, bend client's elbow 90 degrees and support lower arm on chair or on your arm.	____	____	____	_____
(3) Place tips of first two or middle three fingers of hand over groove along radial or thumb side of client's inner wrist. Slightly extend the wrist with palm down until you note the strongest pulse.	____	____	____	_____
(4) Lightly compress against radius, obliterate pulse initially, and then relax pressure so pulse becomes easily palpable.	____	____	____	_____
(5) Determine strength of pulse. Note whether thrust of vessel against fingertips is bounding (+4), full/strong (+3), normal/expected (+2), diminished/barely palpable (+1), or absent (0).	____	____	____	_____
(6) After feeling a regular pulse, look at watch's second hand and begin to count rate: when sweep hand hits number on dial, start counting with zero, then one, two, and so on.	____	____	____	_____
(7) If pulse is regular, count rate for 30 seconds and multiply total by 2.	____	____	____	_____
(8) If pulse is irregular, count rate for 60 seconds. Assess frequency and pattern of irregularity. Compare radial pulses bilaterally.	____	____	____	_____
B. Apical pulse				
(1) Perform hand hygiene, and clean earpieces and diaphragm of stethoscope with alcohol swab.	____	____	____	_____
(2) Draw curtain around bed and/or close room door.	____	____	____	_____
(3) Assist client to supine or sitting position. Move aside bed linen and gown to expose sternum and left side of chest.	____	____	____	_____

Continued

	S	U	NP	Comments

(4) Locate anatomical landmarks to identify the point of maximal impulse (PMI), also called the apical impulse. Heart is located behind and to left of sternum with base at top and apex at bottom. Find angle of Louis just below suprasternal notch between sternal body and manubrium; feels like a bony prominence. Slip fingers down each side of angle to find second intercostal space (ICS). Carefully move fingers down left side of sternum to fifth ICS and laterally to the left midclavicular line (MCL). A light tap felt within an area 1 to 2 cm (½ to 1 inch) of the PMI is reflected from the apex of the heart.

(5) Place diaphragm of stethoscope in palm of hand for 5 to 10 seconds.

(6) Place diaphragm of stethoscope over PMI at the fifth ICS, at left MCL, and auscultate for normal S_1 and S_2 heart sounds (heard as "lub-dub").

(7) When S_1 and S_2 are heard with regularity, use watch's second hand and begin to count rate: when sweep hand hits number on dial, start counting with zero, then one, two, and so on.

(8) If apical rate is regular, count for 30 seconds and multiply by 2.

(9) Note if heart rate is irregular, count for 60 seconds and describe pattern or irregularity (S_1 and S_2 occurring early or later after previous sequence of sounds; for example, every third or every fourth beat is skipped).

(10) Replace client's gown and bed linen; assist client in returning to comfortable position.

(11) Perform hand hygiene.

(12) Clean earpieces and diaphragm of stethoscope with alcohol swab as needed (optional).

8. Perform hand hygiene.
9. Discuss findings with client as needed.
10. Compare readings with previous baseline and/or acceptable range of heart rate for client's age.
11. Compare peripheral pulse rate with apical rate, and note discrepancy.
12. Compare radial pulse equality, and note discrepancy.
13. Correlate pulse rate with data obtained from blood pressure and related signs and symptoms (palpitations, dizziness).

STUDENT: _____   DATE: _____

INSTRUCTOR: _____   DATE: _____

Skill 32-3 Assessing Respirations

	S	U	NP	Comments
1. Determine need to assess client's respirations.				
A. Identify risk factors for respiratory alterations.	___	___	___	_____
B. Assess for signs and symptoms of respiratory alterations such as bluish or cyanotic appearance of nail beds, lips, mucous membranes, and skin; restlessness, irritability, confusion, reduced level of consciousness; pain during inspiration; labored or difficult breathing; adventitious breath sounds, inability to breathe spontaneously; thick, frothy, blood-tinged, or copious sputum produced on coughing.	___	___	___	_____
2. Assess pertinent laboratory values.	___	___	___	_____
A. Arterial blood gases (ABGs): Normal ABGs (values vary slightly among institutions): pH: 7.35–7.45 $PaCO_2$: 35–45 mm Hg PaO_2: 80–100 mm Hg SaO_2: 95%–100%	___	___	___	_____
B. Pulse oximetry (SpO_2): Acceptable SpO_2 ranges from 90% to 100%; however, a range from 85% to 89% is acceptable for certain chronic disease conditions; less than 85% is abnormal.	___	___	___	_____
C. Complete blood count (CBC): Normal CBC for adults (values vary among institutions):	___	___	___	_____
Hemoglobin: 14 to 18 g/100 mL, males; 12 to 16 g/100 mL, females	___	___	___	_____
Hematocrit: 42% to 52%, males; 37% to 47%, females	___	___	___	_____
Red blood cell count: 4.7 to 6.1 million/mm^3, males; 4.2 to 5.4 million/mm^3, females	___	___	___	_____
3. Determine previous baseline respiratory rate (if available) from client's record.	___	___	___	_____
4. Perform hand hygiene. Draw curtain around bed, and/or close door.	___	___	___	_____
5. Be sure client is in comfortable position, preferably sitting or lying with the head of the bed elevated 45 to 60 degrees. Be sure client's chest is visible. If necessary, move bed linen or gown.	___	___	___	_____
6. Place client's arm in relaxed position across the abdomen or lower chest, or place nurse's hand directly over client's upper abdomen.	___	___	___	_____
7. Observe complete respiratory cycle (one inspiration and one expiration).	___	___	___	_____
8. After cycle is observed, look at watch's second hand and begin to count rate: when sweep hand hits number on dial, begin time frame, counting one with first full respiratory cycle.	___	___	___	_____
9. If rhythm is regular, count number of respirations in 30 seconds and multiply by 2. If rhythm is irregular, less than 12, or greater than 20, count for 1 full minute.	___	___	___	_____
10. Note depth of respirations, subjectively assessed by observing degree of chest wall movement while counting rate. Objectively assess depth by palpating chest wall excursion or auscultating the posterior thorax after rate has been counted. Depth is described as shallow, normal, or deep.	___	___	___	_____
11. Note rhythm of ventilatory cycle. Normal breathing is regular and uninterrupted. Do not confuse sighing with abnormal rhythm.	___	___	___	_____

Continued

	S	U	NP	Comments

12. Replace bed linen and client's gown. ____ ____ ____ _____
13. Perform hand hygiene. ____ ____ ____ _____
14. Discuss findings with client as needed. ____ ____ ____ _____
15. If assessing respirations for the first time, establish rate, rhythm, and depth as baseline if within normal range.
16. Compare respirations with client's previous baseline and normal rate, rhythm, and depth. ____ ____ ____ _____

STUDENT: _____ DATE: _____

INSTRUCTOR: _____ DATE: _____

Skill 32-4 Measuring Oxygen Saturation (Pulse Oximetry)

	S	U	NP	Comments
1. Determine need to measure client's oxygen saturation.				
A. Identify risk factors of decreased oxygen saturation.	____	____	____	_____
B. Assess for signs and symptoms of alterations in oxygen saturation such as altered respiratory rate, depth, or rhythm; adventitious breath sounds; cyanotic appearance of nail beds, lips, mucous membranes, and skin; restlessness, irritability, confusion; reduced level of consciousness; labored or difficult breathing.	____	____	____	_____
2. Assess for factors that normally influence measurement of SpO_2 such as oxygen therapy, hemoglobin level, body temperature, and medications such as bronchodilators.	____	____	____	_____
3. Review client's medical record for order, or consult agency policy or procedure manual for standard of care.	____	____	____	_____
4. Determine most appropriate client-specific site (e.g., finger, earlobe) for sensor probe placement by measuring capillary refill. If capillary refill is less than 3 seconds, select alternate site.	____	____	____	_____
A. Site needs to have adequate local circulation and be free of moisture.	____	____	____	_____
B. Choose finger free of polish or artificial nail.	____	____	____	_____
C. If tremors are present, use earlobe as site.	____	____	____	_____
D. If client is obese, clip-on probe may not fit properly, obtain a single-use (tape-on) probe.	____	____	____	_____
5. Determine previous baseline SpO_2 (if available) from client's record.	____	____	____	_____
6. Explain purpose of procedure to client and how you will measure oxygen saturation. Instruct client to breathe normally.	____	____	____	_____
7. Perform hand hygiene.				
8. Position client comfortably. When using finger as monitoring site, support lower arm.	____	____	____	_____
9. Instruct client to breathe normally.	____	____	____	_____
10. When using finger as monitoring site, remove any fingernail polish with acetone.	____	____	____	_____
11. Attach sensor probe to monitoring site. Tell client that clip-on probe will feel like a clothespin on the finger and will not hurt.	____	____	____	_____
12. Once sensor is in place, turn on oximeter by activating power. Observe pulse waveform/intensity display and audible beep. Correlate oximeter pulse rate with client's radial pulse. Differences require reevaluation of oximeter probe placement and may require reassessment of pulse rates.	____	____	____	_____
13. Leave probe in place until oximeter readout reaches constant value and pulse display reaches full strength during each cardiac cycle. Inform client that oximeter will alarm if the probe falls off or if client moves the probe. Read SpO_2 on digital display.	____	____	____	_____
14. If continuous SpO_2 monitoring is necessary, verify SpO_2 alarm limits and alarm volume, which are preset by the manufacturer at a low of 85% and a high of 100%. You determine limits for SpO_2 and pulse rate alarms based on each client's condition. Verify that alarms are on. Assess skin integrity every 2 hours under sensor probe. Relocate sensor probe at least every 24 hours or more frequently if skin integrity is altered or tissue perfusion compromised.	____	____	____	_____
15. Assist client in returning to a comfortable position.	____	____	____	_____
16. Perform hand hygiene.	____	____	____	_____
17. Discuss findings with client as needed.	____	____	____	_____

Continued

	S	U	NP	Comments

18. If planning intermittent or spot-checking SpO$_2$ measurements, remove probe and turn oximeter power off. Store probe in appropriate location.

19. Compare SpO$_2$ reading with client baseline and acceptable values.

20. Correlate SpO$_2$ with SaO$_2$ obtained from arterial blood gas measurements if available.

21. Correlate SpO$_2$ reading with data obtained from respiratory rate, depth, and rhythm assessment.

STUDENT: _____   DATE: _____

INSTRUCTOR: _____   DATE: _____

Skill 32-5 Measuring Blood Pressure

	S	U	NP	Comments
1. Determine need to assess client's blood pressure (BP).				
A. Identify risk factors for BP alterations.	____	____	____	_____
B. Observe for signs and symptoms of BP alterations:	____	____	____	_____
(1) High BP (hypertension): headache (usually occipital), flushing of face, nosebleed, and fatigue in older adults.	____	____	____	_____
(2) Low BP (hypotension): dizziness, mental confusion; restlessness; pale, dusky, or cyanotic skin and mucous membranes; cool, mottled skin over extremities.	____	____	____	_____
2. Determine best site for BP assessment. Avoid applying cuff to extremity when intravenous fluids are infusing; an arteriovenous shunt or fistula is present; breast or axillary surgery has been performed on that side; extremity has been traumatized, diseased, or requires a cast or bulky bandage. Use the lower extremities when the brachial arteries are inaccessible.	____	____	____	_____
3. Determine previous baseline BP (if available) from client's record.	____	____	____	_____
4. Encourage client to avoid caffeine and smoking before BP assessment.	____	____	____	_____
5. Explain to client that you will assess BP. Have client rest at least 5 minutes before measuring client BP sitting or lying down; wait 1 minute if client standing. When possible, have client sit in a chair. Ask client not to speak while measuring BP.	____	____	____	_____
6. Select appropriate cuff size.	____	____	____	_____
7. Perform hand hygiene.	____	____	____	_____
8. Have client assume sitting or lying position. Be sure room is warm, quiet, and relaxing.	____	____	____	_____
9. With client sitting or lying, position client's forearm at heart level, position thigh flat (provide support as needed). For arm, turn palm up; for thigh, position with knee slightly flexed. If sitting, instruct client to keep feet flat on floor without crossing legs.	____	____	____	_____
10. Expose extremity (arm or leg) fully by removing constricting clothing.	____	____	____	_____
11. Palpate brachial artery (arm) or popliteal artery (leg). With cuff fully deflated, apply bladder of cuff above artery by centering arrows marked on cuff over artery. If there are no center arrows on cuff, estimate the center of the bladder and place this center over artery. Position cuff 2.5 cm (1 inch) above site of pulsation (antecubital or popliteal space). Wrap cuff evenly and snugly around extremity.	____	____	____	_____
12. Position aneroid needle no farther that 1 m (approximately 1 yard) away.	____	____	____	_____
13. Measure blood pressure.	____	____	____	_____
A. Two-Step Method				
(1) Relocate brachial pulse. Palpate the artery distal to the cuff with fingertips of nondominant hand while inflating cuff rapidly to pressure 30 mm Hg above point at which pulse disappears. Slowly deflate cuff, and note point when pulse reappears. Deflate cuff fully, and wait 30 seconds.	____	____	____	_____
(2) Place stethoscope earpieces in ears, and be sure sounds are clear, not muffled.	____	____	____	_____

Continued

	S	U	NP	Comments

(3) Relocate brachial or popliteal artery, and place bell or diaphragm chestpiece of stethoscope over it. Do not allow chestpiece to touch cuff or clothing.

(4) Close valve of pressure bulb clockwise until tight.

(5) Quickly inflate cuff to 30 mm Hg above palpated systolic pressure (client's estimated systolic pressure).

(6) Slowly release pressure bulb valve, and allow needle of manometer gauge to fall at rate of 2 to 3 mm Hg/sec. Make sure there are no extraneous sounds

(7) Note point on manometer when you hear the first clear sound. The sound will slowly increase in intensity.

(8) Continue to deflate cuff, noting point at which muffled or dampened sound appears.

(9) Continue to deflate cuff gradually, noting point at which sound disappears in adults. Listen for 10 to 20 mm Hg after the last sound, and then allow remaining air to escape quickly.

B. One-Step Method

(1) Place stethoscope earpieces in ears, and be sure sounds are clear, not muffled.

(2) Relocate brachial or popliteal artery, and place bell or diaphragm chestpiece of stethoscope over it. Do not allow chestpiece to touch cuff or clothing.

(3) Close valve of pressure bulb clockwise until tight. Quickly inflate cuff to 30 mm Hg above palpated systolic pressure.

(4) Slowly release pressure bulb valve, and allow needle of manometer gauge to fall at rate of 2 to 3 mm Hg/sec.

(5) Note point on manometer when you hear the first clear sound. The sound will slowly increase in intensity.

(6) Continue to deflate cuff, noting point at which muffled or dampened sound appears.

(7) While gradually deflating cuff, note point at which sound disappears in adults. Listen for 10 to 20 mm Hg after the last sound, and then allow remaining air to escape quickly.

14. The Joint Commission recommends the average of two sets of BP measurement, 2 minutes apart. Use the second set of BP measurements as the baseline. If readings are different by more than 5 mm Hg, additional readings are necessary.

15. Remove cuff from extremity unless you need to repeat measurement. If this is the first assessment of client, repeat blood pressure assessment on other extremity.

16. Assist client in returning to a comfortable position, and cover upper arm if previously clothed.

17. Discuss findings with client as needed.

18. Perform hand hygiene.

19. Compare reading with previous baseline and/or acceptable BP for client's age-group.

20. Correlate blood pressure with data obtained from pulse assessment and related cardiovascular signs and symptoms.

STUDENT: _____ DATE: _____

INSTRUCTOR: _____ DATE: _____

Skill 34-1 Hand Hygiene

	S	U	NP	Comments
1. Inspect surfaces of hands for breaks or cuts in skin or cuticles. Cover any skin lesions with a dressing before providing client care. If lesions are too large to cover, you may be restricted from direct client care.	____	____	____	_____
2. Inspect hands for visible soiling.	____	____	____	_____
3. Inspect condition of nails. Natural tips should be ¼ inch from fingertip and smooth. DO NOT WEAR artificial nails or extensions.	____	____	____	_____
4. Push wristwatch and long uniform sleeves above wrists. Avoid wearing rings; however, there is not definitive evidence that rings increase microbial load on the hands.	____	____	____	_____
5. Antiseptic hand rub	____	____	____	_____
A. Apply an ample amount of product to palm of one hand.				
B. Rub hands together, covering all surfaces of hands and fingers with antiseptic.	____	____	____	_____
C. Rub hands together for several seconds until alcohol is dry. Allow hands to dry before applying gloves.	____	____	____	_____
6. Hand washing with antiseptic soap				
A. Stand in front of sink, keeping hands and uniform away from sink surface. (If hands touch sink during hand washing, repeat.)	____	____	____	_____
B. Turn on water. Turn faucet on or push knee pedals laterally or press pedals with foot to regulate water flow and temperature.	____	____	____	_____
C. Avoid splashing water against uniform.	____	____	____	_____
D. Regulate flow of water so that temperature is warm.	____	____	____	_____
E. Wet hands and wrists thoroughly under running water. Keep hands and forearms lower than elbows during washing.	____	____	____	_____
F. Apply 3 to 5 mL of antiseptic soap, and rub hands together vigorously, lathering thoroughly. Soap granules and leaflet preparations may be used.	____	____	____	_____
G. Wash hands using plenty of lather and friction for at least 15 seconds. Interlace fingers, and rub palms and back of hands with circular motion at least 5 times each. Keep fingertips down to facilitate removal of microorganisms.	____	____	____	_____
H. Areas under fingernails are often soiled. Clean them with fingernails of other hand and additional soap with an orange stick (optional).	____	____	____	_____
I. Rinse hands and wrists thoroughly, keeping hands down and elbows up.	____	____	____	_____
J. Dry hands thoroughly from fingers to wrists and forearms with paper towel, single-use cloth, or warm air dryer.	____	____	____	_____
K. If used, discard paper towel in proper receptacle.	____	____	____	_____
L. Turn off water with foot or knee pedals. To turn off hand faucet, use clean, dry paper towel; avoid touching handles with hands.	____	____	____	_____

STUDENT: _____ DATE: _____

INSTRUCTOR: _____ DATE: _____

<small>CHECKLIST</small>
Skill 34-2 Preparation of a Sterile Field

	S	U	NP	Comments
1. Apply personal protective equipment as needed (consult agency policy).	___	___	___	_____
2. Select clean work surface above waist level.	___	___	___	_____
3. Assemble necessary equipment, and check dates or labels on supplies for sterility of equipment.				
4. Perform hand hygiene.	___	___	___	_____
5. Prepare sterile field.				
A. Sterile commercial kit or tray containing sterile items				
(1) Place sterile kit or pack containing sterile items on work surface.	___	___	___	_____
(2) Open outside cover, and remove kit from dust cover. Place on work surface.	___	___	___	_____
(3) Grasp outer edge of tip of outermost flap.	___	___	___	_____
(4) Open outermost flap away from body, keeping arm outstretched and away from the sterile field.	___	___	___	_____
(5) Grasp outer edge of first side of flap.	___	___	___	_____
(6) Open side flap, pulling to side and allowing it to lie flat on table surface. Keep arm to the side, and do not extend it over the sterile surface.	___	___	___	_____
(7) Grasp outer edge of second side flap. Repeat for opening second side of package.	___	___	___	_____
(8) Grasp outer edge of last and innermost flap.	___	___	___	_____
(9) Stand away from sterile package, and pull flap back, allowing it to fall flat on work surface.	___	___	___	_____
B. Sterile linen-wrapped package				
(1) Place package on work surface.	___	___	___	_____
(2) Remove tape and seal, and unwrap both layers, following Steps 5A(1) through (9) as with sterile commercial kit.	___	___	___	_____
(3) Use opened package wrapper as a sterile field.	___	___	___	_____
C. Sterile drape				
(1) Place pack containing the sterile drape on work surface.	___	___	___	_____
(2) Apply sterile gloves. (Note: This is an option depending on health care facility policy. You may touch outer 1-inch border of drape without wearing gloves.)	___	___	___	_____
(3) Grasp folded top edge of drape with fingertips of one hand. Gently lift drape up from its wrapper without touching any object.	___	___	___	_____
(4) Allow drape to unfold, keeping it above waist and the work surface and away from the body. (Carefully discard outer wrapper with other hand.)	___	___	___	_____
(5) With other hand, grasp the adjacent corner of drape. Hold drape straight over work surface.	___	___	___	_____
(6) Holding drape, first position the bottom half over top half of the intended work surface.	___	___	___	_____
(7) Allow top half of drape to be placed over bottom half of work surface.	___	___	___	_____
D. Adding sterile items				
(1) Open sterile item (following package directions) while holding outside wrapper in nondominant hand.	___	___	___	_____

Continued

252

	S	U	NP	Comments
(2) Carefully peel wrapper onto nondominant hand.	___	___	___	_____
(3) Being sure wrapper does not fall down on sterile field, place item onto field at angle. Do not hold arm over sterile field.	___	___	___	_____
(4) Dispose of outer wrapper.	___	___	___	_____

STUDENT: _____ DATE: _____

INSTRUCTOR: _____ DATE: _____

Skill 34-3 Surgical Hand Asepsis

	S	U	NP	Comments
1. Consult institutional policy for length of time and antiseptic for hand washing.	___	___	___	_____
2. Remove bracelets, rings, and watches.				
3. Be sure fingernails are short, clean, and healthy. Artificial nails should be removed. Natural nails should be less than 1/4-inch long.	___	___	___	_____
4. Inspect condition of cuticles, hands, and forearms for abrasions, cuts, or open lesions.	___	___	___	_____
5. Apply surgical shoe covers, cap or hood, face mask, and protective eyewear.	___	___	___	_____
6. Turn on water using knee or foot controls, and adjust to comfortable temperature.				
A. Prescrub wash/rinse				
(1) Wet hands and arms under running lukewarm water, and lather with detergent to 5 cm (2 inches) above elbows. (Hands need to be above elbows at all times.)	___	___	___	_____
(2) Rinse hands and arms thoroughly under running water. **Remember to keep hands above** elbows.	___	___	___	_____
(3) Under running water, clean under nails of both hands with nail pick. Discard after use.	___	___	___	_____
B. Surgical hand scrub (with brush)				
(1) Wet clean sponge, and apply antimicrobial agent. Visualize each finger, hand, and arm as having four sides. Wash all four sides effectively. Scrub the nails of one hand with 15 strokes. Scrub the palm, each side of thumb and fingers, and posterior side of hand with 10 strokes each.	___	___	___	_____
(2) Divide the arm mentally into thirds: scrub each third 10 times. Some health care facility policies require scrub by time rather than 10 strokes. Rinse brush, and repeat the sequence for the other arm. A two-brush method may be substituted (check health care facility policy).	___	___	___	_____
(3) Discard brush. Flex arms, and rinse from fingertips to elbows in one continuous motion, allowing water to run off at elbow.	___	___	___	_____
(4) Turn off water with foot or knee control, with hands elevated in front of and away from body. Enter operating room suite by backing into room.	___	___	___	_____
(5) Approach sterile setup, grasp sterile towel, taking care not to drip water onto the sterile setup.	___	___	___	_____
(6) Bending slightly at waist, keeping hands and arms above the waist and outstretched, grasp one end of the sterile towel and dry one hand moving from fingers to elbow in a rotating motion.	___	___	___	_____
(7) Repeat drying method for other hand by carefully reversing towel or using a new sterile towel.	___	___	___	_____
(8) Drop towel into linen hamper or into circulating nurse's hand.	___	___	___	_____
C. Optional: Brushless antiseptic hand rub				
(1) After prescrub wash, dry hands and forearms thoroughly with a paper towel.	___	___	___	_____

Continued

254

	S	U	NP	Comments

(2) Dispense 2 mL of antimicrobial agent hand preparation into the palm of one hand. Dip the fingertips of the opposite hand into the hand preparation, and work it under the nails. Spread the remaining hand preparation over the hand and up to just above the elbow, covering all surfaces. ____ ____ ____ _____

(3) Using another 2 mL of hand preparation, repeat with other hand. ____ ____ ____ _____

(4) Dispense another 2 mL of hand preparation into either hand, and reapply to all aspects of both hands up to the wrist. Allow to dry before donning gloves. ____ ____ ____ _____

STUDENT: _____ DATE: _____

INSTRUCTOR: _____ DATE: _____

CHECKLIST
Skill 34-4 Applying a Sterile Gown and Closed Gloving

	S	U	NP	Comments
1. Applying sterile gown				
A. Before entering operating room or treatment area, apply cap, face mask, and eyewear. Foot covers are also required in operating room.	___	___	___	_____
B. Perform thorough surgical hand wash.	___	___	___	_____
C. Ask circulating nurse to assist by opening sterile pack containing sterile gown (folded inside out).	___	___	___	_____
D. Have circulating nurse prepare glove package by peeling outer wrapper open while keeping inner contents sterile. Place inner glove package on sterile field created by sterile outer wrapper.	___	___	___	_____
E. Reach down to sterile gown package; lift folded gown directly upward and step back away from table.	___	___	___	_____
F. Holding folded gown, locate neckband. With both hands, grasp inside front of gown just below neckband.	___	___	___	_____
G. Allow gown to unfold, keeping inside of gown toward body. Do not touch outside of gown with bare hands.	___	___	___	_____
H. With hands at shoulder level, slip both arms into armholes simultaneously. Ask circulating nurse to bring gown over shoulders by reaching inside to arm seams and pulling gown on, leaving sleeves covering hands.	___	___	___	_____
I. Have circulating nurse securely tie back of gown at neck and waist. (If gown is a wraparound style, do not touch sterile flap to cover gown until you are gloved.)	___	___	___	_____
2. Closed gloving				
A. With hands covered by gown sleeves, open inner sterile glove package.	___	___	___	_____
B. With dominant hand inside gown cuff, pick up glove for nondominant hand by grasping folded cuff.	___	___	___	_____
C. Extend nondominant forearm with palm up, and place palm of glove against palm of nondominant hand. Glove fingers will point toward elbow.	___	___	___	_____
D. Grasp back of glove cuff with covered dominant hand, and turn glove cuff over end of nondominant hand and gown cuff.	___	___	___	_____
E. Grasp top of glove and underlying gown sleeve with covered dominant hand. Carefully extend fingers into glove, being sure glove's cuff covers gown's cuff.	___	___	___	_____
F. Glove dominant hand in same manner, reversing hands. Use gloved nondominant hand to pull on glove. Keep hand inside sleeve.	___	___	___	_____
G. Be sure fingers are fully extended into both gloves.	___	___	___	_____
3. For wraparound sterile gowns: take gloved hand and release fastener or ties in front of gown.	___	___	___	_____
4. Hand tie to sterile team member who stands still. Allowing margin of safety, turn around to the left, covering back with extended gown flap. Take back tie from team member, and secure tie to gown.	___	___	___	_____

STUDENT: _____ DATE: _____

INSTRUCTOR: _____ DATE: _____

Skill 34-5 Open Gloving

	S	U	NP	Comments
1. Perform thorough hand hygiene.				
2. Remove outer glove package wrapper by carefully separating and peeling apart sides.	____	____	____	_____
3. Grasp inner package, and lay it on clean, flat surface just above waist level. Open package, keeping gloves on wrapper's inside surface.	____	____	____	_____
4. If gloves are not prepowdered, take packet of powder and apply lightly to hands over sink or wastebasket.	____	____	____	_____
5. Identify right and left glove.	____	____	____	_____
6. Glove dominant hand first.	____	____	____	_____
7. With thumb and first two fingers of nondominant hand, grasp edge of cuff of glove for dominant hand. Touch only glove's inside surface.	____	____	____	_____
8. Carefully pull glove over dominant hand, leaving cuff and being sure cuff does not roll up wrist. Be sure thumb and fingers are in proper spaces.	____	____	____	_____
9. With gloved hand, slip fingers underneath second glove's cuff to pick it up.	____	____	____	_____
10. Carefully pull second glove over nondominant hand. Do not allow fingers and thumb of gloved dominant hand to touch any part of exposed nondominant hand. Keep thumb of dominant hand abducted back.	____	____	____	_____
11. After second glove is on, interlock hands. The cuffs usually fall down after application. Be sure to touch only sterile sides.	____	____	____	_____
12. Glove disposal				
A. Grasp outside of one cuff with other gloved hand; avoid touching wrist. Pull halfway down palm of hand. Take thumb of half ungloved hand, and place under cuff of the other glove.	____	____	____	_____
B. Pull glove off, turning it inside out. Discard in receptacle.	____	____	____	_____
C. Take fingers of bare hand and tuck inside remaining glove cuff. Peel glove off, inside out. Discard in receptacle.	____	____	____	_____
D. Perform hand hygiene.	____	____	____	_____

STUDENT: _____ DATE: _____

INSTRUCTOR: _____ DATE: _____

CHECKLIST
Skill 35-1 Administering Oral Medications

	S	U	NP	Comments
1. Check accuracy and completeness of each medication administration record (MAR) or computer printout with prescriber's original medication order. Check client's name and medication name, dosage, route, and time for administration. Recopy or re-print any portion of MAR that is difficult to read.	___	___	___	_____
2. Assess for any contraindications to client receiving oral medication.	___	___	___	_____
3. Check the client's swallow, cough, and gag reflexes.	___	___	___	_____
4. Assess client's medical history, history of allergies, medication history, and diet history. List client's food and drug allergies on *each* page of the MAR, and prominently display it on the client's medical record per agency policy.	___	___	___	_____
5. Gather physical examination and laboratory data that influence medication administration (e.g., vital signs, renal and liver function laboratory findings).	___	___	___	_____
6. Assess client's knowledge regarding health and medication use.	___	___	___	_____
7. Assess client's preferences for fluids. Maintain fluid restrictions when applicable. Determine if medication can be given with preferred fluid.	___	___	___	_____
8. Prepare medications:				
A. Perform hand hygiene.	___	___	___	_____
B. If using a medication cart, move it outside client's room.	___	___	___	_____
C. Unlock medicine drawer or cart, or log onto computerized medication dispensing system.	___	___	___	_____
D. Prepare medication for one client at a time. Keep all pages of MARs or computer printouts for one client together, or look at only one client's medication administration computer screen.	___	___	___	_____
E. Select correct medication from stock supply or unit-dose drawer. Compare label of medication with MAR, computer printout, or computer screen. Check expiration date on all medication labels.	___	___	___	_____
F. Calculate medication dose as necessary. Double-check calculation. If needed, have another nurse verify calculations.	___	___	___	_____
G. If preparing a controlled substance, check record for previous medication count and compare current count with supply available.	___	___	___	_____
H. To prepare tablets or capsules from a floor stock bottle, pour required number into bottle cap and transfer medication to medication cup. Do not touch medication with fingers. Return extra tablets or capsules to bottle. Break prescored medications if needed by using a gloved hand or a clean pillating device. Identify prescored tablets by a line placed on the pill by the manufacturer that spans the center of the tablet.	___	___	___	_____
I. To prepare unit-dose tablets or capsules, place packaged tablet or capsule directly into medicine cup. Do not remove wrapper.	___	___	___	_____
J. Place all tablets or capsules for client in one medicine cup, except for those requiring preadministration assessments (e.g., pulse rate or blood pressure); keep medications in their wrappers.	___	___	___	_____

Continued

258

	S	U	NP	Comments

K. If the client has difficulty swallowing and liquid medications are not an option, use pill-crushing device such as a mortar and pestle to grind pills. Before using a mortar and pestle, clean them. If a pill crushing device is not available, place tablet between two medication cups and grind with a blunt instrument. Mix ground tablet in a small amount of soft food (custard or applesauce). ____ ____ ____ _____

L. To prepare liquids:
 (1) Gently shake container. If medication is in a unit-dose container with correct amount to administer, no further preparation is necessary. If medication is in a multidose bottle, remove bottle cap from container and place cap upside down. ____ ____ ____ _____

 (2) Hold multidose bottle with label against palm of hand while pouring. ____ ____ ____ _____

 (3) Hold medication cup at eye level, and fill to desired level on scale. Make sure scale is even with fluid level at its surface or base of meniscus, not edges. Draw up volumes of less than 10 mL in syringe without needle. ____ ____ ____ _____

 (4) Discard any excess liquid into sink. Wipe lip and neck of bottle with paper towel. ____ ____ ____ _____

 (5) Administer liquid medications packaged in single-dose cups directly from the single-dose cup. Do not pour them into medicine cups. ____ ____ ____ _____

M. Compare MAR, computer printout, or computer screen with prepared medication and container. ____ ____ ____ _____

N. Return stock containers or unused unit-dose medications to shelf or drawer, and read label again. ____ ____ ____ _____

O. Do not leave medications unattended. ____ ____ ____ _____

9. Administer medications:
 A. Take medications to client at correct time. ____ ____ ____ _____

 B. Identify client using at least two client identifiers. Compare client's name and one other identifier (e.g., hospital identification number) on MAR, computer printout, or computer screen with information on client's identification bracelet. Ask client to state name if possible for a third identifier. ____ ____ ____ _____

 C. Compare labels of medications with MAR at client's bedside. ____ ____ ____ _____

 D. Explain purpose of each medication and its action to client. Allow client to ask any questions about drugs. ____ ____ ____ _____

 E. Assist client to sitting or side-lying position if sitting is contraindicated. ____ ____ ____ _____

 F. Tablets:
 (1) Some clients want to hold solid medications in hand or cup before placing in mouth. ____ ____ ____ _____

 (2) Offer water or juice to help client swallow medications. Give cold carbonated water if available and not contraindicated. ____ ____ ____ _____

 G. Sublingual-administered medications:
 (1) Have client place medication under tongue and allow it to dissolve completely. ____ ____ ____ _____

 (2) Caution client against swallowing tablet. ____ ____ ____ _____

 H. Buccal medications:
 (1) Have client place medication in mouth against mucous membranes of the cheek until it dissolves. ____ ____ ____ _____

 (2) Avoid administering liquids until buccal medication has dissolved. ____ ____ ____ _____

 I. Powdered medications:
 (1) Mix with liquids at bedside, and give to client to drink. ____ ____ ____ _____

 (2) Give effervescent powders and tablets immediately after dissolving. ____ ____ ____ _____

Continued

	S	U	NP	Comments

J. Lozenges:
   (1) Caution client against chewing or swallowing lozenges. _____ _____ _____ _____

K. If client is unable to hold medications, place medication cup to the lips and gently introduce each drug into the mouth, one at a time. Do not rush. _____ _____ _____ _____

L. If tablet or capsule falls to the floor, discard it and repeat preparation. _____ _____ _____ _____

M. Stay until client has completely swallowed each medication. Ask client to open mouth if uncertain whether medication has been swallowed. _____ _____ _____ _____

N. For highly acidic medications (e.g., aspirin), offer client nonfat snack (e.g., crackers) if not contraindicated by client's condition. _____ _____ _____ _____

O. Assist client in returning to comfortable position. _____ _____ _____ _____

P. Dispose of soiled supplies, and perform hand hygiene. _____ _____ _____ _____

Q. Replenish stock, such as cups and straws, return cart to medication room if used, and clean work area. _____ _____ _____ _____

10. Evaluate client's response to medications at times that correlate with the medication's onset, peak, and duration. _____ _____ _____ _____

11. Ask client or family member to identify medication name and explain purpose, action, dosage schedule, and potential side effects of drug. _____ _____ _____ _____

12. Observe client for adverse effects (side effect, toxic effect, allergic reaction):

A. Assess for symptoms such as urticaria, rash, pruritus, rhinitis, and wheezing that indicate allergic reaction. _____ _____ _____ _____

B. Always notify prescriber and pharmacy when the client exhibits adverse effects. _____ _____ _____ _____

C. Withhold further doses, and add allergy information to client's medical record. _____ _____ _____ _____

13. If client refuses medication:

A. Explore reasons client does not want medication. _____ _____ _____ _____

B. Educate if misunderstandings of medication therapy are apparent. _____ _____ _____ _____

C. Do not force client to take medication; clients have the right to refuse treatment. _____ _____ _____ _____

D. If client continues to refuse medication despite educational attempts, record why the drug was withheld on client's chart and notify prescriber. _____ _____ _____ _____

14. Record administration of oral medications on computerized or paper copy of MAR immediately after administering medications. If using paper copy of MAR, include your initials or signature. _____ _____ _____ _____

15. Record the reason any drug is withheld, and follow agency's policy for proper recording. _____ _____ _____ _____

16. Record and report evaluation of medication effect to prescriber if required (e.g., report urine output following administration of diuretic if ordered by prescriber). _____ _____ _____ _____

STUDENT: _____ DATE: _____

INSTRUCTOR: _____ DATE: _____

Skill 35-2 Administering Ophthalmic Medications

	S	U	NP	Comments
1. Check accuracy and completeness of each medication administration record (MAR) or computer printout with prescriber's medication order. Check client's name and medication name and dosage (e.g., number of drops [if a liquid] and eye [right, left, or both eyes]), route, and time of administration. Recopy or re-print any portion of MAR that is difficult to read.	____	____	____	_____
2. Identify client using at least two client identifiers.	____	____	____	_____
3. Assess condition of external eye structures.	____	____	____	_____
4. Determine whether client has any known allergies to eye medications. Also ask if client has allergy to latex.	____	____	____	_____
5. Determine whether client has any symptoms of visual alterations.	____	____	____	_____
6. Assess client's level of consciousness and ability to follow directions.	____	____	____	_____
7. Assess client's knowledge regarding medication therapy and desire to self-administer medication.	____	____	____	_____
8. Assess client's ability to manipulate and hold dropper.	____	____	____	_____
9. Prepare medication. Be sure to check the label two times while preparing medication.	____	____	____	_____
10. Perform hand hygiene, and take medication to client at correct time.	____	____	____	_____
11. Identify client using at least two client identifiers. Compare client's name and one other identifier (e.g., hospital identification number) on MAR, computer printout, or computer screen with information on client's identification bracelet. Ask client to state name if possible for a third identifier.	____	____	____	_____
12. Compare labels of medications with MAR at client's bedside.	____	____	____	_____
13. Arrange supplies at bedside; apply clean gloves. If eye drops are stored in refrigerator, allow eye drops to come to room temperature before administering eye drops.	____	____	____	_____
14. Gently roll container.	____	____	____	_____
15. Explain procedure to client; include positioning and sensations to expect, such as burning or stinging.	____	____	____	_____
16. Ask client to lie supine or sit back in chair with head slightly hyperextended.	____	____	____	_____
17. If crusts or drainage are present along eyelid margins or inner canthus, gently wash away. Soak any crusts that are dried and difficult to remove by applying damp washcloth or cotton ball over eye for a few minutes. Always wipe clean from inner to outer canthus.	____	____	____	_____
18. Hold cotton ball or clean tissue in nondominant hand on client's cheekbone just below lower eyelid.	____	____	____	_____
19. With tissue or cotton resting below lower lid, gently press downward with thumb or forefinger against bony orbit.	____	____	____	_____
20. Ask client to look at ceiling.	____	____	____	_____
21. Instill eye drops:				
A. With dominant hand resting on client's forehead, hold filled medication eye dropper or ophthalmic solution approximately 1 to 2 cm (½ to ¾ inch) above conjunctival sac.	____	____	____	_____
B. Drop prescribed number of medication drops into conjunctival sac.	____	____	____	_____
C. If client blinks or closes eye or if drops land on outer lid margins, repeat procedure.	____	____	____	_____
D. After instilling drops, ask client to close eye gently.	____	____	____	_____

Continued

	S	U	NP	Comments
E. When administering medications that cause systemic effects, apply gentle pressure with your finger and clean tissue on the client's nasolacrimal duct for 30 to 60 seconds.	____	____	____	_____
22. Instill eye ointment:				
A. Ask client to look at ceiling.	____	____	____	_____
B. Holding ointment applicator above lower lid margin, apply thin stream of ointment evenly along inner edge of lower eyelid on conjunctiva from the inner canthus to outer canthus.	____	____	____	_____
C. Have client close eye and rub lid lightly in circular motion with cotton ball, if rubbing is not contraindicated.	____	____	____	_____
23. Administer intraocular disk:				
A. Application:				
(1) Open package containing the disk. Gently press fingertip against the disk so that it adheres to finger. Position the convex side of the disk on fingertip.	____	____	____	_____
(2) With other hand, gently pull the client's lower eyelid away from the eye. Ask client to look up.	____	____	____	_____
(3) Place the disk in the conjunctival sac, so that it floats on the sclera between the iris and lower eyelid.	____	____	____	_____
(4) Pull the client's lower eyelid out and over the disk.	____	____	____	_____
B. Removal:				
(1) Perform hand hygiene, and apply gloves.	____	____	____	_____
(2) Explain procedure to client.	____	____	____	_____
(3) Gently pull on the client's lower eyelid.	____	____	____	_____
(4) Using forefinger and thumb of opposite hand, pinch the disk and lift it out of the client's eye.	____	____	____	_____
24. If excess medication is on eyelid, gently wipe it from inner to outer canthus.	____	____	____	_____
25. If client had eye patch, apply clean one by placing it over affected eye so entire eye is covered. Tape securely without applying pressure to eye.	____	____	____	_____
26. If client receives eye medication to both eyes at the same time, use a different tissue or cotton ball with each eye.	____	____	____	_____
27. Remove gloves, dispose of soiled supplies in proper receptacle, and perform hand hygiene.	____	____	____	_____
28. Note client's response to instillation; ask if client felt any discomfort.	____	____	____	_____
29. Observe response to medication by assessing visual changes and noting any side effects.	____	____	____	_____
30. Ask client to discuss medication's purpose, action, side effects, and technique of administration.	____	____	____	_____
31. Have client demonstrate self-administration of next dose.				
A. If client cannot instill drops without supervision, reinforce teaching and allow client to self-administer drops as much as possible to enhance confidence.	____	____	____	_____
B. If client cannot self-administer drops, teach others, such as family members, to instill drops into the client's eye.	____	____	____	_____
32. Client displays signs of allergic reaction (e.g., tearing, reddened sclera) or systemic response (e.g., bradycardia) to medication:				
A. Hold medication, and speak with prescriber.	____	____	____	_____
B. Follow institutional policy or guidelines for reporting of adverse or allergic reaction to medications.	____	____	____	_____
C. Add information about allergy to medical record per agency policy.	____	____	____	_____
33. Record medication, concentration, number of drops, time of administration, and eye (left, right, or both) that received medication on electronic or printed MAR.	____	____	____	_____
34. Record appearance of eye in nurses' notes.	____	____	____	_____

STUDENT: _____   DATE: _____

INSTRUCTOR: _____   DATE: _____

Cᴴᴇᴄᴋʟɪsᴛ

Skill 35-3 Using Metered-Dose or Dry Powder Inhalers

	S	U	NP	Comments
1. Check accuracy and completeness of each medication administration record (MAR) or computer printout with prescriber's original medication order. Check client's name and medication name, dosage, route, and time for administration. Recopy or re-print any portion of MAR that is difficult to read.	____	____	____	_____
2. Assess client's respiratory pattern, and auscultate breath sounds.	____	____	____	_____
3. If previously instructed in self-administration, assess client's technique in using inhaler.	____	____	____	_____
4. Assess client's ability to hold, manipulate, and depress canister or strength of inhalation.	____	____	____	_____
5. Assess client's *readiness* to learn: client asks questions about medication, disease, or complications; requests education in use of inhaler; is mentally alert; participates in own care.	____	____	____	_____
6. Assess client's *ability* to learn: make sure client is not fatigued, in pain, or in respiratory distress; assess level of understanding of technical vocabulary terms.	____	____	____	_____
7. Assess client's knowledge and understanding of disease and purpose and action of prescribed medications.	____	____	____	_____
8. Determine medication schedule and number of inhalations prescribed for each dose.	____	____	____	_____
9. Prepare medication. Be sure to compare the label of the medication with the MAR two times while preparing the medication.	____	____	____	_____
10. Identify client using at least two client identifiers. Compare client's name and one other identifier (e.g., hospital identification number) on MAR, computer printout, or computer screen with information on client's identification bracelet. Ask client to state name if possible for a third identifier.	____	____	____	_____
11. Compare labels of medications with MAR at client's bedside.	____	____	____	_____
12. Instruct client in comfortable environment by sitting in chair in hospital room or sitting at kitchen table in home.	____	____	____	_____
13. Provide adequate time for teaching session.	____	____	____	_____
14. Perform hand hygiene, and arrange equipment needed.	____	____	____	_____
15. Allow client opportunity to manipulate inhaler, canister, and spacer device. Explain and demonstrate how canister fits into inhaler.	____	____	____	_____
16. Explain what metered dose is, and warn client about overuse of inhaler, including medication side effects.	____	____	____	_____
17. Explain steps for administering squeeze-and-breathe metered-dose inhaler (MDI) (demonstrate steps when possible):				
A. Insert MDI canister into the holder.	____	____	____	_____
B. Remove mouthpiece cover from inhaler.	____	____	____	_____
C. Shake inhaler vigorously five or six times.	____	____	____	_____
D. Have client take a deep breath and exhale.	____	____	____	_____
E. Instruct the client to position the inhaler in one of two ways.				
(1) Close mouth around MDI with opening toward back of throat.	____	____	____	_____
(2) Position the device 2 to 4 cm (1 to 2 inches) in front of the mouth.	____	____	____	_____
F. With the inhaler properly positioned, have client hold inhaler with thumb at the mouthpiece and the index finger and middle finger at the top. This is called a three-point or lateral hand position.	____	____	____	_____

Continued

	S	U	NP	Comments

G. Instruct client to tilt head back slightly, inhale slowly and deeply through mouth for 3 to 5 seconds while depressing canister fully.

H. Hold breath for approximately 10 seconds.

I. Remove MDI from mouth, and exhale through pursed lips.

18. Explain steps to administer MDI using a spacer such as an Aerochamber (demonstrate when possible):

A. Remove mouthpiece cover from MDI and mouthpiece of spacer. Inspect spacer for foreign objects, and ensure valve is intact if spacer has one.

B. Insert MDI into end of spacer.

C. Shake inhaler vigorously five or six times.

D. Have client exhale completely before closing mouth around mouthpiece of the spacer. Avoid covering small exhalation slots with the lips

E. Have client depress medication canister, spraying one puff into spacer.

F. Instruct client to inhale deeply and slowly through the mouth for 3 to 5 seconds.

G. Have client hold breath for 10 seconds.

H. Remove MDI and spacer before exhaling.

19. Explain steps to administer dry-powder inhaler (DPI) or breath-activated MDI (demonstrate when possible):

A. Remove cover from mouthpiece. Do not shake the inhaler.

B. Prepare the medication as directed by manufacturer (e.g., hold inhaler upright and turn wheel to the right and then to the left until a click is heard, load medication pellet, etc.).

C. Exhale away from inhaler before inhalation.

D. Position mouthpiece between the lips.

E. Inhale deeply and forcefully through the mouth.

F. Hold breath for 5 to 10 seconds.

20. Instruct client to wait at least 20 to 30 seconds between inhalations of the same medication and 2 to 5 minutes between inhalations of different medications.

21. Instruct client against repeating inhalations before next scheduled dose.

22. Explain that client may feel gagging sensation in throat caused by droplets of medication on pharynx or tongue.

23. Instruct client in how to clean inhaler:

A. Once a day, inhaler and cap need to be rinsed in warm running water. Inhaler needs to be completely dry before using.

B. Twice a week, the L-shaped plastic mouthpiece needs to be washed with mild dishwashing soap and warm water. Rinse and dry well before putting canister back inside mouthpiece.

24. Ask if client has any questions.

25. Have client explain and demonstrate steps in use of inhaler.

26. Ask client to explain medication schedule, side effects, and when to call health care provider.

27. Ask client to calculate how many days the inhaler will last.

28. After medication has been taken, assess client's respiratory status, including ease of respirations, auscultation of lungs, and use of pulse oximetry to assess client's oxygenation status.

29. Document skills taught and the client's ability to perform skills.

30. Record medication, time of administration, and the amount of puffs on the MAR.

31. Report any undesirable effects from medication.

CHECKLIST
Skill 35-4 Preparing Injections

	S	U	NP	Comments
1. Check accuracy and completeness of each medication administration record (MAR) or computer printout with prescriber's original medication order. Check client's name and medication name, dosage, route, and time for administration. Recopy or re-print any portion of MAR that is difficult to read.	____	____	____	_____
2. Review pertinent information related to medication, including action, purpose, side effects, and nursing implications.	____	____	____	_____
3. Assess client's body build, muscle size, and weight.	____	____	____	_____
4. Perform hand hygiene, and assemble supplies.	____	____	____	_____
5. Check date of expiration for medication vial or ampule.	____	____	____	_____
6. Prepare medication: Be sure to compare the label of the medication with the MAR two times while preparing the medication.				
A. Ampule preparation				
(1) Tap top of ampule lightly and quickly with finger until fluid moves from neck of ampule.	____	____	____	_____
(2) Place small gauze pad or unopened alcohol swab around neck of ampule.	____	____	____	_____
(3) Snap neck of ampule quickly and firmly away from hands.	____	____	____	_____
(4) Draw up medication quickly, using filter needle long enough to reach bottom of ampule.	____	____	____	_____
(5) Hold ampule upside down, or set it on a flat surface. Insert filter needle into center of ampule opening. Do not allow needle tip or shaft to touch rim of ampule.	____	____	____	_____
(6) Aspirate medication into syringe by gently pulling back on plunger.	____	____	____	_____
(7) Keep needle tip under surface of liquid. Tip ampule to bring all fluid within reach of the needle.	____	____	____	_____
(8) If air bubbles are aspirated, do not expel air into ampule.	____	____	____	_____
(9) To expel excess air bubbles, remove needle from ampule. Hold syringe with needle pointing up. Tap side of syringe to cause bubbles to rise toward needle. Draw back slightly on plunger, and then push plunger upward to eject air. Do not eject fluid.	____	____	____	_____
(10) If syringe contains excess fluid, use sink for disposal. Hold syringe vertically with needle tip up and slanted slightly toward sink. Slowly eject excess fluid into sink. Recheck fluid level in syringe by holding it vertically.	____	____	____	_____
(11) Cover needle with its safety sheath, or scoop needle to recap. Replace filter needle with needle or needleless access device for injection.	____	____	____	_____
B. Vial containing a solution				
(1) Remove cap covering top of unused vial to expose sterile rubber seal, keeping rubber seal sterile. If a multidose vial has been used before, cap is already removed. Firmly and briskly wipe surface of rubber seal with alcohol swab, and allow it to dry.	____	____	____	_____
(2) Pick up syringe, and remove needle cap or cap covering needleless vial access device. Pull back on plunger to draw amount of air into syringe equivalent to volume of medication to be aspirated from vial.	____	____	____	_____

Continued

	S	U	NP	Comments

(3) With vial on flat surface, insert tip of needle with beveled tip entering first through center of rubber seal. Apply pressure to tip of needle during insertion.

(4) Inject air into the vial's airspace, holding on to plunger. Hold plunger with firm pressure; air pressure within the vial sometimes forces the plunger backward.

(5) Invert vial while keeping firm hold on syringe and plunger. Hold vial between thumb and middle fingers of nondominant hand. Grasp end of syringe barrel and plunger with thumb and forefinger of dominant hand to counteract pressure in vial.

(6) Keep tip of needle below fluid level.

(7) Allow air pressure from the vial to fill syringe gradually with medication. If necessary, pull back slightly on plunger to obtain correct amount of solution.

(8) When desired volume is obtained, position needle into vial's airspace; tap side of syringe barrel carefully to dislodge any air bubbles. Eject any air remaining at top of syringe into vial.

(9) Remove needle from vial by pulling back on barrel of syringe.

(10) Hold syringe at eye level, at 90-degree angle, to ensure correct volume and absence of air bubbles. Remove any remaining air by tapping barrel to dislodge any air bubbles. Draw back slightly on plunger; then push plunger upward to eject air. Do not eject fluid. Recheck volume of medication.

(11) If medication will be injected into client's tissue, change needle to appropriate gauge and length according to route of medication.

(12) For multidose vial, make label that includes date of mixing, concentration of medication per milliliter, and your initials.

C. Vial containing a powder (reconstituting medications)

(1) Remove cap covering vial of powdered medication and cap covering vial of proper diluent. Firmly swab both seals with alcohol swab, and allow to dry.

(2) Draw up diluent into syringe following Steps 6B(2) through 6B(10).

(3) Insert tip of needle through center of rubber seal of vial of powdered medication. Inject diluent into vial. Remove needle.

(4) Mix medication thoroughly. Roll in palms. Do not shake.

(5) Reconstituted medication in vial is ready to be drawn into new syringe. Read label carefully to determine dose after reconstitution.

(6) Prepare medication in syringe following Steps 6B(2) through 6B(12).

7. Dispose of soiled supplies. Place broken ampule and/or used vials and used needle in puncture-proof and leakproof container. Clean work area, and perform hand hygiene.

STUDENT: _____ DATE: _____

INSTRUCTOR: _____ DATE: _____

CHECKLIST
Skill 35-5 Administering Injections

	S	U	NP	Comments
1. Check accuracy and completeness of each medication administration record (MAR) or computer printout with prescriber's original medication order. Check client's name and medication name, dosage, route, and time for administration. Recopy or re-print any portion of MAR that is difficult to read.	___	___	___	_____
2. Assess client's medical and medication history.	___	___	___	_____
3. Assess client's history of allergies; know substances client is allergic to and normal allergic reaction.	___	___	___	_____
4. Check date of expiration for medication.	___	___	___	_____
5. Observe verbal and nonverbal responses toward receiving injection.	___	___	___	_____
6. Assess for contraindications.				
A. For subcutaneous injections assess for factors such as circulatory shock or reduced local tissue perfusion. Assess adequacy of client's adipose tissue.	___	___	___	_____
B. For intramuscular injections assess for factors such as muscle atrophy, reduced blood flow, or circulatory shock.	___	___	___	_____
7. Aseptically prepare correct medication dose from ampule or vial. Check label of medication with the MAR two times while preparing medication.	___	___	___	_____
8. Take medication to client at right time, and perform hand hygiene.	___	___	___	_____
9. Close room curtain or door.	___	___	___	_____
10. Identify client using at least two client identifiers. Compare client's name and one other identifier (e.g., hospital identification number) on MAR, computer printout, or computer screen with information on client's identification bracelet. Ask client to state name if possible for a third identifier.	___	___	___	_____
11. Compare the label of the medication with the MAR one more time at the client's bedside.	___	___	___	_____
12. Explain steps of procedure, and tell client injection may cause a slight burning or may sting.	___	___	___	_____
13. Apply disposable gloves.	___	___	___	_____
14. Keep sheet or gown draped over body parts not requiring exposure.	___	___	___	_____
15. Select appropriate injection site. Inspect skin surface over sites for bruises, inflammation, or edema.				
A. Subcutaneous (Sub-Q): Palpate sites for masses or tenderness. Avoid these areas. For daily insulin, rotate site daily. Be sure needle is correct size by grasping skinfold at site with thumb and forefinger. Measure fold from top to bottom. Needle should be one-half length.	___	___	___	_____
B. Intramuscular (IM): Note integrity and size of muscle, and palpate for tenderness or hardness. Avoid these areas. If injections are given frequently, rotate sites. Use ventrogluteal site if possible.	___	___	___	_____
C. Intradermal (ID): Note lesions or discolorations of forearm. Select site three to four finger widths below antecubital space and a hand width above wrist. If you cannot use the forearm, inspect the upper back. If necessary, use sites for Sub-Q injections.	___	___	___	_____
16. Assist client to comfortable position:				
A. Sub-Q: Have client relax arm, leg, or abdomen, depending on site chosen for injection.	___	___	___	_____
B. IM: Position client depending on site chosen (e.g., sit or lie flat, on side, or prone).	___	___	___	_____

Continued

	S	U	NP	Comments

C. ID: Have client extend elbow and support it and forearm on flat surface. ____ ____ ____ _____

D. Have client talk about subject of interest. Ask open-ended questions. ____ ____ ____ _____

17. Relocate site using anatomical landmarks. ____ ____ ____ _____

18. Cleanse site with an antiseptic swab. Apply swab at center of the site, and rotate outward in a circular direction for about 5 cm (2 inches). ____ ____ ____ _____

19. Hold swab or gauze between third and fourth fingers of nondominant hand. ____ ____ ____ _____

20. Remove needle cap or sheath from needle by pulling it straight off. ____ ____ ____ _____

21. Hold syringe between thumb and forefinger of dominant hand.

A. Sub-Q: Hold as dart, palm down, or hold syringe across tops of fingertips. ____ ____ ____ _____

B. IM: Hold as dart, palm down. ____ ____ ____ _____

C. ID: Hold bevel of needle pointing up. ____ ____ ____ _____

22. Administer injection:

A. Subcutaneous

(1) For average-size client, spread skin tightly across injection site, or pinch skin with nondominant hand. ____ ____ ____ _____

(2) Inject needle quickly and firmly at 45- to 90-degree angle. Then release skin, if pinched. ____ ____ ____ _____

(3) For obese client, pinch skin at site and inject needle at 90-degree angle below tissue fold. ____ ____ ____ _____

(4) Inject medication slowly. ____ ____ ____ _____

B. Intramuscular

(1) Position nondominant hand just below site, and pull skin approximately 2.5 to 3.5 cm down or laterally with ulnar side of hand to administer in a Z-track. Hold position until medication is injected. With dominant hand, inject needle quickly at 90-degree angle into muscle. ____ ____ ____ _____

(2) Optional: If client's muscle mass is small, grasp body of muscle between thumb and fingers. ____ ____ ____ _____

(3) Insert needle quickly at 90-degree angle into muscle. After needle pierces skin, grasp lower end of syringe barrel with nondominant hand to stabilize syringe. Continue to hold skin tightly with nondominant hand. Move dominant hand to end of plunger. Do not move syringe. ____ ____ ____ _____

(4) Pull back on plunger 5 to 10 seconds. If no blood appears, inject medicine slowly, at a rate of 1 mL/10 sec. ____ ____ ____ _____

(5) Wait 10 seconds Then smoothly and steadily withdraw needle and release skin. ____ ____ ____ _____

C. Intradermal

(1) With nondominant hand, stretch skin over site with forefinger or thumb. ____ ____ ____ _____

(2) With needle almost against client's skin, insert it slowly with bevel up at a 5- to 15-degree angle until resistance is felt. Then advance needle through epidermis to approximately 3 mm (1/8 inch) below skin surface. You will see needle tip through skin. ____ ____ ____ _____

(3) Inject medication slowly. Normally, you feel resistance. If not, needle is too deep; remove and begin again. Nondominant hand can stabilize the needle during the injection. ____ ____ ____ _____

(4) While injecting medication, notice that small bleb approximately 6 mm (1/4 inch) in diameter (resembling mosquito bite) appears on skin's surface. Instruct client that this is a normal finding. ____ ____ ____ _____

23. Withdraw needle while applying alcohol swab or gauze gently over site. ____ ____ ____ _____

Continued

	S	U	NP	Comments
24. Apply gentle pressure. Do not massage site. Apply bandage if needed.	_____	_____	_____	_____
25. Assist client to comfortable position.	_____	_____	_____	_____
26. Discard uncapped needle or needle enclosed in safety shield and attached syringe into puncture-proof and leakproof receptacle.	_____	_____	_____	_____
27. Remove disposable gloves, and perform hand hygiene.	_____	_____	_____	_____
28. Stay with client, and observe for any allergic reactions.	_____	_____	_____	_____
29. Return to room, and ask if client feels any acute pain, burning, numbness, or tingling at injection site.	_____	_____	_____	_____
30. Inspect site, noting any bruising or induration.	_____	_____	_____	_____
31. Observe client's response to medication at times that correlate with the medication's onset, peak, and duration.	_____	_____	_____	_____
32. Ask client to explain purpose and effects of medication.	_____	_____	_____	_____
33. For ID injections, use skin pencil and draw circle around perimeter of injection site. Read site within appropriate amount of time, designated by type of medication or skin test administered.	_____			
34. Chart medication dose, route, site, time, and date given on MAR immediately after giving medication per agency policy.	_____	_____	_____	_____
35. Document if scheduled medication is withheld, and record the reason per agency policy.	_____	_____	_____	_____
36. Report any undesirable effects from medication to prescriber.	_____	_____	_____	_____
37. Record client's response to medications in nurses' notes, and report to prescriber if required.	_____	_____	_____	_____

STUDENT: _____ DATE: _____

INSTRUCTOR: _____ DATE: _____

Skill 35-6 Adding Medications to Intravenous Fluid Containers

	S	U	NP	Comments
1. Check accuracy and completeness of each medication administration record (MAR) or computer printout with prescriber's original medication order. Check client's name and medication name, dosage, route, and time for administration. Recopy or re-print any portion of MAR that is difficult to read.	___	___	___	_____
2. Assess client's medical history.	___	___	___	_____
3. Collect information necessary to administer drug safely, including action, purpose, side effects, normal dose, time of peak onset, and nursing implications.	___	___	___	_____
4. When adding more than one medication to intravenous (IV) solution, assess for compatibility of medications.	___	___	___	_____
5. Assess client's systemic fluid balance, as reflected by skin hydration and turgor, body weight, pulse, and blood pressure.	___	___	___	_____
6. Assess client's history of medication allergies.	___	___	___	_____
7. Perform hand hygiene.	___	___	___	_____
8. Assess IV insertion site for signs of infiltration or phlebitis, and assess patency of existing IV line.	___	___	___	_____
9. Assess client's understanding of purpose of medication therapy.	___	___	___	_____
10. Prepare medication: Use aseptic technique. Be sure to compare the label of the medication with the MAR two times while preparing the medication.	___	___	___	_____
11. Perform hand hygiene.	___	___	___	_____
12. Compare labels of medication and IV fluid bag with MAR.	___	___	___	_____
13. Add medication to new container (usually done in medication room or at medication cart):				
A. Solution in a bag: Locate medication injection port on plastic IV solution bag (port has small rubber stopper at end). Do not select port for the IV tubing insertion or air vent.	___	___	___	_____
B. Solution in a bottle: Locate injection site on IV solution bottle, which is often covered by a metal or plastic cap.	___	___	___	_____
C. Wipe off port or injection site with alcohol or antiseptic swab.	___	___	___	_____
D. Remove needle cap or sheath from syringe, and insert needle of syringe or needleless device through center of injection port or site; inject medication.	___	___	___	_____
E. Withdraw syringe from bag or bottle.	___	___	___	_____
F. Mix medication and IV solution by holding bag or bottle and turning it gently end to end.	___	___	___	_____
G. Complete medication label with client's name, name and dose of medication, date, time, and nurse's initials. Apply it to bottle or bag.	___	___	___	_____
H. If new tubing is required, spike bag or bottle with IV tubing and prime tubing.	___	___	___	_____
14. Bring assembled items to client's bedside at right time, and perform hand hygiene.	___	___	___	_____
15. Identify client using at least two client identifiers. Compare client's name and one other identifier (e.g., hospital identification number) on MAR, computer printout, or computer screen with information on client's identification bracelet. Ask client to state name if possible for a third identifier.	___	___	___	_____

Continued

	S	U	NP	Comments

16. Prepare client by explaining that medication is to be given through existing IV line or one to be started. Explain that client should feel no discomfort during medication infusion. Encourage client to report symptoms of discomfort. ___ ___ ___ _____

17. Connect new infusion tubing, or spike container with existing tubing. Regulate infusion at ordered rate. ___ ___ ___ _____

18. Add medication to existing container:
   A. Prepare vented IV bottle or plastic bag:
   (1) Check volume of solution remaining in bottle or bag. ___ ___ ___ _____
   (2) Close off IV infusion clamp. ___ ___ ___ _____
   (3) Wipe off medication port with an alcohol or antiseptic swab. ___ ___ ___ _____
   (4) Remove needle cap or sheath from syringe; insert syringe needle or needleless device through injection port and inject medication. ___ ___ ___ _____
   (5) Withdraw syringe from bag or bottle. ___ ___ ___ _____
   (6) Lower bag or bottle from IV pole, and gently mix. Rehang bag. ___ ___ ___ _____
   B. Complete medication label, and apply it to bag or bottle. ___ ___ ___ _____
   C. Regulate infusion to desired rate. Use IV pump if indicated. ___ ___ ___ _____

19. Properly dispose of equipment and supplies. Do not cap needle of syringe. Discard specially sheathed needles as a unit with needle covered. ___ ___ ___ _____

20. Perform hand hygiene. ___ ___ ___ _____

21. Observe client for signs or symptoms of medication reaction. ___ ___ ___ _____

22. Observe for signs and symptoms of fluid volume excess. ___ ___ ___ _____

23. Periodically return to client's room to assess IV insertion site and rate of infusion. ___ ___ ___ _____

24. Observe for signs or symptoms of IV infiltration. ___ ___ ___ _____

25. Ask client to explain purpose and effects of medication therapy. ___ ___ ___ _____

26. Record solution and medication added to parenteral fluid on appropriate form. ___ ___ ___ _____

27. Report any adverse effects to client's health care provider, and document adverse effects according to institutional policy. ___ ___ ___ _____

STUDENT: _____ DATE: _____

INSTRUCTOR: _____ DATE: _____

Skill 35-7 Administering Medications by Intravenous Bolus

	S	U	NP	Comments
1. Check accuracy and completeness of each medication administration record (MAR) or computer printout with prescriber's original medication order. Check client's name and medication name, dosage, route, and time for administration. Recopy or re-print any portion of MAR that is difficult to read.	____	____	____	_____
2. Collect information necessary to administer medication safely, including action, purpose, side effects, normal dose, time of peak onset, how slowly to give the medication, and nursing implications, such as the need to dilute the medication or administer it through the filter.	____	____	____	_____
3. If pushing medication into an intravenous (IV) line, determine the compatibility of the medication with the IV fluids and any additives within the IV solution.	____	____	____	_____
4. Perform hand hygiene. Assess IV or saline (heparin) lock insertion site for signs of infiltration or phlebitis.	____	____	____	_____
5. Check client's medical history and allergies.	____	____	____	_____
6. Check date of expiration for medication vial or ampule.	____	____	____	_____
7. Assess client's understanding of purpose of medication therapy.	____	____	____	_____
8. Prepare ordered medication from vial or ampule using aseptic technique. Check label of medication carefully with MAR two times.	____	____	____	_____
9. Take medication to client at correct time.	____	____	____	_____
10. Identify client using at least two client identifiers. Compare client's name and one other identifier (e.g., hospital identification number) on MAR, computer printout, or computer screen with information on client's identification bracelet. Ask client to state name if possible for a third identifier.	____	____	____	_____
11. Compare label of medication with MAR at client's bedside.	____	____	____	_____
12. Explain procedure to client. Encourage client to report symptoms of discomfort at IV site.	____	____	____	_____
13. Perform hand hygiene. Apply gloves.				
14. Administer medication by IV push (existing line):	____	____	____	_____
A. Select injection port of IV tubing closest to client. Whenever possible, injection port should accept a needleless syringe. Use IV filter if required by medication reference or agency policy.	____	____	____	_____
B. Clean off injection port with antiseptic swab. Allow to dry.	____	____	____	_____
C. Connect syringe to IV line. Insert needleless tip or small-gauge needle of syringe containing prepared drug through center of injection port.	____	____	____	_____
D. Occlude IV line by pinching tubing just above injection port. Pull back gently on syringe's plunger to aspirate blood return.	____	____	____	_____
E. Release tubing, and inject medication within amount of time recommended by institutional policy, pharmacist, or medication reference manual. Use watch to time administration. Intravenous line is sometimes pinched while pushing medication and released when not pushing medication. Allow IV fluids to infuse when not pushing medication.	____	____	____	_____
F. After injecting medication, release tubing, withdraw syringe, and recheck fluid infusion rate.	____	____	____	_____

Continued

272

	S	U	NP	Comments

15. Administering medications by IV push (IV lock or a needleless system):
   A. Prepare flush solutions according to agency policy.
      (1) Saline flush method (preferred method): Prepare two syringes with 2 to 3 mL of normal saline (0.9%) in syringe. ____ ____ ____ _____
      (2) Heparin flush method (traditional method):
         a. Prepare one syringe with ordered amount of heparin flush solution. ____ ____ ____ _____
         b. Prepare two syringes with 2 to 3 mL of normal saline. ____ ____ ____ _____
   B. Administer medication:
      (1) Clean lock's injection port with antiseptic swab. ____ ____ ____ _____
      (2) Insert syringe containing normal saline into injection port of IV lock. ____ ____ ____ _____
      (3) Pull back gently on syringe plunger, and look for blood return. ____ ____ ____ _____
      (4) Flush IV lock with normal saline by pushing slowly on plunger. ____ ____ ____ _____
      (5) Remove saline-filled syringe. ____ ____ ____ _____
      (6) Clean lock's injection port with antiseptic swab. ____ ____ ____ _____
      (7) Insert syringe containing prepared medication into injection port of IV lock. ____ ____ ____ _____
      (8) Inject medication within amount of time recommended by institutional policy, pharmacist, or medication reference manual. Use a watch to time administration. ____ ____ ____ _____
      (9) After administering bolus, withdraw syringe. ____ ____ ____ _____
      (10) Clean lock's injection port with antiseptic swab. ____ ____ ____ _____
      (11) Attach syringe with normal saline, and inject normal saline flush at the same rate the medication was delivered. ____ ____ ____ _____
      (12) Heparin flush option: Insert needle of syringe containing heparin through diaphragm. Inject heparin slowly, and remove syringe. ____ ____ ____ _____
16. Dispose of uncapped needles and syringes in puncture-proof and leakproof container. ____ ____ ____ _____
17. Remove and dispose of gloves. Perform hand hygiene. ____ ____ ____ _____
18. Observe client closely for adverse reaction as drug is administered and for several minutes thereafter. ____ ____ ____ _____
19. Observe IV site during injection for sudden swelling. ____ ____ ____ _____
20. Assess client's status after giving medication to evaluate the effectiveness of the medication. ____ ____ ____ _____
21. Ask client to explain medication's purposes and side effects. ____ ____ ____ _____
22. Record medication, dose, time, route, and time of administration. ____ ____ ____ _____
23. Report any adverse reactions immediately to health care provider because they could be life threatening. Client's response indicates need for additional medical therapy. ____ ____ ____ _____
24. Record client's response to medication in nurses' notes. ____ ____ ____ _____

STUDENT: _____ DATE: _____

INSTRUCTOR: _____ DATE: _____

Skill 35-8 Administering Intravenous Medications by Piggyback, Intermittent Intravenous Infusion Sets, and Miniinfusion Pumps

	S	U	NP	Comments
1. Check accuracy and completeness of each medication administration record (MAR) or computer printout with prescriber's original medication order. Check client's name and medication name, dosage, route, and time for administration. Recopy or re-print any portion of MAR that is difficult to read.	___	___	___	_____
2. Determine client's medical history.	___	___	___	_____
3. Collect information necessary to administer medication safely, including action, purpose, side effects, normal dose, time of peak onset, and nursing implications.	___	___	___	_____
4. Assess compatibility of drug with existing intravenous (IV) solution.	___	___	___	_____
5. Assess patency of client's existing IV infusion line by noting infusion rate of main IV line.	___	___	___	_____
6. Perform hand hygiene. Assess IV insertion site for signs of infiltration or phlebitis: redness, pallor, swelling, tenderness on palpation.	___	___	___	_____
7. Assess client's history of medication allergies.	___	___	___	_____
8. Assess client's understanding of purpose of medication therapy.	___	___	___	_____
9. Prepare medication: Be sure to compare the label of the medication with the MAR two times while preparing the medication.	___	___	___	_____
10. Assemble medication and supplies at bedside. Prepare client by informing client that medication will be given through IV equipment.	___	___	___	_____
11. Perform hand hygiene.	___	___	___	_____
12. Identify client using at least two client identifiers. Compare client's name and one other identifier (e.g., hospital identification number) on MAR, computer printout, or computer screen with information on client's identification bracelet. Ask client to state name if possible for a third identifier.	___	___	___	_____
13. Explain purpose of medication and side effects to client, and explain that medication is to be given through existing IV line. Encourage client to report symptoms of discomfort at site.	___	___	___	_____
14. Administer infusion:				
A. Piggyback or tandem infusion				
(1) Connect infusion tubing to medication bag. Allow solution to fill tubing by opening regulator flow clamp. Once tubing is full, close clamp and cap end of tubing.	___	___	___	_____
(2) Hang piggyback medication bag above level of primary fluid bag (use hook to lower main bag). Hang tandem infusion at same level as primary fluid bag.	___	___	___	_____
(3) Connect tubing of piggyback or tandem infusion to appropriate connector on primary infusion line.				
a. Stopcock: Wipe off stopcock port with alcohol swab, and connect tubing. Turn stopcock to open position.	___	___	___	_____
b. Needleless system: Wipe off needleless port, and insert tip of piggyback or tandem infusion tubing.	___	___	___	_____

Continued

274

	S	U	NP	Comments

c. Tubing port: Connect sterile needle to end of piggyback or tandem infusion tubing, remove cap, cleanse injection port on main IV line, and insert needle through center of port. Secure by taping connection.

(4) Regulate flow rate of medication solution by adjusting regulator clamp. (Infusion times vary. Refer to medication reference or institutional policy for safe flow rate.)

(5) After medication has infused, check flow regulator on primary infusion. The primary infusion automatically begins to flow after the piggyback or tandem solution is empty.

(6) Regulate main infusion line to desired rate, if necessary.

(7) Leave IV piggyback bag and tubing in place for future medication administration, or discard in appropriate containers.

B. Volume-control administration set (e.g., Volutrol)

(1) Fill Volutrol with desired amount of fluid (50 to 100 mL) by opening clamp between Volutrol and main IV bag.

(2) Close clamp, and check to be sure clamp on air vent of Volutrol chamber is open.

(3) Clean injection port on top of Volutrol with antiseptic swab.

(4) Remove needle cap or sheath, and insert syringe needle through port, then inject medication. Gently rotate Volutrol between hands.

(5) Regulate IV infusion rate to allow medication to infuse in time recommended by institutional policy, a pharmacist, or a medication reference manual.

(6) Label Volutrol with name of medication, dosage, total volume including diluent, and time of administration.

(7) Dispose of uncapped needle or needle enclosed in safety shield and syringe in proper container.

(8) Discard supplies in appropriate container, and perform hand hygiene.

C. Miniinfusion administration

(1) Connect prefilled syringe to miniinfusion tubing.

(2) Carefully apply pressure to syringe plunger, allowing tubing to fill with medication.

(3) Place syringe into miniinfusor pump (follow product directions). Be sure syringe is secure.

(4) Connect miniinfusion tubing to main IV line.

a. Stopcock: Wipe off stopcock port with alcohol swab, and connect tubing. Turn stopcock to open position.

b. Needleless system: Wipe off needleless port, and insert tip of miniinfusor tubing.

c. Tubing port: Connect sterile needle to miniinfusion tubing, remove cap, cleanse injection port on main IV line, and insert needle through center of port. Consider placing tape where IV tubing enters port to secure connection.

(5) Hang infusion pump with syringe on IV pole alongside main IV bag. Set pump to deliver medication within time recommended by institutional policy, pharmacist, or medication reference manual. Press button on pump to begin infusion.

(6) After medication has infused, check flow regulator on primary infusion. The infusion should automatically begin to flow once the pump stops. Regulate main infusion line to desired rate as needed. (NOTE: If stopcock is used, turn off miniinfusion line.)

Continued

	S	U	NP	Comments
(7) Observe client for signs of adverse reactions.	___	___	___	_____
(8) During infusion, periodically check infusion rate and condition of IV site.	___	___	___	_____
15. Ask client to explain purpose and side effects of medication.	___	___	___	_____
16. Record medication, dose, route, and time administered on MAR or computer printout.	___	___	___	_____
17. Record volume of fluid in medication bag or Volutrol on intake and output form.	___	___	___	_____
18. Report any adverse reactions to client's health care provider.	___	___	___	_____

STUDENT: _____   DATE: _____

INSTRUCTOR: _____   DATE: _____

Skill 38-1 Applying Restraints

	S	U	NP	Comments
1. Assess client's need for restraint (e.g., continually try to interrupt needed therapy or repeatedly trying to ambulate independently; creating a serious risk for injury to self or others).	____	____	____	_____
2. Assess client's behavior (e.g., confusion, disorientation, agitation, restlessness, combativeness, or inability to follow directions).	____	____	____	_____
3. Review agency policies regarding restraints (e.g., need for a signed consent). Check health care provider's order for purpose, type, location, and duration of restraint.	____	____	____	_____
4. Determine the most appropriate type and size of restraint.	____	____	____	_____
5. Review restraint manufacturer's instructions before entering client's room.	____	____	____	_____
6. Perform hand hygiene, and gather equipment.	____	____	____	_____
7. Introduce yourself. Explain to client and family the need for restraint, that it is temporary, and that is for the client's safety. Attempt to obtain consent if not already secured.	____	____	____	_____
8. Assess the skin underlying area of the client's body where the restraint is to be placed.	____	____	____	_____
9. Approach client in a calm manner, and explain procedure (what you plan to do).	____	____	____	_____
10. Adjust bed to proper height, and lower side rail on side of client contact.	____	____	____	_____
11. Provide privacy. Make sure client is comfortable and in proper body alignment. Drape client as needed.	____	____	____	_____
12. Pad bony prominences (if necessary) before applying restraints.	____	____	____	_____
13. Apply appropriate-size restraint, making sure it is not over an intravenous (IV) line or other device (e.g., dialysis shunt).				
A. Belt restraint: Apply over clothes or gown. Remove wrinkles from front and back of restraint while placing it around client's waist. Bring ties through slots in belt. Avoid placing belt across the chest or too tightly across the abdomen.	____	____	____	_____
B. Extremity (ankle or wrist) restraint: Restraint designed to immobilize one or all extremities. Wrap limb restraint around wrist or ankle with soft part toward skin and secured snugly in place by Velcro straps.	____	____	____	_____
C. Mitten restraint: Place hand in mitten, being sure to bring end all the way up over the wrist.	____	____	____	_____
D. Elbow restraint: Piece of fabric with slots in which tongue blades are placed so that elbow remains rigid.	____	____	____	_____
E. Mummy restraint: Open blanket or sheet on bed or crib with one corner folded toward center. Place child on blanket with shoulders at fold and feet toward opposite corner. With child's right arm straight down against body, pull right side of blanket firmly across right shoulder and chest and secure beneath left side of body. Place left arm straight against body, and bring left side of blanket across shoulder and chest and lock it beneath child's body on right side. Fold lower corner and bring it over body, and tuck or fasten it securely with safety pins.	____	____	____	_____

Continued

	S	U	NP	Comments

14. Attach restraints to movable part of the bed frame, which moves when the head of bed is raised or lowered. ___ ___ ___ _____

15. When client is in a chair, secure jacket restraint by placing ties under armrests and securing them at the back of the chair. ___ ___ ___ _____

16. Secure restraints with a quick-release tie. Do not tie in a knot. ___ ___ ___ _____

17. Make sure two fingers will fit under secured restraint. ___ ___ ___ _____

18. Assess proper placement of restraint, skin integrity, pulses, temperature, color, and sensation of the restrained body part at least every 2 hours or according to agency policy. ___ ___ ___ _____

19. Restraints should be removed at least every 2 hours. If client is violent and noncompliant, remove one restraint at a time and/or have staff assistance while removing restraints. Do not leave clients unattended at this time. ___ ___ ___ _____

20. Secure call bell or intercom within client's reach. ___ ___ ___ _____

21. Leave client's bed or chair with wheels locked. Bed should be in lowest position. ___ ___ ___ _____

22. Perform hand hygiene before leaving room. ___ ___ ___ _____

23. While restraints are in use:
   A. Inspect client for any injury. ___ ___ ___ _____
   B. Observe IV catheters and urinary catheters to determine that they are positioned correctly and that therapy remains uninterrupted. ___ ___ ___ _____
   C. Frequently reassess client's need for continued use of restraint with the intent of discontinuing restraint at the earliest possible time. ___ ___ ___ _____
   D. Provide sensory stimulation and reorient client as needed. ___ ___ ___ _____

24. Record/Document:
   A. Client behaviors that may place client at risk for injury. ___ ___ ___ _____
   B. Client's response and expected or unexpected outcomes after restraint is applied. ___ ___ ___ _____
   C. Restraint alternatives attempted and client's response. ___ ___ ___ _____
   D. Client's and/or family's understanding of and consent to restraint application. ___ ___ ___ _____
   E. Type and location of restraint and time applied ___ ___ ___ _____
   F. Time of assessments and releases. ___ ___ ___ _____
   G. Document client's behavior after application of restraint. ___ ___ ___ _____
   H. Document specific assessments related to orientation, oxygenation, skin integrity, circulation, and positioning. ___ ___ ___ _____
   I. Describe client's response when restraints were removed. ___ ___ ___ _____

STUDENT: _____ DATE: _____

INSTRUCTOR: _____ DATE: _____

Skill 38-2 Seizure Precautions

	S	U	NP	Comments
1. Assess seizure history, noting frequency of seizures, presence of aura, and sequence of events, if known. Assess for medical and surgical conditions that will lead to seizures or exacerbate existing seizure condition. Assess medication history.	____	____	____	_____
2. Inspect client's environment for potential safety hazards if risk for seizure exists: bedside stand or table, intravenous (IV) pole or other medical equipment.	____	____	____	_____
3. Perform hand hygiene, and prepare bed with padded side rails and headboard, bed in low position, and client positioned in side-lying position when possible.	____	____	____	_____
4. For clients with a history of seizures have airway, suction equipment, clean gloves, and pillows available in room.	____	____	____	_____
5. When a seizure begins, position client safely. If client is standing or sitting, guide client to floor and protect head by cradling in nurse's lap or placing a pillow under head. Clear surrounding area of furniture. If client is in bed, raise side rails, add padding, and put bed in low position.	____	____	____	_____
6. Provide privacy.	____	____	____	_____
7. Turn client on side, if possible, with head flexed slightly forward.	____	____	____	_____
8. Do not restrain client. Loosen client's clothing.	____	____	____	_____
9. Do not place anything in client's mouth (e.g., fingers, tongue depressor, medicine).	____	____	____	_____
10. Stay with client. Observe sequence and timing of seizure activity. Note aura, level of consciousness, mobility, incontinence, sleep patterns, or confusion afterward.	____	____	____	_____
11. After the seizure is over, explain what happened and answer client's questions. Foster an atmosphere of acceptance and respect.	____	____	____	_____
12. Following seizure, perform hand hygiene and assist client to position of comfort in bed with padded side rails up and bed in low position. Place call light within reach, and provide a quiet, nonstimulating environment.	____	____	____	_____
13. For status epilepticus:				
A. Apply clean gloves.	____	____	____	_____
B. Insert airway when client's jaw is relaxed between seizure activity. Hold airway with curved side up, insert downward until airway reaches back of throat, then rotate and follow natural curve of the tongue.	____	____	____	_____
C. Obtain oxygen and suction equipment.	____	____	____	_____
D. Prepare for IV insertion.				
E. Pad side rails and headboard. Use pillows/pads to protect client from injuring self.	____	____	____	_____
F. Do not place fingers near or in client's mouth.	____	____	____	_____
14. Record and report:				
A. The timing of seizure activity, sequence of events, and interventions. Record presence of aura (if any), level of consciousness, posture, color, movements of extremities, incontinence, and patterns of sleep following the seizure.	____	____	____	_____
B. Document client's response and expected or unexpected outcomes.	____	____	____	_____
C. Report to health care provider immediately as seizure begins. Status epilepticus is an emergency situation requiring immediate medical management.	____	____	____	_____

CHECKLIST
Skill 39-1 Bathing a Client

	S	U	NP	Comments

1. Assess client's tolerance for bathing, activity tolerance, comfort level, cognitive ability, musculoskeletal function, and presence of shortness of breath.
2. Assess client's visual status, ability to sit without support, hand grasp, range of motion (ROM) of extremities.
3. Assess client's bathing preferences: frequency and time of day preferred for bathing, type of hygiene products, and other facts related to client preferences.
4. Ask if client has noticed any problems or unusual marks on skin: excessive moisture, inflammation, drainage or excretions from lesions or body cavities, rashes or other skin lesions.
5. Assess condition of client's skin. Note the presence of dryness, indicated by flaking, redness, scaling, and cracking.
6. Review orders for specific precautions concerning client's movement or positioning.
7. Explain procedure, and ask client for suggestions on how to prepare supplies. If partial bath, ask how much of bath client wishes to complete.
8. Adjust room temperature and ventilation, close room doors and windows, and draw room divider curtain.
9. Prepare equipment and supplies.
10. Offer client bedpan or urinal. Provide towel and washcloth.
11. Perform hand hygiene. If client's skin is soiled with drainage or body secretions, apply clean gloves. Ensure client is not allergic to latex.
12. Bathe client.
    A. Complete or partial bed bath
       (1) Validate that the bed is in locked position, and raise bed to your comfort level. If raised, lower side rail closest to you, and assist client in assuming comfortable position, maintaining body alignment. Bring client toward side closest to nurse.
       (2) Loosen top covers at foot of bed. Place bath blanket over top sheet. Fold and remove top sheet from under blanket. If possible, have client hold bath blanket while withdrawing sheet. Optional: Use top sheet when bath blanket is not available.
       (3) If top sheet is to be reused, fold it for replacement later. If not, dispose in laundry bag, taking care not to allow linen to contact uniform.
       (4) Remove client's gown or pajamas.
          a. If an extremity is injured or has reduced mobility, begin removal from unaffected side.
          b. If client has intravenous (IV) tube, remove gown from arm *without* IV first; then lower IV container or remove from pump and slide gown covering affected arm over tubing and container. Rehang IV container, and check flow rate.

Continued

280

	S	U	NP	Comments

c. If IV pump is in use, turn pump off, clamp tubing, remove tubing from pump, proceed as in Step b. Insert tubing into pump, unclamp tubing, and turn pump on at correct rate. Observe flow rate, and regulate if necessary.

d. Do not disconnect tubing.

(5) Pull side rail up. Fill washbasin two thirds full with warm water. Have client place fingers in water to test temperature tolerance. Place plastic container of bath lotion in bath water to warm, if desired.

(6) Remove pillow if allowed, and raise head of bed 30 to 45 degrees. Place bath towel under client's head. Place second bath towel over client's chest.

(7) Immerse washcloth in water, and wring thoroughly. If desired, fold washcloth around fingers of nurse's hand to form mitt.

(8) Inquire if client is wearing contact lenses. Wash client's eyes with plain warm water, and perform eye care as needed. Wash client's eyes using a. different section of mitt for each eye. Move mitt from inner to outer canthus. Soak any crusts on eyelid for 2 to 3 minutes with damp cloth before attempting removal. Dry eye thoroughly but gently.

(9) Ask if client prefers to use soap on face. Wash, rinse, and dry well forehead, cheeks, nose, neck, and ears. (Men often wish to shave at this point or after bath.)

(10) Remove bath blanket from client's arm that is closest to nurse. Place bath towel lengthwise under arm.

(11) Bathe arm with soap and water using long, firm strokes from distal to proximal areas (fingers to axilla). Raise and support arm as needed while thoroughly washing axilla.

(12) Rinse and dry arm and axilla thoroughly. If client uses deodorant or talcum powder, apply it.

(13) Fold bath towel in half, and lay it on bed beside client. Place basin on towel. Immerse client's hand in water. Allow hand to soak for 3 to 5 minutes before washing hand and fingernails. Remove basin, and dry hand well.

(14) Raise side rail, and move to other side of bed. Lower side rail, and repeat Steps 10 through 13 for other arm.

(15) Check temperature of bath water, and change water if necessary.

(16) Cover client's chest with bath towel, and fold bath blanket down to umbilicus. With one hand, lift edge of towel away from chest. With washcloth or mitted hand, bathe chest using long, firm strokes. Take special care to wash skin folds under female client's breasts. It is often necessary to lift breast upward while bathing underneath it. Keep client's chest covered between wash and rinse periods. Dry well.

(17) Place bath towel lengthwise over chest and abdomen. (Two towels may be needed.) Fold blanket down to just above pubic region.

(18) With one hand, lift bath towel. With mitted hand, bathe abdomen, giving special attention to bathing umbilicus and abdominal folds. Stroke from side to side. Keep abdomen covered between washing and rinsing. Dry well.

Continued

	S	U	NP	Comments

(19) Apply clean gown or pajama top. If one extremity is injured or immobilized, always dress affected side first. You may omit this step until completion of bath; make sure gown does not become damp or soiled during remainder of bath.

(20) Cover chest and abdomen with top of bath blanket. Expose near leg by folding blanket toward midline. Be sure other leg and perineum are draped.

(21) Bend client's leg at knee by positioning nurse's arm under leg. While grasping client's heel, elevate leg from mattress slightly, and slide bath towel lengthwise under leg. Ask client to hold foot still. Place bath basin on towel on bed, and secure its position next to foot to be washed.

(22) With one hand supporting lower leg, raise it and slide basin under lifted foot. Make sure foot is firmly placed on bottom of basin. Allow foot to soak while washing leg. If client is unable to hold leg, do not immerse; simply wash with washcloth.

(23) Unless contraindicated, use long, firm strokes in washing from ankle to knee and from knee to thigh. Dry well.

(24) Cleanse foot, making sure to bathe between toes. Clean and clip nails as per health care provider's orders. Dry well. If skin is dry, apply lotion.

(25) Raise side rail, and move to other side of the bed. Lower side rail, and repeat Steps 20 through 24 for other leg and foot.

(26) Cover client with bath blanket, raise side rail for client's safety, and change bath water.

(27) Lower side rail. Assist client in assuming prone or side-lying position (as applicable). Place towel lengthwise along client's side.

(28) Keep client draped by sliding bath blanket over shoulders and thighs. Wash, rinse, and dry back from neck to buttocks using long, firm strokes. Pay special attention to folds of buttocks and anus. Give a back rub. Change bath water.

(29) Apply clean gloves if not done previously.

(30) Assist client in assuming side-lying or supine position. Cover chest and upper extremities with towel and lower extremities with bath blanket. Expose only genitalia. (If client is able to wash, covering entire body with bath blanket is preferable.) Provide perineal care. Pay special attention to skin folds. Apply water-repellent ointment to area exposed to moisture.

(31) Dispose of gloves in receptacle.

(32) Apply moisturizing lotion as desired.

(33) Assist client in dressing. Comb client's hair. Some women will want to apply makeup.

(34) Make client's bed.

(35) Remove soiled linen, and place in dirty-linen bag. Clean and replace bathing equipment. Replace call light and personal possessions. Leave room as clean and comfortable as possible.

(36) Perform hand hygiene.

B. Commercial cleansing pack

(1) The cleansing pack contains 8 to 10 premoistened towels for cleansing. Warm the package contents in a microwave following package instructions.

(2) Use a single towel for each general body part cleansed. Follow the same order of cleansing as the total or partial bed bath.

Continued

282

	S	U	NP	Comments

(3) Allow the skin to air dry for 30 seconds. It is permissible to lightly cover the client with a bath towel to prevent chilling.

(4) NOTE: If there is excessive soiling (e.g., in the perineal region), use an extra Bag Bath or conventional washcloths, soap, water, and towels.

C. Tub or whirlpool bath or shower; verify with agency policy if a health care provider's order is necessary.

  (1) Consider client's condition, and review orders for precautions concerning client's movement or positioning.

  (2) Check tub or shower for cleanliness. Use cleaning techniques outlined in agency policy. Place rubber mat on tub or shower bottom. Place disposable bath mat or towel on floor in front of tub or shower.

  (3) Collect all hygienic aids, toiletry items, and linens requested by client. Place within easy reach of tub or shower.

  (4) Assist client to bathroom if necessary. Have client wear robe and nonslip footwear to bathroom.

  (5) Demonstrate how to use call signal for assistance.

  (6) Place "occupied" sign on bathroom door.

  (7) Provide shower seat or tub chair if needed. Fill bathtub halfway with warm water. If sensation is normal, ask client to test water, and adjust temperature if water is too warm. Explain which faucet controls hot water. If client is taking shower, turn shower on, and adjust water temperature before client enters shower stall.

  (8) Instruct client to use safety bars when getting in and out of tub or shower. Caution client against use of bath oil in tub water.

  (9) Instruct client not to remain in tub longer than 20 minutes. Check on client every 5 minutes.

  (10) Return to bathroom when client signals, and knock before entering.

  (11) For client who is unsteady, drain tub of water before client attempts to get out of it. Place bath towel over client's shoulders. Assist client in getting out of tub as needed, and assist with drying. If client is weak or unstable, have another person assist.

  (12) Assist client as needed in dressing in clean gown or pajamas, slippers, and robe. (In home setting, client will dress in regular clothing.)

  (13) Assist client to room and comfortable position in bed or chair.

  (14) Clean tub or shower according to agency policy. Whirlpool baths often require special cleansing. Remove soiled linen, and place in dirty-linen bag. Discard disposable equipment in proper receptacle. Place "unoccupied" sign on bathroom door. Return supplies to storage area.

  (15) Perform hand hygiene.

13. Observe skin, paying particular attention to areas that were previously soiled, reddened, or showed early signs of breakdown.

Continued

	S	U	NP	Comments

14. Observe or perform ROM during bath. _____ _____ _____ _____
15. Ask client to rate level of comfort. _____ _____ _____ _____
16. Recording and reporting:
   A. Record procedure on flow sheet if appropriate and amount of assistance, client participation. _____ _____ _____ _____
   B. Record condition of skin and any significant findings (e.g., reddened areas, bruises, nevi, joint or muscle pain). _____ _____ _____ _____
   C. Report evidence of alterations in skin integrity, break in suture line, or increased wound secretions to nurse in charge or health care provider. _____ _____ _____ _____

CHECKLIST
Skill 39-2 Perineal Care

	S	U	NP	Comments
1. Identify clients at risk for developing infection of genitalia, urinary tract, or reproductive tract (e.g., uncircumcised male, presence of indwelling catheter, fecal incontinence).	___	___	___	_____
2. Assess client's cognitive, visual, and musculoskeletal function and activity tolerance.	___	___	___	_____
3. Apply clean gloves, and assess genitalia for signs of inflammation, skin breakdown, or infection. Discard gloves. Perform hand hygiene.	___	___	___	_____
4. Assess client's knowledge of importance of perineal hygiene.	___	___	___	_____
5. Explain procedure and its purpose to client.	___	___	___	_____
6. Prepare necessary equipment and supplies.	___	___	___	_____
7. Pull curtain around client's bed, or close room door. Assemble supplies at bedside.	___	___	___	_____
8. Raise bed to comfortable working position. If raised, lower side rail, and assist client in assuming side-lying position, placing towel lengthwise along client's side and keeping client covered with bath blanket or top sheet.				
9. Apply clean gloves.	___	___	___	_____
10. If fecal material is present, enclose in a fold of underpad or toilet tissue, and remove with disposable wipes or tissue. Cleanse buttocks and anus, washing front to back. Cleanse, rinse, and dry area thoroughly. If needed, place an absorbent pad under client's buttocks. Remove and discard underpad, and replace with clean one.	___	___	___	_____
11. Change gloves when they are soiled. Perform hand hygiene.	___	___	___	_____
12. Fold top bed linen down toward foot of bed, and raise client's gown above genital area. Prepare bed linen to protect client's privacy.	___	___	___	_____
13. "Diamond" drape client by placing bath blanket with one corner between client's legs, one corner pointing toward each side of bed, and one corner over client's chest. Tuck side corners around client's legs and under hips.	___	___	___	_____
14. Raise side rail. Fill washbasin with warm water.	___	___	___	_____
15. Place washbasin and toilet tissue on over-bed table. Place washcloths in basin.	___	___	___	_____
16. Provide perineal care.				
A. Female perineal care.				
(1) Assist client to dorsal recumbent position.	___	___	___	_____
(2) Lower side rail, and help client flex knees and spread legs. Note restrictions or limitations in client's positioning.	___	___	___	_____
(3) Fold lower corner of bath blanket up between client's legs onto abdomen. Wash and dry client's upper thighs.	___	___	___	_____
(4) Wash labia majora. Use nondominant hand to gently retract labia from thigh; with dominant hand, wash carefully in skin folds. Wipe in direction from perineum to rectum (front to back). Repeat on opposite side using separate section of washcloth. Rinse and dry area thoroughly.	___	___	___	_____
(5) Separate labia with nondominant hand to expose urethral meatus and vaginal orifice. With dominant hand, wash downward from pubic area toward rectum in one smooth stroke. Use separate section of cloth for each stroke. Cleanse thoroughly around labia minora, clitoris, and vaginal orifice.	___	___	___	_____

Continued

	S	U	NP	Comments

(6) If client uses bedpan, pour warm water over perineal area. Dry perineal area thoroughly, using front-to-back method. ____ ____ ____ _____

(7) Fold lower corner of bath blanket back between client's legs and over perineum. Assist client to lower legs and assume comfortable position. ____ ____ ____ _____

B. Male perineal care

(1) Lower side rails, and assist client to supine position. Note restriction in mobility. ____ ____ ____ _____

(2) Fold lower corner of bath blanket up between client's legs and onto abdomen. Wash and dry client's upper thighs. ____ ____ ____ _____

(3) Gently raise penis, and place bath towel underneath. Gently grasp shaft of penis. If client is uncircumcised, retract foreskin. If client has an erection, defer procedure until later. ____ ____ ____ _____

(4) Wash tip of penis at urethral meatus first. Using circular motion, cleanse from meatus outward. Discard washcloth, and repeat with clean cloth until penis is clean. Rinse and dry gently. ____ ____ ____ _____

(5) Return foreskin to its natural position. ____ ____ ____ _____

(6) Wash shaft of penis with gentle but firm downward strokes. Pay special attention to underlying surface of penis. Rinse and dry penis thoroughly. Instruct client to spread legs apart slightly. ____ ____ ____ _____

(7) Gently cleanse scrotum. Lift it carefully, and wash underlying skin folds. Rinse and dry. ____ ____ ____ _____

(8) Fold bath blanket back over client's perineum, and assist client in turning to side-lying position. ____ ____ ____ _____

(9) If client has had urinary or bowel incontinence, apply thin layer of skin barrier containing petrolatum or zinc oxide over anal and perineal skin. ____ ____ ____ _____

(10) Remove gloves, dispose in proper receptacle, and perform hand hygiene. ____ ____ ____ _____

(11) Assist client in assuming a comfortable position, and cover with sheet. ____ ____ ____ _____

(12) Remove bath blanket, and dispose of all soiled bed linen. Return unused equipment to storage area. ____ ____ ____ _____

(13) Inspect surface of external genitalia and surrounding skin after cleansing. ____ ____ ____ _____

(14) Ask if client feels sense of cleanliness.

(15) Observe for abnormal drainage or discharge from genitalia. ____ ____ ____ _____

17. Record procedure and presence of any abnormal findings (e.g., character and amount of discharge, condition of genitalia). ____ ____ ____ _____

CHECKLIST
Skill 39-3 Performing Nail and Foot Care

	S	U	NP	Comments
1. Inspect all surfaces of fingers, toes, feet, and nails. Pay particular attention to areas of dryness, inflammation, or cracking. Also inspect areas between toes, heels, and soles of feet.	___	___	___	_____
2. Assess color and temperature of toes, feet, and fingers. Assess capillary refill of nails. Palpate radial and ulnar pulse of each hand and dorsalis pedis pulse of foot; note character of pulses.	___	___	___	_____
3. Observe client's walking gait. Have client walk down hall or walk straight line (if able).				
4. Ask female clients about whether they use nail polish and polish remover frequently.	___	___	___	_____
5. Assess type of footwear worn by client: Does client wear socks? Are shoes tight or ill fitting? Does client wear garters or knee-high nylons? Is footwear clean?	___	___	___	_____
6. Identify client's risk for foot or nail problems.	___	___	___	_____
7. Assess type of home remedies client uses for existing foot problems.	___	___	___	_____
8. Assess client's ability to care for nails or feet: visual alterations, fatigue, and musculoskeletal weakness.	___	___	___	_____
9. Assess client's knowledge of foot and nail care practices.	___	___	___	_____
10. Explain procedure to client, including fact that proper soaking requires several minutes.	___	___	___	_____
11. Obtain health care provider's order for cutting nails if agency policy requires it.	___	___	___	_____
12. Perform hand hygiene.	___	___	___	_____
13. Arrange equipment on over-bed table.	___	___	___	_____
14. Pull curtain around bed, and close room door.	___	___	___	_____
15. Assist ambulatory client with sitting in bedside chair. Help bed-bound client to supine position with head of bed elevated.				
16. Place disposable bath mat on floor under client's feet, or place towel on mattress.	___	___	___	_____
17. Fill washbasin with warm water. Test water temperature.	___	___	___	_____
18. Place basin on bath mat or towel, and help client place feet in basin. Place call light within client's reach.	___	___	___	_____
19. Adjust over-bed table to low position, and place it over client's lap. (Client sits in chair or lies in bed.)	___	___	___	_____
20. Fill emesis basin with warm water, and place basin on paper towels on over-bed table.	___	___	___	_____
21. Instruct client to place fingers in emesis basin and place arms in comfortable position.	___	___	___	_____
22. Allow client's feet and fingernails to soak for 10 to 20 minutes. (Rewarm after 10 minutes.)	___	___	___	_____
23. Clean gently under fingernails with orange stick or wooden end of cotton-tipped swab while fingers are immersed. Remove emesis basin, and dry fingers thoroughly.	___	___	___	_____
24. Using nail clippers, clip fingernails straight across and even with tops of fingers; check agency policy. Shape nails with emery board or file. (If client has circulatory problems, do not cut nail; file the nail only.)	___	___	___	_____
25. Use a soft cuticle brush or nail brush around cuticles.	___	___	___	_____
26. Move over-bed table away from client.	___	___	___	_____

Continued

	S	U	NP	Comments
27. Put on clean gloves, and scrub callused areas of feet with washcloth.	____	____	____	_____
28. Clean gently under nails with orange stick. Remove feet from basin, and dry thoroughly.	____	____	____	_____
29. Clean and trim toenails using procedures in Steps 24 and 25. Do not file corners of toenails. Check agency policy for trimming client's nails.	____	____	____	_____
30. Apply lotion to feet and hands, and assist client back to bed and into comfortable position.	____	____	____	_____
31. Remove clean gloves, and place in receptacle. Clean and return equipment and supplies to proper place. Dispose of soiled linen in hamper.	____	____	____	_____
32. Perform hand hygiene.	____	____	____	_____
33. Inspect nails and surrounding skin surfaces after soaking and nail trimming.	____	____	____	_____
34. Ask client to explain or demonstrate nail care.	____	____	____	_____
35. Observe client's walk after toenail care.	____	____	____	_____
36. Record procedure and observations (e.g., breaks in skin, inflammation, ulcerations).	____	____	____	_____
37. Report any breaks in skin or ulcerations to nurse in charge or health care provider.	____	____	____	_____

STUDENT: _____ DATE: _____

INSTRUCTOR: _____ DATE: _____

Skill 39-4 Providing Oral Hygiene

	S	U	NP	Comments
1. Perform hand hygiene, and apply clean gloves.	___	___	___	_____
2. Instruct client not to bite down. Inspect integrity of lips, teeth, buccal mucosa, gums, palate, and tongue.	___	___	___	_____
3. Identify presence of common oral problems (dental caries, gingivitis, periodontitis, halitosis, cheilosis, stomatitis).	___	___	___	_____
4. Remove gloves, and perform hand hygiene.	___	___	___	_____
5. Assess client's risk for aspiration: impaired swallowing, reduced gag reflex.	___	___	___	_____
6. Determine client's oral hygiene practices.	___	___	___	_____
7. Assess client's ability to grasp and manipulate toothbrush.	___	___	___	_____
8. Prepare equipment at bedside.	___	___	___	_____
9. Explain procedure to client, and discuss preferences regarding use of hygiene aids.	___	___	___	_____
10. Place paper towels on over-bed table, and arrange other equipment within easy reach.	___	___	___	_____
11. Raise bed to comfortable working position. Raise head of bed (if allowed), and lower side rail. Move client, or help client move closer. Use side-lying position if needed.	___	___	___	_____
12. Place towel over client's chest.	___	___	___	_____
13. Apply gloves.	___	___	___	_____
14. Apply toothpaste to brush, holding brush over emesis basin. Pour small amount of water over toothpaste.	___	___	___	_____
15. Client may assist by brushing. Have client:				
A. Hold toothbrush bristles at 45-degree angle to gum line. Be sure tips of bristles rest against and penetrate under gum line.	___	___	___	_____
B. Brush inner and outer surfaces of upper and lower teeth by brushing from gum to crown of each tooth.	___	___	___	_____
C. Clean biting surfaces of teeth by holding top of bristles parallel with teeth and brushing gently back and forth.	___	___	___	_____
D. Brush sides of teeth by moving bristles back and forth	___	___	___	_____
16. Have client hold brush at 45-degree angle and lightly brush over surface and sides of tongue. Avoid initiating gag reflex.	___	___	___	_____
17. Allow client to rinse mouth thoroughly by taking several sips of water, swishing water across all tooth surfaces, and spitting into emesis basin.	___	___	___	_____
18. Allow client to gargle to rinse mouth with mouthwash as desired.	___	___	___	_____
19. Assist in wiping client's mouth.	___	___	___	_____
20. Allow client to floss.	___	___	___	_____
21. Allow client to rinse mouth thoroughly with cool water and spit into emesis basin. Assist in wiping client's mouth.	___	___	___	_____
22. Assist client to comfortable position, remove emesis basin and over-bed table, raise side rail, and lower bed to original position.	___	___	___	_____
23. Wipe off over-bed table, discard soiled linen and paper towels in appropriate containers, remove soiled gloves, and return equipment to proper place.	___	___	___	_____
24. Perform hand hygiene.	___	___	___	_____
25. Ask client if any area of oral cavity feels uncomfortable or irritated.	___	___	___	_____

Continued

	S	U	NP	Comments
26. Apply gloves, and inspect condition of oral cavity.	_____	_____	_____	_____
27. Ask client to describe proper hygiene techniques.	_____	_____	_____	_____
28. Observe client brushing.	_____	_____	_____	_____
29. Record procedure on flow sheet. Note condition of oral cavity in nurses' notes.	_____	_____	_____	_____
30. Report bleeding or presence of lesions to nurse in charge or health care provider.	_____	_____	_____	_____

STUDENT: _____ DATE: _____

INSTRUCTOR: _____ DATE: _____

Skill 39-5 Performing Mouth Care for an Unconscious or Debilitated Client

	S	U	NP	Comments
1. Perform hand hygiene. Apply clean gloves.	___	___	___	_____
2. Assess client's risk for oral hygiene problems.	___	___	___	_____
3. Test for presence of gag reflex by placing tongue blade on back half of client's tongue.	___	___	___	_____
4. Inspect condition of oral cavity.	___	___	___	_____
5. Remove gloves. Perform hand hygiene.	___	___	___	_____
6. Explain procedure to client.	___	___	___	_____
7. Apply clean gloves.	___	___	___	_____
8. Place paper towels on over-bed table, and arrange equipment. If needed, turn on suction machine, and connect tubing to suction catheter.	___	___	___	_____
9. Pull curtain around bed, or close room door.	___	___	___	_____
10. Raise bed to the appropriate height for nurse; lower head of bed, and then lower side rail.	___	___	___	_____
11. Position client close to side of bed; turn client's head toward mattress. Client can also be placed on side (Sims' position).	___	___	___	_____
12. Place towel under client's head and emesis basin under chin.	___	___	___	_____
13. If client is unconscious, uncooperative, or having difficulty keeping mouth open, insert an oral airway. Insert upside down, then turn the airway sideways and then over tongue to keep teeth apart. Insert with client is relaxed. Do not use force.	___	___	___	_____
14. Clean mouth using brush moistened with dental cleansing agent, such as commercial diluted hydrogen peroxide and sodium bicarbonate solution or chlorhexidine, if prescribed.				
A. Clean chewing and inner tooth surfaces first.	___	___	___	_____
B. Clean outer tooth surfaces.	___	___	___	_____
C. Use swab or toothette to clean roof of mouth, gums, and inside cheeks.	___	___	___	_____
D. Gently swab or brush tongue but avoid stimulating gag reflex (if present).	___	___	___	_____
E. Moisten clean swab or toothette with water to rinse. (Use bulb syringe to rinse.)	___	___	___	_____
F. Repeat rinse several times.	___	___	___	_____
15. Suction oral secretions as they accumulate, if necessary.	___	___	___	_____
16. Apply thin layer of water-soluble jelly to lips.	___	___	___	_____
17. Inform client that procedure is completed.	___	___	___	_____
18. Reposition client comfortably, raise side rail as appropriate or as ordered, and return bed to original position.	___	___	___	_____
19. Clean equipment and return to its proper place. Place soiled linen in proper receptacle.	___	___	___	_____
20. Remove and discard gloves. Perform hand hygiene.	___	___	___	_____
21. Apply clean gloves, and inspect oral cavity.	___	___	___	_____
22. Ask debilitated client if mouth feels clean.	___	___	___	_____
23. Assess client's respirations on an ongoing basis.	___	___	___	_____
24. Record procedure, including pertinent observations (e.g., presence of bleeding gums, dry mucosa, ulcerations, crusts on tongue).				
25. Report any unusual findings to nurse in charge or health care provider.	___	___	___	_____

CHECKLIST
Skill 39-6 Making an Occupied Bed

	S	U	NP	Comments
1. Assess potential for client incontinence or for excess drainage on bed linen.	___	___	___	_____
2. Check chart for orders or specific precautions concerning movement and positioning.	___	___	___	_____
3. Explain procedure to the client, noting that the client will be asked to turn on side and roll over linen.	___	___	___	_____
4. Perform hand hygiene, and apply gloves (wear gloves only if linen is soiled or there is risk for contact with body secretions).	___	___	___	_____
5. Assemble equipment, and arrange on bedside chair or table. Remove unnecessary equipment such as a dietary tray or items used for hygiene.	___	___	___	_____
6. Draw room curtain around bed, or close door.	___	___	___	_____
7. Adjust bed height to comfortable working position. Lower any raised side rail on one side of bed. Remove call light.	___	___	___	_____
8. Loosen top linen at foot of bed.	___	___	___	_____
9. Remove bedspread and blanket separately. If spread and blanket are soiled, place them in linen bag. Keep soiled linen away from uniform.	___	___	___	_____
10. If blanket and spread are to be reused, fold them by bringing the top and bottom edges together. Fold farthest side over onto nearer bottom edge. Bring top and bottom edges together again. Place folded linen over back of chair.	___	___	___	_____
11. Cover client with bath blanket in the following manner: unfold bath blanket over top sheet. Ask client to hold top edge of bath blanket. If client is unable to help, tuck top of bath blanket under shoulder. Grasp top sheet under bath blanket at client's shoulders, and bring sheet down to foot of bed. Remove sheet, and discard in linen bag.	___	___	___	_____
12. With assistance from another nurse, slide mattress toward head of bed.	___	___	___	_____
13. Position client on the far side of the bed, turned onto side and facing away from you. Be sure side rail in front of client is up. Adjust pillow under client's head.	___	___	___	_____
14. Loosen bottom linens, moving from head to foot. With seam side down (facing the mattress), fanfold bottom sheet and drawsheet toward client—first drawsheet, then bottom sheet. Tuck edges of linen just under buttocks, back, and shoulders. Do not fanfold mattress pad if it is to be reused.	___	___	___	_____
15. Wipe off any moisture on exposed mattress with towel and appropriate disinfectant. Make sure mattress surface is dry before applying linens.	___	___	___	_____
16. Apply clean linen to exposed half of bed:	___	___	___	_____
A. Place clean mattress pad on bed by folding it lengthwise with center crease in middle of bed. Fanfold top layer over mattress. (If pad is reused, simply smooth out any wrinkles.)	___	___	___	_____
B. Unfold bottom sheet lengthwise so that center crease is situated lengthwise along center of bed. Fanfold sheet's top layer toward center of bed alongside the client. Smooth bottom layer of sheet over mattress, and bring edge over closest side of mattress. Pull fitted sheet smoothly over mattress ends. Allow edge of flat unfitted sheet to hang about 25 cm (10 inches) over mattress edge. Make sure lower hem of bottom flat sheet lies seam down and even with bottom edge of mattress.	___	___	___	_____

Continued

292

	S	U	NP	Comments

17. Miter bottom flat sheet at head of bed:
    A. Face head of bed diagonally. Place hand away from head of bed under top corner of mattress, near mattress edge, and lift. _____ _____ _____ _____
    B. With other hand, tuck top edge of bottom sheet smoothly under mattress so that side edges of sheet above and below mattress meet when brought together. _____ _____ _____ _____
    C. Face side of bed, and pick up top edge of sheet at approximately 45 cm (18 inches) from top of mattress. _____ _____ _____ _____
    D. Lift sheet, and lay it on top of mattress to form a neat triangular fold, with lower base of triangle even with mattress side edge. _____ _____ _____ _____
    E. Tuck lower edge of sheet, which is hanging free below the mattress, under mattress. Tuck with palms down, without pulling triangular fold. _____ _____ _____ _____
    F. Hold portion of sheet covering side of mattress in place with one hand. With the other hand, pick up top of triangular linen fold and bring it down over side of mattress. Tuck this portion under mattress. _____ _____ _____ _____
18. Tuck remaining portion of sheet under mattress, moving toward foot of bed. Keep linen smooth. _____ _____ _____ _____
19. Optional: Open drawsheet so that it unfolds in half. Lay centerfold along middle of bed lengthwise, and position sheet so that it will be under the client's buttocks and torso. Fanfold top layer toward client, with edge along client's back. Smooth bottom layer out over mattress, and tuck excess edge under mattress (keep palms down). _____ _____ _____ _____
20. Place waterproof pad over drawsheet, with centerfold against client's side. Fanfold top layer toward client. _____ _____ _____ _____
21. Advise client that he or she will be rolling over thick layer of linens and will feel a lump. Have client roll slowly toward you, over the layers of linen. Raise side rail on working side, and go to other side of bed. _____ _____ _____ _____
22. Lower side rail. Assist client in positioning on other side, over folds of linen. Loosen edges of soiled linen from under mattress. _____ _____ _____ _____
23. Remove soiled linen by folding it into a bundle or square, with soiled side turned in. Discard in linen bag. If necessary, wipe mattress with antiseptic solution, and dry mattress surface before applying new linen. _____ _____ _____ _____
24. Pull clean, fanfolded linen smoothly over edge of mattress from head to foot of bed. _____ _____ _____ _____
25. Assist client in rolling back into supine position. Reposition pillow. _____ _____ _____ _____
26. Pull fitted sheet smoothly over mattress ends. Miter top corner of bottom sheet. When tucking corner, be sure that sheet is smooth and free of wrinkles. _____ _____ _____ _____
27. Facing side of bed, grasp remaining edge of bottom flat sheet. Lean back, keep back straight, and pull while tucking excess linen under mattress. Proceed from head to foot of bed. (Avoid lifting mattress during tucking to ensure fit.) _____ _____ _____ _____
28. Smooth fanfolded drawsheet out over bottom sheet. Grasp edge of sheet with palms down, lean back, and tuck sheet under mattress. Tuck from middle to top and then to bottom. _____ _____ _____ _____
29. Place top sheet over client with centerfold lengthwise down middle of bed. Open sheet from head to foot, and unfold over client. _____ _____ _____ _____
30. Ask client to hold clean top sheet, or tuck sheet around client's shoulders. Remove bath blanket, and discard in linen bag. _____ _____ _____ _____

Continued

	S	U	NP	Comments

31. Place blanket on bed, unfolding it so that crease runs lengthwise along middle of bed. Unfold blanket to cover client. Make sure top edge is parallel with edge of top sheet and 15 to 20 cm (6 to 8 inches) from top sheet's edge.

32. Place spread over bed according to Step 31. Be sure that top edge of spread extends about 2.5 cm (1 inch) above blanket's edge. Tuck top edge of spread over and under top edge of blanket.

33. Make cuff by turning edge of top sheet down over top edge of blanket and spread.

34. Standing on one side at foot of bed, lift mattress corner slightly with one hand and tuck linens under mattress. Top sheet and blanket are tucked under together. Be sure that linens are loose enough to allow movement of client's feet. Making a horizontal toe pleat is an option.

35. Make modified mitered corner with top sheet, blanket, and spread.
   A. Pick up side edge of top sheet, blanket, and spread approximately 45 cm (18 inches) from foot of mattress. Lift linen to form triangular fold, and lay it on bed.
   B. Tuck lower edge of sheet, which is hanging free below mattress, under mattress. Do not pull triangular fold.
   C. Pick up triangular fold, and bring it down over mattress while holding linen in place along side of mattress. Do not tuck tip of triangle.

36. Raise side rail. Make other side of bed; spread sheet, blanket, and bedspread out evenly. Fold top edge of spread over blanket and make cuff with top sheet (see Step 33); make modified mitered corner at foot of bed.

37. Change pillowcase:
   A. Have client raise head. While supporting neck with one hand, remove pillow. Allow client to lower head.
   B. Remove soiled case by grasping pillow at open end with one hand and pulling case back over pillow with the other hand. Discard case in linen bag.
   C. Grasp clean pillowcase at center of closed end. Gather case, turning it inside out over the hand holding it. With the same hand, pick up middle of one end of the pillow. Pull pillowcase down over pillow with the other hand.
   D. Be sure pillow corners fit evenly into corners of pillowcase. Place pillow under client's head.

38. Place call light within client's reach, and return bed to comfortable position.

39. Open room curtains, and rearrange furniture. Place personal items within easy reach on over-bed table or bedside stand. Return bed to a comfortable height.

40. Discard dirty linen in hamper or chute, and perform hand hygiene.

41. Ask if client feels comfortable.

42. Inspect skin for areas of irritation.

43. Observe client for signs of fatigue, dyspnea, pain, or discomfort.

STUDENT: _____ DATE: _____

INSTRUCTOR: _____ DATE: _____

Skill 40-1 Suctioning

	S	U	NP	Comments
1. Assess client for signs and symptoms of airway obstruction.	____	____	____	_____
2. Assess client for signs and symptoms associated with hypoxia and hypercapnia.	____	____	____	_____
3. Assess client for risk factors for upper or lower airway obstruction.	____	____	____	_____
4. Identify contraindications to nasotracheal suctioning.	____	____	____	_____
5. Obtain sputum microbiology data.	____	____	____	_____
6. Assess client's understanding of procedure.	____	____	____	_____
7. Explain to client how procedure will help clear airway and relieve breathing problems and that temporary coughing, sneezing, gagging, or shortness of breath is normal.	____	____	____	_____
8. Encourage client to cough out secretions.	____	____	____	_____
9. Instruct client to practice coughing, if able.	____	____	____	_____
10. Instruct client to splint surgical incisions, if necessary.	____	____	____	_____
11. Assist client with assuming position comfortable for nurse and client.	____	____	____	_____
12. Place pulse oximeter on client's finger. Take reading, and leave pulse oximeter in place.	____	____	____	_____
13. Place towel across client's chest.	____	____	____	_____
14. Perform hand hygiene, and apply face shield if splashing is likely.	____	____	____	_____
15. Connect one end of connecting tubing to suction machine, and place other end in convenient location near client. Turn suction device on, and set vacuum regulator to appropriate negative pressure.	____	____	____	_____
16. If indicated, increase supplemental oxygen therapy to 100% or as ordered by health care provider. Encourage client to deep breathe.	____	____	____	_____
17. Preparation for all types of suctioning:				
A. Open appropriate suction kit or catheter with use of aseptic technique. If sterile drape is available, place it across client's chest or on the over-bed table. Do not allow the suction catheter to touch any nonsterile surfaces.	____	____	____	_____
B. Unwrap or open sterile basin, and place on bedside table. Fill basin or cup with approximately 100 mL of sterile normal saline solution or water.	____	____	____	_____
C. Connect one end of connecting tubing to suction machine. Place other end in convenient location near client. Check that equipment is functioning properly by suctioning a small amount of water from basin.	____	____	____	_____
D. Turn on suction device. Set regulator to appropriate negative pressure: 100 to 150 mm Hg for adults.	____	____	____	_____
18. Suction airway.				
A. Oropharyngeal suctioning				
(1) Apply clean disposable glove to dominant hand.	____	____	____	_____
(2) Remove oxygen mask if present. Nasal cannula remains in place.	____	____	____	_____
(3) Insert catheter into client's mouth. With suction applied, move catheter around mouth, including pharynx and gum line, until secretions are cleared.	____	____	____	_____

Continued

295

	S	U	NP	Comments

(4) Encourage client to cough, and repeat suctioning if needed. Replace oxygen mask if used.

(5) Suction water from basin through catheter until catheter is cleared of secretions.

(6) Place catheter in a clean, dry area for reuse with suction turned off or within client's reach, with suction on, if client is capable of suctioning self.

B. Nasopharyngeal and nasotracheal suctioning

(1) If indicated, increase supplemental oxygen therapy to 100% or as ordered by health care provider. Encourage client's deep breathing.

(2) Open lubricant. Squeeze small amount onto open sterile catheter package without touching package.

(3) Apply sterile glove to each hand, or apply nonsterile glove to nondominant hand and sterile glove to dominant hand.

(4) Pick up suction catheter with dominant hand without touching nonsterile surfaces. Pick up connecting tubing with nondominant hand. Secure catheter to tubing.

(5) Check that the equipment is functioning properly by suctioning small amount of normal saline solution from basin.

(6) Lightly coat distal 6 to 8 cm (2 to 3 inches) of catheter with water-soluble lubricant.

(7) Remove oxygen delivery device, if applicable, with nondominant hand. Without applying suction and using dominant thumb and forefinger, gently insert catheter into naris during inhalation.

a. Nasopharyngeal

i. Follow natural course of naris; slightly slant catheter downward, and advance to back of pharynx. In adults insert catheter about 16 cm; in older children, 8 to 12 cm (3 to 5 inches); in infants and young children, 4 to 8 cm (2 to 3 inches). (Rule of thumb is to insert catheter distance from tip of nose [or mouth] to base of earlobe.)

ii. Apply intermittent suction for up to 10 to 15 seconds by placing and releasing nondominant thumb over catheter vent. Slowly withdraw catheter while rotating it back and forth between thumb and forefinger.

b. Nasotracheal

i. Follow natural course of naris, and advance catheter slightly slanted and downward to just above entrance into trachea.

ii. Allow client to take a breath.

iii. Quickly insert catheter about 16 to 20 cm (6 to 8 inches in adult) into trachea. Client will begin to cough. NOTE: In older children advance 14 to 20 cm (5 1/2 to 8 inches); in young children and infants, 8 to 14 cm (3 to 5 1/2 inches).

Continued

296

	S	U	NP	Comments

iv. Positioning option for nasotracheal suctioning: In some instances turning client's head to right helps suction the left mainstem bronchus; turning head to left helps suction the right mainstem bronchus. If you feel resistance after insertion of catheter for maximum recommended distance, catheter has probably hit carina. Pull catheter back 1 cm before applying suction. _____ _____ _____ _____

v. Apply intermittent suction for up to 10 to 15 seconds by placing and releasing nondominant thumb over vent of catheter and slowly withdrawing catheter while rotating it back and forth between dominant thumb and forefinger. _____ _____ _____ _____

vi. Encourage client to cough. _____ _____ _____ _____

vii. Replace oxygen device, if applicable. _____ _____ _____ _____

(8) Rinse catheter and connecting tubing with normal saline or water until cleared. _____ _____ _____ _____

(9) Assess for need to repeat suctioning procedure. Allow adequate time between suction passes for ventilation and oxygenation. When possible ask client to deep breathe and cough, or preoxygenate with 100% supplemental oxygen. _____ _____ _____ _____

C. Performing artificial airway suctioning

(1) Apply face shield. _____ _____ _____ _____

(2) Prepare proper suction catheter. _____ _____ _____ _____

(3) Apply one sterile glove to each hand, or apply nonsterile glove to nondominant hand and sterile glove to dominant hand. _____ _____ _____ _____

(4) Pick up suction catheter with dominant hand without touching nonsterile surfaces. Pick up connecting tubing with nondominant hand. Secure catheter to tubing. _____ _____ _____ _____

(5) Check that equipment is functioning properly by suctioning small amount of saline from basin. _____ _____ _____ _____

(6) Hyperinflate and/or hyperoxygenate client before suctioning, using manual resuscitation Ambu-bag connected to oxygen source or sigh mechanism on mechanical ventilator. Some mechanical ventilators have a button that when pushed delivers 100% oxygen for a few minutes and then resets to the previous value. _____ _____ _____ _____

(7) If client is receiving mechanical ventilation, open swivel adapter or if necessary remove oxygen or humidity delivery device with nondominant hand. _____ _____ _____ _____

(8) Without applying suction, gently but quickly insert catheter using dominant thumb and forefinger into artificial airway (best to time catheter insertion with inspiration) until you meet resistance or client coughs; then pull back 1 cm (½ inch). _____ _____ _____ _____

(9) Apply intermittent suction by placing and releasing nondominant thumb over vent of catheter; slowly withdraw catheter while rotating it back and forth between dominant thumb and forefinger. Encourage client to cough. Watch for respiratory distress. _____ _____ _____ _____

Continued

	S	U	NP	Comments

(10) If client is receiving mechanical ventilation, close swivel adapter or replace oxygen delivery device. ____ ____ ____ _____

(11) Encourage client to deep breathe, if able. Some clients respond well to several manual breaths from the mechanical ventilator or Ambu-bag. ____ ____ ____ _____

(12) Rinse catheter and connecting tubing with normal saline until clear. Use continuous suction. ____ ____ ____ _____

(13) Assess client's cardiopulmonary status for secretion clearance and complications. Repeat Steps 18C(6) through 18C(12) once or twice more to clear secretions. Allow adequate time (at least 1 full minute) between suction passes for ventilation and hyperoxygenation. ____ ____ ____ _____

(14) Perform nasopharyngeal and oropharyngeal suctioning (Steps 18A, 18B). ____ ____ ____ _____

(15) After performing nasopharyngeal and oropharyngeal suctioning, catheter is contaminated; do not reinsert into endotracheal tube or tracheostomy tube.

19. Complete procedure.

A. Disconnect catheter from connecting tubing. Roll catheter around fingers of dominant hand. Pull glove off inside out so that catheter remains in glove. Pull off other glove over first glove in same way to contain contaminants. Discard into appropriate receptacle. Turn off suction device. ____ ____ ____ _____

B. Remove towel and place in laundry, or remove drape and discard in appropriate receptacle. ____ ____ ____ _____

C. Reposition client as indicated by condition. Reapply clean gloves for client's personal care (e.g., oral hygiene). ____ ____ ____ _____

D. If indicated, readjust oxygen to original level. ____ ____ ____ _____

E. Discard remainder of normal saline into appropriate receptacle. If basin is disposable, discard into appropriate receptacle. If basin is reusable, rinse and place in soiled utility room. ____ ____ ____ _____

F. Remove and discard face shield, and perform hand hygiene. ____ ____ ____ _____

G. Place unopened suction kit on suction machine table or at head of bed according to institution preference. ____ ____ ____ _____

20. Compare client's vital signs and pulse oximetry saturation before and after suctioning. ____ ____ ____ _____

21. Ask client if breathing is easier and if congestion is decreased. ____ ____ ____ _____

22. Auscultate lungs for change in adventitious lung sounds. ____ ____ ____ _____

23. Observe airway secretions. ____ ____ ____ _____

24. Record the amount, consistency, color, and odor of secretions and client's response to procedure; document client's presuctioning and postsuctioning cardiopulmonary status. ____ ____ ____ _____

STUDENT: _____ DATE: _____

INSTRUCTOR: _____ DATE: _____

Skill 40-2 Care of an Artificial Airway

	S	U	NP	Comments
1. Perform cardiopulmonary assessment.	___	___	___	_____
2. Explain procedure to client.	___	___	___	_____
3. Position client.	___	___	___	_____
4. Place towel across client's chest.	___	___	___	_____
5. Perform hand hygiene.	___	___	___	_____
6. Perform airway care.	___	___	___	_____
A. Endotracheal tube (ET) care				
(1) Assess client for signs and symptoms indicating the need to perform care of the artificial airway.	___	___	___	_____
(2) Identify factors that increase risk for complications from ET tubes.	___	___	___	_____
(3) Suction endotracheal tube:				
a. Instruct client not to bite or move ET tube with tongue or pull on tubing.	___	___	___	_____
b. Leave Yankauer suction catheter connected to suction source.	___	___	___	_____
(4) Prepare method to secure ET tube.				
a. Tape method:				
i. Cut piece of tape long enough to go completely around client's head from naris to naris plus 15 cm (6 inches).	___	___	___	_____
ii. Lay adhesive side up on bedside table.	___	___	___	_____
iii. Cut and lay 8 to 16 cm (3 to 6 inches) of tape, adhesive sides together, in center of long strip to prevent tape from sticking to hair.	___	___	___	_____
b. Commercially available endotracheal tube holder:	___	___	___	_____
i. Open package per manufacturer's instructions.	___	___	___	_____
ii. Set device aside with the head guard in place and the Velcro strips open.	___	___	___	_____
(5) Apply gloves, and instruct assistant to apply gloves and hold ET tube firmly at client's lips. Note the number marking on the ET tube at the gum line.	___	___	___	_____
(6) Remove old tape or device.				
a. Tape: Carefully remove tape from ET tube and client's face. If tape is difficult to remove, moisten with water or adhesive tape remover. Discard tape in appropriate receptacle if nearby.	___	___	___	_____
b. Commercially available device: Remove Velcro strips from ET tube, and remove ET tube holder from client.	___	___	___	_____
(7) Remove excess secretions or adhesive left on client's face.	___	___	___	_____
(8) Remove oral airway or bite block if present.	___	___	___	_____
(9) Clean mouth, gums, and teeth opposite ET tube with mouthwash solution and 4 × 4 gauze, sponge-tipped applicators, or saline swabs. Brush teeth as indicated. If necessary, administer oropharyngeal suctioning with Yankauer catheter.	___	___	___	_____
(10) Note "cm" ET tube marking at lips or gums. With help of assistant, move ET tube to opposite side or center of mouth. Do not change tube depth.	___	___	___	_____
(11) Repeat oral cleaning as in Step (9) on opposite side of mouth.	___	___	___	_____

Continued

	S	U	NP	Comments

(12) Clean face and neck with soapy
washcloth; rinse and dry. Shave male
client as necessary.

(13) Use small amount of skin protectant or
liquid adhesive on clean 2 × 2 gauze, and
dot on upper lip (oral ET tube) or across
nose (nasal ET tube) and cheeks to ear.
Allow tincture to dry completely.

(14) Secure ET tube.
   a. Tape method
      i. Slip tape under client's head and
      neck, adhesive side up. Take care
      not to twist tape or catch hair. Do
      not allow tape to stick to itself. It
      helps to stick tape gently to
      tongue blade, which serves as a
      guide as tape is passed behind the
      client's head. Center tape so that
      double-faced tape extends around
      back of neck from ear to ear.
      ii. On one side of face, secure tape
      from ear to naris (nasal ET tube)
      or edge of mouth (oral ET tube).
      Tear remaining tape in half
      lengthwise, forming two pieces
      that are ½- to ¾-inch wide.
      Secure bottom half of tape across
      upper lip (oral ET tube) or across
      top of nose (nasal ET tube). Wrap
      top half of tape around tube. Tape
      encircles the tube at least two
      times for security.
      iii. Gently pull other side of tape
      firmly to pick up slack, and secure
      to remaining side of face. Have
      assistant release hold when tube is
      secure. You need an assistant to
      help reinsert oral airway.
   b. Commercially available device
      i. Thread ET tube through the
      opening designed to secure the
      ET tube. Be sure that the pilot
      balloon is accessible.
      ii. Place strips of ET holder under
      the client at the occipital region
      of the head.
      iii. Verify that the ET tube is at the
      established position using the lip
      or gum line marker as a guide.
      iv. Attach the Velcro strips at the
      base of the client's head. Leave
      1 cm (½ inch) slack in the strips.
      v. Verify that the tube is secure, it
      does not move forward from the
      client's mouth or backward down
      into the client's throat, and there
      are no pressure areas on the oral
      mucosa or the occipital region
      of the head.

(15) Clean oral airway in warm soapy water,
and rinse well. Hydrogen peroxide can
aid in removal of crusted secretions.
Shake excess water from oral airway.

(16) For unconscious client, reinsert oral
airway without pushing tongue into
oropharynx.

B. Tracheostomy Care:
   (1) Observe for signs and symptoms of need
   to perform tracheostomy care:

Continued

	S	U	NP	Comments

a. Soiled/loose ties or dressing.

b. Nonstable tube.

c. Excessive secretions.

(2) Suction tracheostomy. Before removing gloves, remove soiled tracheostomy dressing and discard in glove with coiled catheter.

(3) Prepare equipment.

a. Open two packages of cotton-tipped swabs, and pour normal saline (NS) on one package and hydrogen peroxide on the other. Do not recap hydrogen peroxide and NS.

b. Open sterile tracheostomy package.

c. Unwrap sterile basin, and pour about 2 cm (3/4 inch) of hydrogen peroxide into it.

d. Open small sterile brush package, and place aseptically into sterile basin.

e. If using large roll of twill tape, cut appropriate length of tape and lay aside in dry area.

f. Apply gloves. Keep dominant hand sterile throughout procedure.

g. Remove oxygen source. Apply oxygen source loosely over tracheostomy if client desaturates during procedure.

h. Tracheostomy with *inner cannula* care:

  i. While touching only the outer aspect of the tube, remove the inner cannula with nondominant hand. Drop inner cannula into hydrogen peroxide basin.

  ii. Place tracheostomy collar or T tube and ventilator oxygen source over or near outer cannula. (NOTE: T tube and ventilator oxygen devices cannot be attached to all outer cannulas when inner cannula is removed.)

  iii. To prevent oxygen desaturation in affected clients, quickly pick up inner cannula and use small brush to remove secretions inside and outside cannula.

  iv. Hold inner cannula over basin, and rinse with NS, using nondominant hand to pour.

  v. Replace inner cannula, and secure "locking" mechanism. Reapply ventilator or oxygen sources.

i. Tracheostomy with *disposable inner cannula* care:

  i. Remove cannula from manufacturer's packaging.

  ii. While touching only the outer aspect of the tube, withdraw inner cannula and replace with new cannula. Lock into position.

  iii. Dispose of contaminated cannula in appropriate receptacle, and apply oxygen source.

(4) Using hydrogen peroxide–prepared cotton-tipped swabs and 4 × 4 gauze, clean exposed outer cannula surfaces and stoma under faceplate, extending 5 to 10 cm (2 to 4 inches) in all directions from stoma. Clean in circular motion from stoma site outward, using dominant hand to handle sterile supplies.

Continued

	S	U	NP	Comments

(5) Using NS-prepared cotton-tipped swabs and 4 × 4 gauze, rinse hydrogen peroxide from tracheostomy tube and skin surfaces. ____ ____ ____ _____

(6) Using dry 4 × 4 gauze, pat lightly at skin and exposed outer cannula surfaces. ____ ____ ____ _____

(7) Secure tracheostomy.

　a. Tracheostomy tie method:

　　i. Instruct assistant, if available, to hold tracheostomy tube securely in place while ties are cut. ____ ____ ____ _____

　　ii. Cut length of twill tape long enough to go around client's neck two times, about 60 to 75 cm (24 to 30 inches) for an adult. ____ ____ ____ _____

　　iii. Cut ends on a diagonal. ____ ____ ____ _____

　　iv. Take prepared tie, and insert one end of tie through faceplate eyelet and pull ends even. ____ ____ ____ _____

　　v. Slide both ends of tie behind head and around neck to other eyelet, and insert one tie through second eyelet. ____ ____ ____ _____

　　vi. Pull snugly. ____ ____ ____ _____

　　vii. Tie ends securely in double square knot, allowing space for only one finger in tie. ____ ____ ____ _____

　b. Tracheostomy tube holder method:

　　i. While wearing gloves, maintain a secure hold on the tracheostomy tube. You can do this with an assistant or, when an assistant is not available, by leaving the old trach tube holder in place until the new device is secure. ____ ____ ____ _____

　　ii. Align strap under client's neck. Be sure that the Velcro attachments are positioned on either side of the tracheostomy tube. ____ ____ ____ _____

　　iii. Place narrow end of the ties under and through the faceplate eyelets. Pull ends even, and secure with the Velcro closures. ____ ____ ____ _____

　　iv. Verify that there is space for only one loose or two snug finger width(s) under neck strap. ____ ____ ____ _____

(8) Insert fresh tracheostomy dressing under clean ties and faceplate. ____ ____ ____ _____

(9) Position client comfortably, and assess respiratory status. ____ ____ ____ _____

7. Replace any oxygen delivery devices. ____ ____ ____ _____

8. Remove and discard gloves. Perform hand hygiene. ____ ____ ____ _____

9. Compare respiratory assessments before and after procedure. ____ ____ ____ _____

10. Observe depth and position of tubes. ____ ____ ____ _____

11. Assess security of tape or commercial ET or tracheostomy tube holder by tugging at tube.

12. Assess skin around mouth and oral mucosa (ET tube) and tracheostomy stoma for drainage, pressure, and signs of irritation. ____ ____ ____ _____

13. Record respiratory assessments before and after care.

　A. Record ET tube care: depth of ET tube, frequency and extent of care, client tolerance, and any complications related to presence of the tube. ____ ____ ____ _____

　B. Record tracheostomy care: type and size of tracheostomy tube, frequency and extent of care, client tolerance, and any complications related to presence of the tube. ____ ____ ____ _____

STUDENT: _____ DATE: _____

INSTRUCTOR: _____ DATE: _____

Skill 40-3 Care of Clients With Chest Tubes

	S	U	NP	Comments
1. Perform hand hygiene, and assess client.				
A. Pulmonary status: Assess for respiratory distress, chest pain, breath sounds over affected lung area.	____	____	____	_____
B. Signs and symptoms of increased respiratory distress and/or chest pain are decreased breath sounds over the affected and nonaffected lungs, marked cyanosis, asymmetrical chest movements, presence of subcutaneous emphysema around tube insertion site or neck, hypotension, and tachycardia.	____	____	____	_____
C. Chest pain on inspiration.	____	____	____	_____
D. Vital signs and pulse oximetry (SpO_2).	____	____	____	_____
E. If possible, ask client to rate level of comfort on a scale of 0 to 10.	____	____	____	_____
2. Observe:				
A. Chest tube dressing and site surrounding tube insertion.	____	____	____	_____
B. Tubing for kinks, dependent loops, or clots.	____	____	____	_____
C. Chest drainage system remains upright and below level of tube insertion.	____	____	____	_____
3. Provide two rubber-tipped hemostats or approved clamps for each chest tube, attached to top of client's bed with adhesive tape. Chest tubes are only clamped under specific circumstances per health care provider's order or nursing policy and procedure:				
A. To assess air leak	____	____	____	_____
B. To quickly empty or change disposable systems; performed by a nurse who has received education in the procedure.	____	____	____	_____
C. If there is an accidental disconnection of drainage tubing from the drainage collection device or damage to the device.	____	____	____	_____
D. To assess if client is ready to have chest tube removed (which is done by health care provider's order).	____	____	____	_____
4. Position client.				
A. Semi-Fowler's position to evacuate air (pneumothorax).	____	____	____	_____
B. High-Fowler's position to drain fluid (hemothorax, effusion).	____	____	____	_____
5. Be sure tube connection between chest and drainage tube is intact and taped.				
A. Determine that water-seal vent is not occluded.	____	____	____	_____
B. Be sure suction-control chamber vent is not occluded when using suction. Waterless systems have relief valves without caps.	____	____	____	_____
6. Avoid excess tubing; lay the tubing horizontally across the client bed or chair before dropping vertically into the drainage bottle. If the client is in a chair and the tubing is coiled, lift the tubing every 15 minutes to promote drainage.	____	____	____	_____
7. Adjust tubing to hang in straight line from top of mattress to drainage chamber. If chest tube is draining fluid, indicate time (e.g., 0900) that drainage was begun on drainage bottle's adhesive tape or on write-on surface of disposable commercial system.	____	____	____	_____

Continued

	S	U	NP	Comments

8. Strip or milk chest tube only if indicated
(this means compressing the tube to encourage
clots to pass through the tube).
   A. Stripping—apply pressure along length of the
   tubing beginning at client and continuing until
   you reach the drainage unit.
   B. Milking—compress and release the tube
   sequentially.
9. Perform hand hygiene.
10. Evaluation
   A. Monitor vital signs and pulse oximetry as
   ordered or if client's condition changes.
   B. Observe appearance of chest tube dressing.
   C. Observe that tubing is free of kinks and
   dependent loops.
   D. Verify that the chest drainage system is upright
   and below level of tube insertion. Note
   presence of clots or debris in tubing.
   E. Observe water seal for fluctuations with client's
   inspiration and expiration.
      (1) Observe waterless system: The suction control
      (float ball) indicates the amount of suction the
      client's intrapleural space is receiving.
      (2) Observe water seal system: bubbling in the
      water seal chamber.
      (3) Observe water-seal system: bubbling in the
      suction-control chamber (when using suction).
   F. Observe type of fluid, and measure fluid
   drainage: Note color and amount of drainage,
   client's vital signs, and skin color.
      (1) In the adult: less than 50 to 200 mL/hr
      immediately after surgery in a mediastinal
      chest tube; approximately 500 mL in first
      24 hours.
      (2) Between 100 and 300 mL of fluid drain in
      pleural chest tube in an adult during first
      3 hours after insertion. This rate will decrease
      after 2 hours; expect 500 to 1000 mL in first
      24 hours. Drainage is grossly bloody during
      first several hours after surgery and then
      changes to serous. Remember that a sudden
      gush of drainage is often retained blood and
      not active bleeding. This increase in drainage
      often results from client position changes.
   G. Observe client for decreased respiratory distress
   and chest pain, auscultate lung sounds over
   affected lung area, and monitor SpO_2.
   H. Ask client to evaluate pain on a level of 0 to 10.
   I. Record patency of chest tube; presence, type, and
   amount of drainage; presence of fluctuations;
   client's vital signs; chest dressing status, amount
   of suction and/or water seal; and level of comfort.

STUDENT: _____ DATE: _____

INSTRUCTOR: _____ DATE: _____

Skill 40-4 Applying a Nasal Cannula or an Oxygen Mask

	S	U	NP	Comments
1. Inspect client for signs and symptoms associated with hypoxia and presence of airway secretions.	____	____	____	_____
2. Obtain client's most recent pulse oximetry (SpO$_2$) or arterial blood gas (ABG) values.	____	____	____	_____
3. Explain to client and family what happens during the procedure and purpose of oxygen therapy.	____	____	____	_____
4. Perform hand hygiene.	____	____	____	_____
5. Attach nasal cannula or mask to oxygen tubing, and attach to humidified oxygen source adjusted to prescribed flow rate.	____	____	____	_____
6. Place tips of cannula into client's nares, and adjust elastic headband or plastic slide until cannula fits snugly and comfortably. If using an oxygen mask, adjust elastic headband until mask fits comfortably over client's face and mouth.	____	____	____	_____
7. Maintain sufficient slack on oxygen tubing, and secure to client's clothes.	____	____	____	_____
8. Check cannula at least 8 hours or with changes in client's cardiopulmonary status. Keep humidification jar filled at all times.	____	____	____	_____
9. Observe client's nares and superior surface of both ears for skin breakdown.	____	____	____	_____
10. Check oxygen flow rate and health care provider's orders at least every 8 hours or with changes in client's cardiopulmonary status.	____	____	____	_____
11. Perform hand hygiene.	____	____	____	_____
12. Inspect client for relief of symptoms associated with hypoxia.	____	____	____	_____
13. Record oxygen delivery device and liter flow in medical record; document client and family education; report oxygen delivery device, liter flow, and response to changes in therapy to oncoming shift.	____	____	____	_____

STUDENT: _____ DATE: _____

INSTRUCTOR: _____ DATE: _____

CHECKLIST
Skill 40-5 Using Home Oxygen Equipment

	S	U	NP	Comments
1. While client is still in the hospital, determine client's or family's ability to use oxygen equipment correctly. In the home setting reassess for appropriate use of equipment.	____	____	____	_____
2. Assess home environment for adequate electrical service if oxygen concentrator is ordered.	____	____	____	_____
3. Assess client's and family's ability to observe for signs and symptoms of hypoxia: apprehension, anxiety, decreased ability to concentrate, decreased level of consciousness, increased fatigue, dizziness, behavioral changes, increased pulse, increased respiratory rate, pallor, or cyanosis of the mucous membranes.	____	____	____	_____
4. Determine appropriate resources in the community for equipment and assistance, including maintenance and repair services, and medical equipment supplier.	____	____	____	_____
5. In case there is a power failure, determine appropriate backup systems when using compressor. Have a spare oxygen tank available.	____	____	____	_____
6. Perform hand hygiene.	____	____	____	_____
7. Place oxygen delivery system in a clutter-free environment that is well ventilated, away from walls, drapes, bedding, combustible materials, and at least 8 feet from heat source.	____	____	____	_____
8. Demonstrate each step for preparation and completion of oxygen therapy.				
A. Compressed oxygen system:				
(1) Turn cylinder valve counterclockwise two or three turns with wrench. Store wrench with oxygen tank	____	____	____	_____
(2) Check cylinders by reading amount on pressure gauge.	____	____	____	_____
B. Oxygen concentrator system:				
(1) Plug in concentrator into appropriate outlet.	____	____	____	_____
(2) Turn on power switch.	____	____	____	_____
(3) Alarm will sound for a few seconds.	____	____	____	_____
C. Refilling oxygen tank:				
(1) Wipe both filling connectors with a clean, dry, lint-free cloth.	____	____	____	_____
(2) Turn off flow selector of ambulatory unit.	____	____	____	_____
(3) Attach ambulatory unit to stationary reservoir by inserting adapter from ambulatory tank into adapter of stationary reservoir.	____	____	____	_____
(4) Open fill valve on ambulatory tank, and apply firm pressure to top of stationary reservoir. Stay with unit while it is filling. You will hear a loud hissing noise. Tank fills in about 2 minutes.	____	____	____	_____
(5) Disengage ambulatory unit from stationary reservoir when hissing noise changes and vapor cloud begins to form from stationary unit.	____	____	____	_____
(6) Wipe both filling connectors with clean, dry, lint-free cloth.	____	____	____	_____
9. Connect oxygen delivery device to oxygen system.	____	____	____	_____
10. Adjust to prescribed flow rate (L/min).	____	____	____	_____
11. Place oxygen delivery device on client.	____	____	____	_____
A. Perform hand hygiene	____	____	____	_____

Continued

	S	U	NP	Comments

B. Instruct client and family not to change oxygen flow rate. _____ _____ _____ _____

C. Guide the client and family as they perform each step. Provide written material for reinforcement and review. _____ _____ _____ _____

D. Instruct client and family to notify health care provider if signs or symptoms of hypoxia or respiratory tract infection (e.g., fever, increased sputum, change in color of sputum, odor) occur. _____ _____ _____ _____

E. Discuss emergency plan for power loss, natural disaster, and acute respiratory distress. Have client or family/caregiver call 911 and notify health care provider and home care agency. _____ _____ _____ _____

F. Instruct client in safe home oxygen practices, including not allowing smoking in the house, keeping oxygen tanks away from open flame, and storing tanks upright. _____ _____ _____ _____

G. Monitor oxygen delivery rate. _____ _____ _____ _____

H. Ask client and family about ease or problems associated with home oxygen. _____ _____ _____ _____

I. Ask client and family to state safety guidelines, emergency precautions, and emergency plan. _____ _____ _____ _____

12. Record the teaching plan, the client's and family's ability to safely use the home oxygen equipment; report the type of home oxygen equipment to be used, the client's and family's understanding of how to use the equipment, knowledge of safety guidelines and unexpected outcomes, and ability to return demonstrate proper use of the oxygen delivery device. _____ _____ _____ _____

STUDENT: _____ DATE: _____

INSTRUCTOR: _____ DATE: _____

Skill 41-1 Initiating Intravenous Therapy

	S	U	NP	Comments
1. Review health care provider's order for type and amount of intravenous (IV) fluid, rate of fluid administration, and purpose of infusion. Follows six rights for administration of medications.	___	___	___	_____
2. Assess for clinical factors/conditions that will respond to or be affected by IV fluid administration:				
A. Peripheral edema can be rated for severity by assessing pitting over bony prominences; 1+ indicates barely detectable edema to 4+ for deep persistent pitting.	___	___	___	_____
B. Body weight.	___	___	___	_____
C. Dry skin and mucous membranes.	___	___	___	_____
D. Distended neck veins.	___	___	___	_____
E. Blood pressure changes.	___	___	___	_____
F. Irregular pulse rhythm; increased pulse rate (tachycardia).	___	___	___	_____
G. Auscultation of crackles or rhonchi in lungs.	___	___	___	_____
H. Inelastic skin turgor (after pinching, fails to return to normal position within 3 seconds).	___	___	___	_____
I. Anorexia, nausea, and vomiting.	___	___	___	_____
J. Thirst.	___	___	___	_____
K. Decreased urine output.	___	___	___	_____
L. Behavioral changes (i.e., confusion, restlessness).	___	___	___	_____
M. Decreased capillary refill.	___	___	___	_____
3. Assess client's previous or perceived experience with IV therapy and arm placement preference.	___	___	___	_____
4. Obtain information from drug reference books or pharmacist about composition of IV fluids, purposes of administration, potential incompatibilities, and side effects for monitoring guidelines.	___	___	___	_____
5. Determine if client is to undergo any planned surgeries or is to receive blood infusion later.	___	___	___	_____
6. Assess for the following risk factors: child or older adult; presence of heart failure or renal failure; skin lesions; infection; low platelet count; or receiving anticoagulants.	___	___	___	_____
7. Assess laboratory data and client's history of allergies to iodine, adhesive, or latex.	___	___	___	_____
8. Explain to client and family the procedure, its purpose, and what is expected of client. Explain what sensations client is to expect.	___	___	___	_____
9. Assist client to comfortable sitting or supine position. Be positioned at a level position with client. Provide adequate lighting.	___	___	___	_____
10. Check client's identification using two identifiers.	___	___	___	_____
11. Perform hand hygiene. Organize equipment on clean, clutter-free bedside stand or over-bed table.	___	___	___	_____
12. Change client's gown to the more easily removed gown with snaps at the shoulder, if available.	___	___	___	_____
13. Open sterile packages using sterile aseptic technique.	___	___	___	_____
14. Prepare IV tubing and solution.				
A. Check IV solution, using six rights of medication administration. Make sure prescribed additives, such as potassium and vitamins, have been added. Check solution for color, clarity, and expiration date. Check bag for leaks, which is best if done before reaching the bedside.	___	___	___	_____
B. Open infusion set, maintaining sterility of both ends of tubing. Many sets allow for priming of tubing without removal of cap end.	___	___	___	_____

Continued

308

	S	U	NP	Comments

C. Place roller clamp about 2 to 5 cm (1 to 2 inches) below drip chamber, and move roller clamp to "off" position. ___ ___ ___ _____

D. Remove protective sheath over IV tubing port on plastic IV solution bag. ___ ___ ___ _____

E. Insert infusion set into fluid bag or bottle: Remove protector cap from tubing insertion spike, not touching spike, and insert spike into opening of IV bag. Cleanse rubber stopper on glass bottled solution with antiseptic, and insert spike into black rubber stopper of IV bottle. ___ ___ ___ _____

F. Prime infusion tubing by filling with IV solution: Compress the drip chamber and release, allowing it to fill one-third to one-half full. ___ ___ ___ _____

G. Remove protector cap on end of tubing (some tubing can be primed without removal), and slowly open roller clamp to allow fluid to travel from drip chamber through tubing to needle adapter. Return roller clamp to "off" position after priming tubing (filled with IV fluid). ___ ___ ___ _____

H. Be certain tubing is clear of air and air bubbles by tapping IV tubing where air bubbles are located. Check entire length of tubing to ensure that all air bubbles are removed. If using multiple-port tubing, turn port upside down, and tap to fill and remove air. Optional: Add an extension tubing to IV tubing to allow for more length, enabling client to move freely while keeping IV line stable. ___ ___ ___ _____

I. Replace cap protector on end of infusion tubing. ___ ___ ___ _____

15. Optional: Prepare heparin or normal saline lock for infusion:

A. If a loop or short extension tubing is needed because of awkward IV site placement, use sterile technique to connect the IV plug to the loop or short extension tubing. Inject 1 to 3 mL normal saline through the plug and through the loop or short extension tubing before connecting it to IV site. ___ ___ ___ _____

16. Apply clean gloves. Eye protection and mask may be worn (see agency policy) if splash or spray of blood is possible. ___ ___ ___ _____

17. Identify accessible vein for IV cannula. Apply tourniquet 4 to 6 inches (10 to 15 cm) above the proposed insertion site. Do not apply tourniquet too tightly to avoid injury or bruising the skin. Check for presence of radial pulse. You may apply tourniquet on top of a thin layer of clothing such as a gown sleeve, to protect fragile skin or excess hair. It may become necessary to remove tourniquet and move lower down arm. Optional: Apply blood pressure cuff instead of tourniquet. Inflate to a level just below client's normal diastolic pressure. Maintain inflation at that pressure until venipuncture is completed. ___ ___ ___ _____

18. Select the vein for IV insertion. Veins found on the dorsal and ventral surfaces of upper extremities (e.g., cephalic, basilic, and metacarpal veins) are preferred in adults.

A. Use the most distal site in the nondominant arm, if possible. Clip arm hair with scissors if necessary. ___ ___ ___ _____

B. Avoid areas that are painful to palpation. ___ ___ ___ _____

C. Select a vein large enough for cannula placement. ___ ___ ___ _____

D. Choose a site that will not interfere with client's activities of daily living (ADLs) or planned procedures. ___ ___ ___ _____

E. With the index finger, palpate the vein by pressing downward. Note the resilient, soft, bouncy feeling while releasing the pressure. ___ ___ ___ _____

Continued

	S	U	NP	Comments

F. If possible, place extremity in dependent position.

G. Select well-dilated vein. Other methods to foster venous distention include the following:

  (1) Stroking the extremity from distal to proximal below the proposed venipuncture site.

  (2) Applying warmth to the extremity for several minutes, for example, with a warm washcloth.

H. Avoid sites distal to previous venipuncture site, sclerosed or hardened cordlike veins, infiltrate site or phlebotic vessels, bruised areas, and areas of venous valves or bifurcation.

I. Avoid fragile dorsal veins in older adult clients and vessels in an extremity with compromised circulation (e.g., in cases of mastectomy, dialysis graft, or paralysis).

19. Release tourniquet temporarily and carefully. Optional: At this point of the procedure there is the option of applying a local anesthetic to site. Monitor client for allergic reaction.

20. Place connection of infusion set or IV plug nearby, maintaining sterility of system.

21. If area of insertion appears to need cleansing, use soap and water first. Use antiseptic swab to cleanse insertion site using friction in a horizontal plane, then a vertical plane followed with a circular motion (middle to outward); allow antiseptic to dry completely. Refrain from touching the cleansed site unless using sterile technique.

22. Reapply tourniquet 10 to 12 cm (4 to 5 inches) above anticipated insertion site. Check presence of distal pulse.

23. Perform venipuncture. Anchor vein by placing thumb over vein, and gently tighten the skin distal to the site 1 ½ to 2 inches (4 to 5 cm). Warn client of a sharp, quick stick.

A. Over-the-needle (ONC) cannula with safety device: Insert with the bevel up at 10- to 30-degree angle slightly distal to actual site of venipuncture in the direction of the vein.

B. Winged needle: Hold needle at 10- to 30-degree angle with bevel up, slightly distal to actual site of venipuncture.

24. Observe for blood return through flashback cannula or tubing of winged needle, indicating that needle has entered vein. Lower cannula/winged needle until almost flush with skin. (*Advance cannula approximately ¼ inch into vein, and then loosen stylet*). Continue to hold skin taut, and advance cannula/winged needle into vein until hub rests at venipuncture site. *Do not reinsert the stylet once it is loosened.*

25. Stabilize the cannula with one hand, and release tourniquet with other. Apply gentle pressure with the middle finger of nondominant hand ¼ inches (3 cm) above insertion site. Keep cannula stable with index finger. For a safety device, glide the protective guard over the stylet, or retract stylet by pressing safety tab. A click indicates the device is locked over the stylet. (NOTE: Techniques will vary with each IV device.) Remove the stylet. Place directly into sharps container.

26. Continuous infusion: Quickly connect end of infusion tubing set to end of ONC cannula. Do not touch point of entry of adapter.

27. Intermittent infusion: Quickly connect adapter of heparin lock to hub of ONC cannula. Clean hub of heparin lock with alcohol. Insert prefilled syringe containing flush solution into injection cap. Flush injection cap slowly with flush solution. Use positive flow adapter, or withdraw the syringe while still flushing.

Continued

310

	S	U	NP	Comments

28. Continuous infusion: Begin infusion by slowly opening the clamp of the IV tubing.

29. Secure cannula (procedures can differ; follow agency policy):
   a. Transparent dressing: Secure cannula with non-dominant hand while preparing to apply dressing.
   b. Sterile gauze dressing: Place narrow piece (1/2 inch) of tape under cannula hub with sticky side up, and criss-cross tape over cannula hub to make a chevron. Place tape only on the cannula, never over the insertion site. Secure site to allow easy visual inspection. Avoid applying tape around arm.

30. Apply sterile dressing over site:
   a. Transparent dressing:
      (1) Carefully remove adherent backing. Apply one edge of dressing, and then gently smooth remaining dressing over IV site, leaving connection between IV tubing and cannula hub uncovered. Remove outer covering, and smooth dressing gently over site.
      (2) Take a 1-inch piece of transparent tape, and place it from end of hub of cannula to insertion site, over transparent dressing.
      (3) Apply chevron to infusion tubing, and place only over tape, not the transparent dressing.
   b. Sterile gauze dressing:
      (1) Fold a 2 × 2 gauze in half, and cover with a 1-inch-wide tape extending about an inch from each side. Place under the tubing/cannula hub junction. Curl a loop of tubing alongside the arm, and place a second piece of tape directly over the tubing and padded 2 × 2, securing tubing in two places.
      (2) Pace a gauze pad over insertion site and cannula hub. Secure all edges with tape. Do not cover connection between IV tubing and cannula hub.

31. Loop tubing alongside the arm, and place a second piece of tape directly over the tape covering the transparent dressing or over the padded 2 × 2.

32. For IV fluid administration, recheck flow rate to correct drops per minute or connect to electronic infusion device as per agency policy.

33. Write date and time of IV placement, cannula gauge size and length, and nurse's initials on dressing.

34. Dispose of stylet or other sharps in appropriate sharps container. Discard supplies. Remove gloves, and perform hand hygiene.

35. Instruct client on how to move or turn without pulling on IV cannula.

36. Change peripheral IV access every 72 hours or per health care provider's orders or immediately upon suspected contamination or complication.

37. When solution has less than 100 mL remaining, have next solution available at client's bedside.

38. Observe client every 1 to 2 hours:
   a. Check if correct amount of IV solution has infused by comparing the time tape on IV container or EID record.
   b. Count drip rate (if gravity drip), or check rate on infusion pump.
   c. Check patency of IV cannula.
   d. Observe client during palpation of vessel for signs of discomfort.
   e. Inspect insertion site, note color (e.g., redness, pallor). Inspect for presence of swelling, infiltration, and phlebitis. Palpate temperature of skin above dressing.

39. Evaluate client's response to therapy (i.e., measure intake and output [I&O], weights, vital signs).

Copyright © 2009, 2005, 2001, 1997 by Mosby, Inc., an affiliate of Elsevier Inc. All rights reserved.

STUDENT: _____ DATE: _____

INSTRUCTOR: _____ DATE: _____

Skill 41-2 Regulating Intravenous Flow Rate

	S	U	NP	Comments
1. Check client's medical record for order of solution and additives. Follow six rights of medication administration. Usual order includes name of solution, additives or medications (if included), and time over which each liter is to infuse or an hourly infusion rate or volume in specified time period. Occasionally, an intravenous (IV) order calls for 1 L to keep vein open (KVO).	____	____	____	_____
2. Perform hand hygiene. Observe for patency of IV line and cannula.	____	____	____	_____
3. Assess client's knowledge of how positioning of the IV site affects flow rate.	____	____	____	_____
4. Inspect IV site, and verify with client how venipuncture site feels; determine if there is pain or burning. Palpate site for tenderness.	____	____	____	_____
5. Have paper and pencil or calculator to calculate flow rate.	____	____	____	_____
6. Know calibration (drop factor) in drops per milliliter (gtt/mL) of infusion set currently in use: *Microdrip*: 60 gtt/mL *Macrodrip*: Abbott: 15 gtt/mL Travenol: 10 gtt/mL McGaw: 15 gtt/mL	____	____	____	_____
7. Review how long each liter of fluid should run. Calculate mL/hr. Determine hourly rate by dividing volume by hours, for example: mL/hr = total infusion (mL) / hours of infusion 1000 mL/8 hr = 125 mL/hr or if 3 L is ordered for 24 hours 3000 mL/24 hr = 125 mL/hr	____	____	____	_____
8. Select one of the following formulas to calculate minute flow rate (drops/min) based on drop factor of infusion set: A. mL/hr/60 min = mL/min and Drop factor × mL/min = drops/min Or	____	____	____	_____
B. mL/hr × drop factor/60 min = drops/min Using formula B above, calculate minute flow rate for bottle 1:1000 mL with 20 mEq KCl @ 125 mL/hr. Microdrip: 125 mL/hr × 60 gtt/mL = 7500 gtt/hr 7500 gtt ÷ 60 minutes = 125 gtt/min Macrodrip: 125 mL/hr × 15 gtt/mL = 1875 gtt/hr 1875 gtt ÷ 60 minutes = 31–32 gtt/min	____	____	____	_____
9. Place marked adhesive tape or commercial fluid indicator tape on IV container next to volume markings.	____	____	____	_____
10. Regulate flow rate by counting drops in drip chamber for 1 minute by watch, then adjust roller clamp to increase or decrease rate of infusion.	____	____	____	_____
11. Set up and regulate infusion gravity controller or electronic infusion device (EID) pump. A. Consult manufacturer's directions for setup of the infusion. Place electronic eye over drip chamber. If a gravity controller is used, ensure that IV container is 36 inches above the IV site.	____	____	____	_____

Continued

	S	U	NP	Comments
B. Insert IV tubing into chamber of control mechanism (see manufacturer's directions).	____	____	____	_____
C. Select required drops per minute or volume per hour, close door to control chamber, turn on power button, and press start button.	____	____	____	_____
D. Open drip regulator completely while EID is in use.	____	____	____	_____
E. Monitor infusion rate and IV site for infiltration according to agency policy. Check rate of infusion by comparing volume in the container with the calculated amount that should have been infused even when EID is used.	____	____	____	_____
F. Assess patency of system when alarm signals.	____	____	____	_____
12. Follow this procedure for gravity volume-control device:				
A. Place volume-control device between IV bag and insertion spike of infusion set using aseptic technique.	____	____	____	_____
B. Place no more than 2 hours' allotment of fluid into device by opening clamp between IV bag and device.	____	____	____	_____
C. Assess system at least hourly; add fluid to volume-control device. Regulate flow rate.	____	____	____	_____
13. Monitor IV infusion at least every hour, noting volume of IV fluid infused and rate.	____	____	____	_____
14. Observe client for signs of overhydration or dehydration to determine response to therapy and restoration of fluid and electrolyte balance.	____	____	____	_____
15. Evaluate for signs of infiltration, inflammation at site, clot in cannula, kink or knot in infusion tubing.	____	____	____	_____

STUDENT: _____ DATE: _____

INSTRUCTOR: _____ DATE: _____

Skill 41-3 Maintenance of an Intravenous System

	S	U	NP	Comments
1. Assemble equipment, and position client to make intravenous (IV) site accessible.	____	____	____	_____
2. Determine client's/family member's understanding of need for IV therapy.	____	____	____	_____
3. Explain to client/family member each procedure, its purpose, and what is expected of client.	____	____	____	_____
4. Change intravenous solution:	____	____	____	_____
A. Check health care provider's order for type of fluid and infusion rate. Follow the six rights of medication administration.	____	____	____	_____
B. If order is written for keep vein open (KVO) or to keep open (TKO), note date and time when solution was last changed.	____	____	____	_____
C. Determine the compatibility of all IV fluids and additives by consulting appropriate literature or the pharmacy.	____	____	____	_____
D. Determine if current IV access is patent by carefully adjusting the roller clamp to see an increase in flow rate then regulating back to ordered rate. *Lowering IV container below level of IV site for presence of blood return (retrograde) is an unreliable indicator.* Assess swelling, coolness to touch, or tenderness around IV site.	____	____	____	_____
E. Have next solution prepared and accessible at least 1 hour before needed. Check that solution is correct and properly labeled. Check solution expiration date. Observe for precipitate, discoloration, and leakage.	____	____	____	_____
F. Check client's identification by checking identification band and asking client to state name and birth date.	____	____	____	_____
G. Prepare to change solution when less than 25 to 50 mL of fluid remains in container.	____	____	____	_____
H. Be sure drip chamber is at least half full.	____	____	____	_____
I. Perform hand hygiene.	____	____	____	_____
J. Prepare new solution for changing. If using plastic bag, remove protective cover from IV tubing port. If using glass bottle, remove metal cap and metal and rubber disks.	____	____	____	_____
K. Move roller clamp to stop flow rate on existing infusion.	____	____	____	_____
L. Remove old IV fluid container from IV pole.	____	____	____	_____
M. Quickly remove spike from old solution container and, without touching tip, insert spike into new container.	____	____	____	_____
N. Hang new container of solution.	____	____	____	_____
O. Check for air in tubing. If bubbles form, they can be removed by closing the roller clamp below the bubbles, stretching the tubing downward, and tapping the tubing with the finger (bubbles rise in the fluid to the drip chamber). For larger amounts of air, remove using a needleless syringe: swab port with alcohol, allow to dry, insert needleless syringe into port below the air, and aspirate the air into the syringe.	____	____	____	_____
P. Make sure drip chamber is one-third to one-half full. If the drip chamber is too full, pinch off tubing below the drip chamber, invert container, squeeze the drip chamber, release tubing, and hang bag.	____	____	____	_____

Continued

314

	S	U	NP	Comments

Q. Regulate flow to prescribed rate. _____ _____ _____ _____

R. Place time label on side of container, and label with the time hung, the time of anticipated completion, and appropriate intervals. If using polyvinylchloride (PVC) containers, mark only on the label and not the container.

S. Observe client for signs of overhydration or dehydration. _____ _____ _____ _____

T. Periodically check infusion rate. _____ _____ _____ _____

5. Changing infusion tubing:

  A. Determine when new infusion set is needed:

    (1) Agency policy will indicate frequency of routine change for IV administration sets and heparin/saline flushes. _____ _____ _____ _____

    (2) Puncture of infusion tubing requires immediate change. _____ _____ _____ _____

    (3) Contamination of tubing requires immediate change. _____ _____ _____ _____

    (4) Occlusions in tubing following infusion of packed red cells, whole blood, albumin, or other blood components, or administration of incompatible mixtures requires an immediate change. _____ _____ _____ _____

  B. Perform hand hygiene. _____ _____ _____ _____

  C. Open new infusion set, keeping protective coverings over infusion spike and connector site for cannula. Secure all connections. _____ _____ _____ _____

  D. Apply clean gloves. _____ _____ _____ _____

  E. If cannula hub is not visible, remove IV dressing. Do not remove tape securing cannula to skin. _____ _____ _____ _____

  F. Continuous infusion:

    (1) Move roller clamp on new IV tubing to "off" position. _____ _____ _____ _____

    (2) Slow rate of infusion by regulating drip rate on old tubing. Be sure rate is at KVO rate. _____ _____ _____ _____

    (3) Compress drip chamber of old tubing, and fill chamber. _____ _____ _____ _____

    (4) Remove container from IV pole. _____ _____ _____ _____

    (5) Invert container, and remove old tubing from container: keep spike sterile until new tubing connected. Optional: Tape old drip chamber to IV pole without contaminating spike. _____ _____ _____ _____

    (6) Place insertion spike of new tubing into old solution container opening, and hang solution container on IV pole. _____ _____ _____ _____

    (7) Compress and release drip chamber on new tubing; slowly fill drip chamber one-third to one-half full. _____ _____ _____ _____

    (8) Slowly open roller clamp, remove protective cap from adapter (if necessary), and flush new tubing with solution. Stop infusion. Replace cap. Place end of adapter near client's IV site. _____ _____ _____ _____

    (9) Turn roller clamp on old tubing to "off" position. _____ _____ _____ _____

  G. Saline/heparin lock:

    (1) If a loop or short extension tubing is needed because of an awkward IV site placement, use sterile technique to connect the new injection cap to the loop or tubing. _____ _____ _____ _____

    (2) Swab injection cap with antiseptic swab. Insert syringe with 1 to 3 mL saline or heparin flush solution, and inject through the injection cap into the loop or short extension tubing. _____ _____ _____ _____

  H. Optional: Place 2 × 2 gauze under cannula hub. _____ _____ _____ _____

Continued

	S	U	NP	Comments

I. Stabilize cannula hub, and apply pressure over vein just above cannula tip (at least 1½ inches above insertion site). Gently disconnect old tubing from cannula hub, and quickly insert adapter of new tubing into cannula hub.

J. For continuous infusion, open roller clamp on new tubing, allowing solution to run rapidly for 30 to 60 seconds, then regulating IV drip according to health care provider's orders, and monitor rate hourly. Optional: Connect new tubing to electronic infusion device (EID) and regulate.

K. Attach a piece of tape or a preprinted label with date and time of tubing change onto tubing below the drip chamber.

L. Form a loop of tubing, and secure it to client's arm with a strip of tape.

M. If necessary, apply new dressing.

6. Discontinuing peripheral IV access:

A. Observe IV site for signs and symptoms of infection, infiltration, or phlebitis.

B. Review health care provider's order for discontinuation of IV.

C. Explain to client that burning sensation might be felt when catheter is removed. Explain that affected extremity must be held still and how long procedure will take (about 5 minutes or less).

D. Perform hand hygiene. Apply clean gloves.

E. Turn IV tubing roller clamp to "off" position, or turn EID off and then turn roller clamp to "off" position.

F. Remove IV site dressing, stabilizing IV device. Then remove tape securing cannula.

G. Hold cannula, and clean site with antimicrobial swab. Allow to dry completely.

H. Place clean sterile gauze over venipuncture site, apply light pressure, and remove cannula by pulling straight away from insertion site in a slow, steady motion. Keep the cannula parallel to the skin during withdrawal. Do not raise or lift catheter before it is completely out of the vein. Inspect catheter for intactness after removal.

I. Keep gauze in place, and apply continuous pressure to site for 2 to 3 minutes.

J. Apply clean folded gauze dressing over insertion site, and secure with tape.

K. Continue to inspect site for redness, edema, and tenderness for 48 hours.

7. Discard all used supplies, remove gloves, and perform hand hygiene.

STUDENT: _____ DATE: _____

INSTRUCTOR: _____ DATE: _____

CHECKLIST

Skill 41-4 Changing a Peripheral Intravenous Dressing

	S	U	NP	Comments
1. Determine when dressing was last changed. Many institutions require the date and time written on the dressing and date the device was first placed.	___	___	___	_____
2. Perform hand hygiene. Observe present dressing for moisture and intactness.	___	___	___	_____
3. Observe intravenous (IV) system for proper functioning or complications: current flow rate, presence of kinks in infusion tubing or IV catheter. Palpate the skin around the cannula site through the intact dressing for inflammation or subjective complaints of pain or burning.	___	___	___	_____
4. Assess client's body temperature.	___	___	___	_____
5. Assess client's understanding of need for continued IV infusion.	___	___	___	_____
6. Explain procedure and purpose to client and family. Explain that affected extremity must be held still and how long procedure will take.	___	___	___	_____
7. Apply clean gloves.	___	___	___	_____
8. Remove tape, gauze, and/or transparent dressing from old dressing one layer at a time by pulling toward the insertion site, leaving tape that secures IV cannula in place. Be cautious if cannula tubing becomes tangled between two layers of dressing. When removing transparent dressing, hold cannula hub and tubing with nondominant hand.	___	___	___	_____
9. Observe insertion site for signs and/or symptoms of infection: tenderness, redness, swelling, and exudate.	___	___	___	_____
10. If complication exists or if ordered by health care provider, discontinue infusion.	___	___	___	_____
11. If IV is infusing properly, gently remove tape securing cannula. Stabilize cannula with one hand. Use adhesive remover to cleanse skin and remove adhesive residue, if needed.	___	___	___	_____
12. Cleanse insertion site with antiseptic swab using friction. Use the first swab in a horizontal plane, cleansing the skin from side to side. Apply the second swab on a vertical plane, up and down. Apply the final swab in a circular pattern moving outward from the insertion site. Allow each swab to dry completely.	___	___	___	_____
13. Optional: Apply skin protectant solution to the area where the tape or dressing will be applied. Allow to dry.	___	___	___	_____
14. Tape or secure catheter. A. Secure cannula with nondominant hand. B. Apply chevron to stabilize catheter.	___	___	___	_____
15. Apply sterile dressing over site. A. Transparent dressing B. Gauze dressing	___	___	___	_____
16. Remove and discard gloves.	___	___	___	_____
17. Optional: Apply hand board securement device if insertion site is affected by motion of the joint or a protective device if client is active and uses hand freely.	___	___	___	_____
18. Anchor IV tubing with additional pieces of tape if necessary. When using transparent dressing, avoid placing tape over dressing.	___	___	___	_____
19. Place date and time of dressing change and size and gauge of cannula directly on dressing.	___	___	___	_____
20. Discard equipment, and perform hand hygiene.	___	___	___	_____
21. Ensure flow rate is accurate.	___	___	___	_____
22. Monitor client's body temperature.	___	___	___	_____

STUDENT: _____ DATE: _____

INSTRUCTOR: _____ DATE: _____

Skill 44-1 Aspiration Precautions

	S	U	NP	Comments
1. Perform nutritional screening.				
2. Assess clients who are at increased risk for aspiration for signs and symptoms of dysphagia (e.g., cough, pharyngeal pooling, change in voice after swallowing).	___	___	___	_____
3. Observe client during mealtime for signs of dysphagia, and allow client to attempt to feed self. Observe client eat various consistencies of foods and liquids. Note at end of meal if client becomes tired.	___	___	___	_____
4. Ask client about any difficulties with chewing or swallowing various textures of food.	___	___	___	_____
5. Report signs and symptoms of dysphagia to the health care provider.	___	___	___	_____
6. Place identification on client's chart or Kardex indicating that dysphagia is present.	___	___	___	_____
7. Explain to client why you are observing him or her while he or she eats.	___	___	___	_____
8. Perform hand hygiene.				
9. Using penlight and tongue blade, gently inspect mouth for pockets of food.	___	___	___	_____
10. Elevate head of client's bed so that hips are flexed at a 90-degree angle and head is flexed slightly forward, or help client to same position in a chair.	___	___	___	_____
11. Observe client consume various consistencies of foods and liquids.	___	___	___	_____
12. Add thickener to thin liquids to create the consistency of mashed potatoes, or serve client pureed foods.	___	___	___	_____
13. Place ½ to 1 teaspoon of food on unaffected side of the mouth, allowing utensil to touch the mouth or tongue.	___	___	___	_____
14. Place hand on throat to gently palpate swallowing event as it occurs. Swallowing twice is often necessary to clear the pharynx.	___	___	___	_____
15. Provide verbal coaching while feeding client and positive reinforcement to client:				
A. Open your mouth.	___	___	___	_____
B. Feel the food in your mouth.	___	___	___	_____
C. Chew and taste the food.	___	___	___	_____
D. Raise your tongue to the roof of your mouth.	___	___	___	_____
E. Think about swallowing.	___	___	___	_____
F. Close your mouth and swallow.	___	___	___	_____
G. Swallow again.	___	___	___	_____
H. Cough to clear airway.	___	___	___	_____
16. Observe for coughing, choking, gagging, and drooling of food; suction airway as necessary.	___	___	___	_____
17. Provide rest periods as necessary during meal to avoid rushed or forced feeding.	___	___	___	_____
18. Ask client to remain sitting upright for at least 30 minutes after the meal.	___	___	___	_____
19. Help client to perform hand hygiene and perform mouth care.	___	___	___	_____
20. Return client's tray to appropriate place, and perform hand hygiene.	___	___	___	_____
21. Observe client's ability to ingest foods of various textures and thickness.	___	___	___	_____
22. Monitor client's food and fluid intake.				
23. Weigh client weekly at the same time on the same scale.	___	___	___	_____

Continued

318

	S	U	NP	Comments
24. Observe client's oral cavity after meal to detect pockets of food.	___	___	___	_____
25. Document the following in the client's chart: client's tolerance of various food textures, amount of assistance required, position during meal, absence or presence of any symptoms of dysphagia, and amount eaten.	___	___	___	_____
26. Report any coughing, gagging, choking, or swallowing difficulties to nurse in charge or health care provider.	___	___	___	_____

STUDENT: _____ DATE: _____

INSTRUCTOR: _____ DATE: _____

Skill 44-2 Inserting a Small-Bore Nasoenteric Tube for Enteral Feedings

	S	U	NP	Comments
1. Assess client for the need for enteral tube feeding: nothing by mouth (NPO) or insufficient intake for more than 5 days, functional gastrointestinal (GI) tract, unable to ingest sufficient nutrients.	___	___	___	_____
2. Perform hand hygiene. Assess patency of nares. Have client close each nostril alternately and breathe. Examine each naris for patency and skin breakdown.	___	___	___	_____
3. Assess for gag reflex. Place tongue blade in client's mouth, touching uvula to induce a gag response.	___	___	___	_____
4. Review client's medical history for nasal problems (e.g., nosebleeds, oral facial surgery, facial trauma, past history of aspiration, or anticoagulation therapy).	___	___	___	_____
5. Review health care provider's order for type of tube and enteral feeding schedule.	___	___	___	_____
6. Auscultate abdomen for bowel sounds.	___	___	___	_____
7. Perform hand hygiene.	___	___	___	_____
8. Explain procedure to client and how to communicate during intubation by raising index finger to indicate gagging or discomfort.	___	___	___	_____
9. Stand on same side of bed as naris for insertion, and assist client to high-Fowler's position unless contraindicated. Place pillow behind head and shoulders.	___	___	___	_____
10. Place bath towel over chest. Keep facial tissues within reach.	___	___	___	_____
11. Determine length of tube to be inserted, and mark with tape. (Traditional method: Measure distance from tip of nose to earlobe to xiphoid process of sternum.)	___	___	___	_____
12. Prepare nasogastric or nasointestinal tube for intubation:				
A. Do not ice plastic tubes.	___	___	___	_____
B. Inject 10 mL of water from 30-mL or larger Luer-Lok or catheter-tip syringe into the tube.	___	___	___	_____
C. Make certain that guide wire is securely positioned against weighted tip and that both Luer-Lok connections are snugly fitted together.	___	___	___	_____
13. Cut tape 10 cm (4 inches) long, or prepare tube fixation device.	___	___	___	_____
14. Put on clean gloves.	___	___	___	_____
15. Dip tube with surface lubricant into glass of water.	___	___	___	_____
16. Insert tube through nostril to back of throat (posterior nasopharynx). Aim back and down toward ear.	___	___	___	_____
17. Have client flex head toward chest after tube has passed through nasopharynx.	___	___	___	_____
18. Emphasize need to mouth breathe and swallow during the procedure.	___	___	___	_____
19. When tip of tube reaches the carina (about 25 cm [10 inches] in an adult), stop, hold end of tube near ear and listen for air exchange from the distal portion of the tube.	___	___	___	_____
20. Advance tube each time client swallows until desired length has been passed.	___	___	___	_____
21. Check for position of tube in back of throat with penlight and tongue blade.	___	___	___	_____

Continued

	S	U	NP	Comments

22. Perform measures to verify placement of tube. ____ ____ ____ _____

23. After gastric aspirates are obtained, anchor tube ____ ____ ____ _____
to nose and avoid pressure on nares. Mark exit site
with indelible ink. Select one of the following options:
   A. Apply tape:
     (1) Apply tincture of benzoin or other skin ____ ____ ____ _____
       adhesive on tip of client's nose and tube
       and allow it to become "tacky."
     (2) Remove gloves, and split one end of ____ ____ ____ _____
       tape lengthwise 5 cm (2 inches).
     (3) Place the intact end of tape over bridge ____ ____ ____ _____
       of client's nose. Wrap each of the
       5-cm strips around tube as it exits nose
   B. Apply tube fixation device using shaped
     adhesive patch:
     (1) Apply wide end of patch to bridge of nose. ____ ____ ____ _____
     (2) Slip connector around tube as it exits nose. ____ ____ ____ _____

24. Fasten end of nasogastric tube to client's gown ____ ____ ____ _____
using a piece of tape. Do not use safety pins
to fasten the tube to the gown.

25. For intestinal placement, position client on right ____ ____ ____ _____
side when possible until radiological confirmation
of correct placement has been verified.

26. Remove gloves, perform hand hygiene, and assist ____ ____ ____ _____
client to a comfortable position.

27. Obtain x-ray film of abdomen. ____ ____ ____ _____

28. Apply clean gloves, and administer oral hygiene. ____ ____ ____ _____
Cleanse tubing at nostril.

29. Remove gloves, dispose of equipment, and perform ____ ____ ____ _____
hand hygiene.

30. Inspect naris and oropharynx for any irritation ____ ____ ____ _____
after insertion.

31. Ask if client feels comfortable. ____ ____ ____ _____

32. Observe client for any difficulty breathing, ____ ____ ____ _____
coughing, or gagging.

33. Auscultate lung sounds. ____ ____ ____ _____

34. Record and report type and size of tube placed, ____ ____ ____ _____
location of distal tip of tube, client's tolerance of
procedure, pH value, and confirmation of tube
position by x-ray examination.

STUDENT: _____ DATE: _____

INSTRUCTOR: _____ DATE: _____

Skill 44-3 Administering Enteral Feedings via Nasoenteric, Gastrostomy, or Jejunostomy Tubes

	S	U	NP	Comments
1. Assess client's need for enteral tube feedings: impaired swallowing, decreased level of consciousness, head or neck surgery, facial trauma, surgeries of upper alimentary canal.	____	____	____	_____
2. Evaluate client's nutritional status. Obtain baseline weight and laboratory values. Assess client for fluid volume excess or deficit, electrolyte abnormalities, and metabolic abnormalities such as hyperglycemia.	____	____	____	_____
3. Verify health care provider's order for formula, rate, route, and frequency. Laboratory data and bedside assessments, such as finger-stick blood glucose measurement, are also ordered by the health care provider.	____	____	____	_____
4. For feeding tubes placed through the abdominal wall, assess tube site for breakdown, irritation, or drainage.	____	____	____	_____
5. Explain procedure to client.	____	____	____	_____
6. Perform hand hygiene.	____	____	____	_____
7. Auscultate for bowel sounds before feeding.	____	____	____	_____
8. Prepare feeding container to administer formula:				
A. Check expiration date on formula and integrity of container.	____	____	____	_____
B. Have tube feeding at room temperature.	____	____	____	_____
C. Connect tubing to container as needed or prepare ready-to-hang container.	____	____	____	_____
D. Shake formula container well, and fill container with formula. Open stopcock on tubing and fill with formula to remove air. Hang on intravenous (IV) pole.	____	____	____	_____
9. For intermittent feeding have syringe ready and be sure formula is at room temperature.	____	____	____	_____
10. Place client in high-Fowler's position, or elevate head of bed at least 30 degrees.	____	____	____	_____
11. Apply gloves and verify tube placement:				
A. Gastrostomy tube: Attach syringe and aspirate gastric secretions; observe their appearance and check pH. Return aspirated contents to stomach unless the volume exceeds 200 mL. If the volume is greater than 200 mL on two consecutive assessments, hold feeding and notify health care provider.	____	____	____	_____
B. Jejunostomy tube: Aspirate intestinal secretions, observe their appearance and check pH.	____	____	____	_____
12. Check for gastric residual:				
A. Draw up 30 mL of air with syringe. Connect to end of feeding tube. Flush tube with air.	____	____	____	_____
B. Pull back evenly to aspirate gastric contents	____	____	____	_____
C. Return aspirated contents to stomach unless the volume exceeds 200 mL (check agency policy).	____	____	____	_____
13. Flush tubing with 30 mL water.	____	____	____	_____
14. Initiate feeding:				
A. Syringe or intermittent feeding				
(1) Pinch proximal end of the feeding tube.	____	____	____	_____
(2) Remove plunger from syringe and attach barrel of syringe to end of tube.	____	____	____	_____

Continued

322

	S	U	NP	Comments

(3) Fill syringe with measured amount of formula. Release tube and hold syringe high enough to allow it to empty gradually by gravity, refill; repeat until prescribed amount has been delivered to the client. ___ ___ ___ _____

(4) If feeding bag is used, hang feeding bag on an IV pole. Fill bag with prescribed amount of formula and prime tubing. Allow bag to empty gradually over 30 to 60 minutes by setting rate by adjusting roller clamp on tubing or placing on a feeding pump. ___ ___ ___ _____

B. Continuous drip method:

(1) Prime and hang feeding bag and tubing on IV pole. ___ ___ ___ _____

(2) Connect distal end of tubing to the proximal end of the feeding tube. ___ ___ ___ _____

(3) Connect tubing through infusion pump and set rate. ___ ___ ___ _____

15. Advance tube feeding gradually. ___ ___ ___ _____

16. Administer water via feeding tube as ordered with or between feedings. ___ ___ ___ _____

17. Following intermittent infusion or at end of continuous infusion, flush feeding tubing with 30 mL of water. Repeat every 4 to 6 hours. Remove gloves, or perform hand hygiene. ___ ___ ___ _____

18. When tube feedings are not being administered, cap or clamp the proximal end of the feeding tube. ___ ___ ___ _____

19. Rinse bag and tubing with warm water whenever feedings are interrupted. ___ ___ ___ _____

20. Change bag, and use a new administration set every 24 hours. ___ ___ ___ _____

21. Measure amount of aspirate (residual) every 4 to 6 hours. ___ ___ ___ _____

22. Monitor finger-stick blood glucose every 6 hours until maximum administration rate is reached and maintained for 24 hours. ___ ___ ___ _____

23. Monitor intake and output every 8 hours, and calculate daily totals every 24 hours. ___ ___ ___ _____

24. Weigh client daily until maximum administration rate is reached and maintained for 24 hours; then weigh client 3 times per week at the same time using the same scale. ___ ___ ___ _____

25. Monitor laboratory values.

26. For tubes placed through the abdominal wall, inspect insertion site for signs of impaired skin integrity. ___ ___ ___ _____

27. Auscultate bowel sounds. ___ ___ ___ _____

28. Record amount and type of feeding, client's response to tube feeding, patency of tube, condition of skin at tube site for tubes placed in abdominal wall, and any side effects. ___ ___ ___ _____

29. Report client's tolerance and adverse effects. ___ ___ ___ _____

STUDENT: _____ DATE: _____

INSTRUCTOR: _____ DATE: _____

Skill 45-1 Collecting Midstream (Clean-Voided) Urine Specimen

	S	U	NP	Comments
1. Assess client's voiding status:				
A. When client last voided.	___	___	___	_____
B. Level of awareness or developmental stage.	___	___	___	_____
C. Mobility, balance, and physical limitations.	___	___	___	_____
2. Assess client's understanding of purpose of test and method of collection.	___	___	___	_____
3. Provide fluids to drink ½ hour before collection unless contraindicated (i.e., fluid restriction) if client does not feel urge to void.	___	___	___	_____
4. Explain procedure to client:				
A. Reason midstream specimen is necessary.	___	___	___	_____
B. Ways for client and family to assist.	___	___	___	_____
C. Ways to obtain specimen free of feces.	___	___	___	_____
D. Use visual aids (if applicable) to explain procedure.				
5. Identify client, and perform hand hygiene	___	___	___	_____
6. Provide privacy for client by closing door or bed curtain:				
A. Give client or family members cleansing towelette, soap, washcloth, and towel to cleanse perineal area, or assist client as needed.	___	___	___	_____
B. Assist nonambulatory or incapacitated client onto bedpan. Raise head of bed.	___	___	___	_____
C. Using surgical asepsis, open sterile kit or prepare sterile supplies.	___	___	___	_____
D. Apply sterile gloves after opening sterile specimen cup, placing cap with sterile inside surface up, and do not touch inside of container or cap.	___	___	___	_____
E. Pour antiseptic solution over cotton balls or gauze pads unless kit contains prepared gauze pads in antiseptic solution.	___	___	___	_____
F. Perform urine collection by assisting or allowing client to independently cleanse perineum and collect specimen:	___	___	___	_____
(1) Female				
a. Spread labia with thumb and forefinger of nondominant hand.	___	___	___	_____
b. Cleanse area with cotton ball or gauze, moving from front (above urethral orifice) to back (toward anus). Using a fresh swab each time, repeat front-to-back motion three times (begin with center, then left side, then right side).	___	___	___	_____
c. If agency policy indicates, rinse area with sterile water, and dry with dry cotton ball or gauze.	___	___	___	_____
d. While continuing to hold labia apart, have client initiate stream. After client achieves a stream, pass container into stream and collect 30 to 60 mL.	___	___	___	_____
(2) Male				
a. Hold penis with one hand, and using circular motion and antiseptic swab, cleanse end of penis, moving from center to outside. In uncircumcised men, retract the foreskin before cleansing.	___	___	___	_____
b. If agency procedure indicates, rinse area with sterile water, and dry with cotton or gauze.	___	___	___	_____

Continued

324

	S	U	NP	Comments
c. After client has initiated urine stream, pass specimen collection container into stream, and collect 30 to 60 mL.	_____	_____	_____	_____
7. Remove specimen container before flow of urine stops and before releasing labia or penis. Client finishes voiding in bedpan or toilet.	_____	_____	_____	_____
8. Replace cap securely on specimen container (touch outside only).	_____	_____	_____	_____
9. Cleanse any urine from exterior surface of container, and place in a plastic specimen bag as required by agency.	_____	_____	_____	_____
10. Remove and empty bedpan (if applicable), and assist client to comfortable position.	_____	_____	_____	_____
11. Label specimen, and attach laboratory requisition.	_____	_____	_____	_____
12. Remove gloves, dispose of them in proper receptacle, and perform hand hygiene.	_____	_____	_____	_____
13. Transport specimen to laboratory within 15 to 30 minutes, or refrigerate immediately.	_____	_____	_____	_____
14. Record date and time urine specimen was obtained in nurses' notes.	_____	_____	_____	_____
15. Notify health care provider of any significant abnormalities.	_____	_____	_____	_____

STUDENT: _____ DATE: _____

INSTRUCTOR: _____ DATE: _____

CHECKLIST
Skill 45-2 Inserting a Straight or Indwelling Catheter

	S	U	NP	Comments
1. Review client's medical record, including health care provider's order and nurses' notes.	___	___	___	_____
2. Identify client using two client identifiers.	___	___	___	_____
3. Assess status of client:				
A. Ask client when last voided, or check input and output (I&O) flow sheet, or palpate bladder.	___	___	___	_____
B. Level of awareness or developmental stage.	___	___	___	_____
C. Mobility and physical limitations of client.	___	___	___	_____
D. Client's gender and age.	___	___	___	_____
E. Perform hand hygiene. Apply clean gloves. Inspect perineum for erythema, drainage, and odor.	___	___	___	_____
F. Note any pathological condition that will impair passage of catheter (e.g., enlarged prostate in men).	___	___	___	_____
G. Allergies.	___	___	___	_____
4. Assess client's knowledge of the purpose for catheterization.	___	___	___	_____
5. Explain procedure to client.	___	___	___	_____
6. Arrange for extra nursing personnel to assist as necessary.	___	___	___	_____
7. Perform hand hygiene.	___	___	___	_____
8. Close curtain or door.	___	___	___	_____
9. Raise bed to appropriate working height.	___	___	___	_____
10. Facing client, stand on left side of bed if right-handed (on right side of bed if left-handed). Clear the bedside table, and arrange equipment.	___	___	___	_____
11. If side rails are in use, raise side rail on opposite side of bed, and put side rail down on working side.	___	___	___	_____
12. Place waterproof pad under client.	___	___	___	_____
13. Position client:				
A. Female client:				
(1) Assist to dorsal recumbent position (supine with knees flexed). Ask client to relax thighs so you can rotate the hips.	___	___	___	_____
(2) Position female client in side-lying (Sims') position with upper leg flexed at hip if unable to assume dorsal recumbent position.	___	___	___	_____
B. Male client:				
(1) Assist to supine position with thighs slightly abducted.	___	___	___	_____
14. Drape client:				
A. Female client: Drape with bath blanket. Place blanket diamond fashion over client, with one corner at client's midsection, side corners over each thigh and abdomen, and last corner over perineum.	___	___	___	_____
B. Male client: Drape upper trunk with bath blanket, and cover lower extremities with bed sheets, exposing only genitalia.	___	___	___	_____
15. Wearing disposable gloves, wash perineal area with soap and water as needed; dry thoroughly. Remove and discard gloves; perform hand hygiene.	___	___	___	_____
16. Position light source to illuminate perineal area. (Have an assistant hold flashlight if necessary.)	___	___	___	_____
17. Open package containing drainage system; place drainage bag over edge of bottom bed frame, and bring drainage tube up between side rails and mattress.	___	___	___	_____

Continued

326

	S	U	NP	Comments

18. Open catheterization kit according to directions, keeping bottom of container sterile.

19. Place plastic bag that contained kit within reach of work area to use as a waterproof bag to dispose of used supplies.

20. Apply sterile gloves.

21. Organize supplies on sterile field. Open inner sterile package containing catheter. Pour sterile antiseptic solution into correct compartment containing sterile cotton balls. Open packet containing lubricant. Remove specimen container (lid should be placed loosely on top) and prefilled syringe from collection compartment of tray, and set them aside on sterile field.

22. Generously lubricate 2.5 to 5 cm (1 to 2 inches) of catheter for women and 12.5 to 17.7 cm (5 to 7 inches) for men.

23. Apply sterile drape:
   A. Female client:
      (1) Allow top edge of drape to form a cuff over both gloved hands. Place drape down on bed between client's thighs. Slip cuffed edge just under buttocks, taking care not to touch contaminated surface with gloves. If using Sims' position (side-lying), take extra precautions to cover rectal area with a sterile drape.
      (2) Pick up fenestrated sterile drape, and allow it to unfold without touching an unsterile object. Apply drape over perineum, exposing labia and being sure not to touch contaminated surface.
   B. Male client (There are two methods for draping depending on preferences.):
      (1) First method: Apply drape over thighs and under penis without completely opening fenestrated drape.
      (2) Second method: Apply drape over thighs just below penis. Pick up fenestrated sterile drape, allow it to unfold, and drape it over penis with fenestrated slit resting over penis.

24. Place sterile tray and contents on sterile drape. Open specimen container. Actual positioning of sterile tray will depend on client size and positioning. This method works best with flexible, average-size clients.

25. Cleanse urethral meatus:
   A. Female client:
      (1) With nondominant hand, carefully retract labia to fully expose urethral meatus. Maintain position of nondominant hand throughout procedure.
      (2) Using forceps in sterile dominant hand, pick up cotton ball saturated with antiseptic solution and clean perineal area, wiping from front to back from clitoris toward anus. Using a new cotton ball for each area, wipe along the far labial fold, near labial fold, and directly over center of urethral meatus.
   B. Male client:
      (1) If client is not circumcised, retract foreskin with nondominant hand. Grasp penis at shaft just below glans. Retract urethral meatus between thumb and forefinger. Maintain nondominant hand in this position throughout procedure.

Continued

	S	U	NP	Comments

(2) With dominant hand, pick up cotton ball with forceps and clean penis. Move in a circular motion from urethral meatus down to base of glans. Repeat cleansing three more times, using a clean cotton ball each time.

26. Pick up catheter with gloved dominant hand 7.5 to 10 cm (3 to 4 inches) from catheter tip. Hold end of catheter loosely coiled in palm of dominant hand. (Optional: May grasp catheter with forceps.) Place distal end of catheter in urine tray receptacle if straight catheterization is ordered.

27. Insert catheter:
   A. Female client:
      (1) Ask client to bear down gently as if to void, and slowly insert catheter through urethral meatus.
      (2) Advance catheter a total of 5 to 7.5 cm (2 to 3 inches) in adult or **until urine flows out of catheter's end.** When urine appears, advance catheter another 2.5 to 5 cm (1 to 2 inches). **Do not use force to insert a catheter.**
      (3) Release labia, and hold catheter securely with nondominant hand. Slowly inflate balloon if using retention catheter.
   B. Male client:
      (1) Lift penis to position perpendicular to client's body, and apply light traction
      (2) Ask client to bear down as if to void, and slowly insert catheter through urethral meatus.
      (3) Advance catheter 17 to 22.5 cm (7 to 9 inches) in adult **or until urine flows out catheter's end.** If you feel resistance, withdraw catheter; do not force it through urethra. When urine appears, advance catheter another 2.5 to 5 cm (1 to 2 inches). **Do not use force to insert a catheter.**
      (4) Lower penis, and hold catheter securely in nondominant hand. Place end of catheter in urine tray. Inflate balloon if using retention catheter.
      (5) Reduce (or reposition) the foreskin.

28. Collect urine specimen as needed. Fill specimen cup or jar to desired level (20 to 30 mL) by holding end of catheter in dominant hand over cup.

29. Allow bladder to empty fully (about 800 to 1000 mL) unless institution policy restricts maximal volume of urine to drain with each catheterization. Check institution policy before beginning catheterization. If a restriction is in place, the range is often 800 to 1000 mL.

30. Inflate balloon fully per manufacturer's recommendation, and then release catheter with nondominant hand and pull gently.

31. Attach end of retention catheter to collecting tube of drainage system. Make sure drainage bag is below level of bladder; attach bag to bed frame; do not place bag on side rails of bed.

32. Anchor catheter:
   A. Female client: Secure catheter tubing to inner thigh with strip of nonallergenic tape (or multipurpose tube holders with a Velcro strap). Allow for slack so movement of thigh does not create tension on catheter.

Continued

328

	S	U	NP	Comments
B. Male client: Secure catheter tubing to top of thigh or lower abdomen (with penis directed toward chest). Allow slack in catheter so movement does not create tension on catheter.	____	____	____	_____
33. Assist client to comfortable position. Wash and dry perineal area as needed.	____	____	____	_____
34. Remove gloves, and dispose of equipment, drapes, and urine in proper receptacles.	____	____	____	_____
35. Perform hand hygiene.	____	____	____	_____
36. Palpate bladder.	____	____	____	_____
37. Ask about client's comfort.	____	____	____	_____
38. Observe character and amount of urine in drainage system.	____	____	____	_____
39. Determine that there is no urine leaking from catheter or tubing connections.	____	____	____	_____
40. Report and record type and size of catheter inserted, amount of fluid used to inflate the balloon, characteristics of urine, amount of urine, reasons for catheterization, specimen collection if appropriate, and client's response to procedure and teaching concepts.	____	____	____	_____
41. Initiate I&O record.	____	____	____	_____
42. If catheter is definitely in bladder and no urine is produced within an hour, immediately report absence of urine to health care provider.	____	____	____	_____

STUDENT: _____ DATE: _____

INSTRUCTOR: _____ DATE: _____

Skill 45-3 Indwelling Catheter Care

	S	U	NP	Comments
1. Assess for episode of bowel incontinence or client discomfort, or provide care as per agency routine as part of hygiene measures.	____	____	____	_____
2. Explain procedure to client. Offer opportunity to perform self-care to able client.	____	____	____	_____
3. Close door or bedside curtain.	____	____	____	_____
4. Perform hand hygiene.	____	____	____	_____
5. Position client:				
A. Female: Dorsal recumbent position	____	____	____	_____
B. Male: Supine or Fowler's position	____	____	____	_____
6. Place waterproof pad under client.	____	____	____	_____
7. Drape bath blanket on client so that only perineal area is exposed.	____	____	____	_____
8. Apply clean gloves.	____	____	____	_____
9. Remove anchor device to free catheter tubing.	____	____	____	_____
10. With nondominant hand:				
A. Female: Gently retract labia to fully expose urethral meatus and catheter insertion site, maintaining position of hand throughout procedure.	____	____	____	_____
B. Male: Retract foreskin if not circumscribed, and hold penis at shaft just below glans, maintaining position throughout procedure.	____	____	____	_____
11. Assess urethral meatus and surrounding tissue for inflammation, swelling, and discharge. Note amount, color, odor, and consistency of discharge. Ask client if any burning or discomfort is felt.	____	____	____	_____
12. Cleanse perineal tissue:				
A. Female: Use clean cloth, soap, and water. Cleanse around urethral meatus and catheter. Cleaning from pubis toward anus, clean labia minora. Use a clean side of cloth for each wipe. Clean around anus last. Dry each area well.	____	____	____	_____
B. Male: While spreading urethral meatus, cleanse around catheter first, and then wipe in circular motion around meatus and glans.	____	____	____	_____
13. Reassess urethral meatus for discharge.	____	____	____	_____
14. While stabilizing the catheter with nondominant hand, cleanse length of the catheter from meatus to tubing in a circular motion. Follow agency guidelines.	____	____	____	_____
15. In male client reduce (or reposition) the foreskin after care.	____	____	____	_____
16. Place client in a safe, comfortable position.	____	____	____	_____
17. Dispose of contaminated supplies, remove gloves, and perform hand hygiene.	____	____	____	_____
18. Report and record presence and characteristics of drainage, condition of perineal tissue, and any discomfort reported by client.	____	____	____	_____
19. If infection is suspected, report findings to health care provider.	____	____	____	_____

STUDENT: _____   DATE: _____

INSTRUCTOR: _____   DATE: _____

Skill 45-4 Closed Catheter Irrigation

	S	U	NP	Comments

1. Assess client's record to determine:
   A. Purpose of bladder irrigation.
   B. Prescriber's order for type and amount of irrigant (e.g., saline).
   C. Type of irrigation: continuous or intermittent.
   D. Type of catheter used. (NOTE: Appropriate catheter should be inserted during the original catheterization.)
      (1) Single lumen (single use) for open intermittent irrigation only.
      (2) Double lumen (one lumen to inflate balloon, one to allow outflow of urine).
      (3) Triple lumen (one lumen to inflate balloon, one to instill irrigation solution, one to allow outflow of urine).
2. Assess the following:
   A. Color of urine and presence of, mucus, clots, or sediment.
   B. Palpate bladder.
   C. Existing closed irrigation system.
      (1) Note if fluid entering bladder and fluid draining from bladder are in approximate proportions.
      (2) Determine that drainage tubing is not kinked, clamped off incorrectly, or looped below bladder level.
      (3) Note amount of fluid remaining in existing irrigating solution container.
3. Review intake and output (I&O) record.
4. Assess client for presence of bladder spasms and discomfort.
5. Identify client using two client identifiers.
6. Assess client's knowledge regarding purpose of performing catheter irrigations.
7. Perform hand hygiene, and apply clean gloves for closed methods.
8. Provide privacy by pulling bed curtains closed. Fold back covers so that catheter is exposed. Cover client's upper torso with bath blanket.
9. Position client in dorsal recumbent or supine position.
10. Closed intermittent irrigation or instillation with double-lumen catheter:
    A. Prepare prescribed sterile solution in sterile graduated cup.
    B. Clamp indwelling retention catheter just below the specimen port.
    C. Draw sterile solution into syringe using aseptic technique.
    D. Apply gloves, and cleanse injection port with antiseptic swab (same port used for specimen collection).
    E. Insert hub of syringe through port at 30-degree angle toward bladder using needleless or blunt needle syringe system.
    F. Slowly inject fluid into catheter and bladder.
    G. Withdraw syringe, remove clamp, and allow solution to drain into drainage bag. If an instillation, keep catheter clamped to allow solution to remain in bladder for ordered time.

Continued

	S	U	NP	Comments

11. Closed continuous irrigation:
    A. Apply gloves, and using aseptic technique, insert spike of sterile irrigation tubing into bag of sterile irrigating solution. _____ _____ _____ _____
    B. Close clamp on tubing, and hang bag of solution on intravenous (IV) pole. _____ _____ _____ _____
    C. Open clamp, and allow solution to flow through tubing, keeping end of tubing sterile. Close clamp. _____ _____ _____ _____
    D. Use aseptic technique to wipe off irrigation port of triple-lumen catheter, or attach sterile Y connector to double-lumen catheter and then attach to irrigation tubing. _____ _____ _____ _____
    E. Be sure that drainage bag and tubing are securely connected to drainage port of triple-lumen catheter or other arm of Y connector. _____ _____ _____ _____
    F. For continuous drainage, calculate drip rate and adjust clamp on irrigation tubing accordingly. Be sure that clamp on drainage tubing is open, and check volume of drainage in drainage bag. Make sure drainage tubing is patent, and avoid kinks. _____ _____ _____ _____
    G. For intermittent flow, clamp tubing on drainage system, open clamp on irrigation tubing, and allow prescribed amount of fluid to enter bladder (100 mL is normal for adults). Close irrigation clamp, and then open drainage tubing clamp. (Optional: Leave clamp closed for 20 to 30 minutes if ordered.) _____ _____ _____ _____
12. When procedure completed, dispose of contaminated supplies, remove gloves, and perform hand hygiene. _____ _____ _____ _____
13. Calculate amount of irrigation or instillation fluid, and subtract from total output. _____ _____ _____ _____
14. Assess characteristics of output: viscosity, color, and presence of matter (e.g., sediment, clots, blood). _____ _____ _____ _____
15. Record type and amount of irrigation solution used, amount returned as drainage, and the character of drainage. _____ _____ _____ _____
16. Record and report any findings such as complaints of bladder spasms, inability to instill fluid into bladder, and/or presence of blood clots. _____ _____ _____ _____

STUDENT: _____ DATE: _____

INSTRUCTOR: _____ DATE: _____

CHECKLIST
Skill 46-1 Administering a Cleansing Enema

	S	U	NP	Comments
1. Assess status of client: last bowel movement, normal bowel patterns, hemorrhoids, mobility, external sphincter control, and abdominal pain.	___	___	___	_____
2. Assess for presence of increased intracranial pressure, glaucoma, or recent rectal or prostate surgery.	___	___	___	_____
3. Check client's medical record to clarify the rationale for the enema.	___	___	___	_____
4. Review health care provider's order for enema.	___	___	___	_____
5. Inspect for abdominal distension, and auscultate for bowel sounds.	___	___	___	_____
6. Determine client's level of understanding of purpose of enema.	___	___	___	_____
7. Correctly identify client, and explain procedure.	___	___	___	_____
8. Collect appropriate equipment, and arrange at bedside.	___	___	___	_____
9. Assemble enema bag with appropriate solution and rectal tube.	___	___	___	_____
10. Perform hand hygiene, and apply gloves.				
11. Provide privacy by closing curtains around bed or closing door.	___	___	___	_____
12. Raise bed to appropriate working height: raise side rail on client's left.	___	___	___	_____
13. Assist client into left side-lying (Sims') position with right knee flexed. You can also place children in dorsal recumbent position.	___	___	___	_____
14. Place waterproof pad under hips and buttocks.	___	___	___	_____
15. Cover client with bath blanket, exposing only rectal area, clearly visualizing anus.	___	___	___	_____
16. Place bedpan or commode in easily accessible position. If client will be expelling contents in toilet, ensure that toilet is free. (If client will be getting up to bathroom to expel enema, place client's slippers and bathrobe in easily accessible position.)	___	___	___	_____
17. Administer enema:				
A. Enema bag:				
(1) Add warmed solution to enema bag: warm tap water as it flows from faucet; place saline container in basin of hot water before adding saline to enema bag; check temperature of solution by pouring small amount of solution over inner wrist.	___	___	___	_____
(2) Raise container, release clamp, and allow solution to flow long enough to fill tubing.	___	___	___	_____
(3) Reclamp tubing.	___	___	___	_____
(4) Lubricate 6 to 8 cm (2 ½ to 3 inches) of tip of rectal tube with lubricating jelly.	___	___	___	_____
(5) Gently separate buttocks, and locate anus. Instruct client to relax by breathing out slowly through mouth.	___	___	___	_____
(6) Insert tip of rectal tube slowly by pointing tip in direction of client's umbilicus.	___	___	___	_____
(7) Hold tubing in rectum constantly until end of fluid instillation.	___	___	___	_____
(8) Open regulating clamp, and allow solution to enter slowly with container at client's hip level.	___	___	___	_____

Continued

	S	U	NP	Comments

(9) Raise height of enema container slowly to appropriate level above anus: 30 to 45 cm (12 to 18 inches) for high enema, 30 cm (12 inches) for regular enema, 7.5 cm (3 inches) for low enema. Instillation time varies with the volume of solution administered. ____ ____ ____ _____

(10) Lower container or clamp tubing if client complains of cramping or if fluid escapes around rectal tube. ____ ____ ____ _____

(11) Clamp tubing after all solution is instilled. ____ ____ ____ _____

B. Prepackaged disposable container:

(1) Remove plastic cap from rectal tip. Tip is already lubricated, but you can apply more jelly as needed. ____ ____ ____ _____

(2) Gently separate buttocks, and locate rectum. Instruct client to relax by breathing out slowly through mouth. ____ ____ ____ _____

(3) Insert tip of bottle gently into rectum. ____ ____ ____ _____

(4) Squeeze bottle until all of solution has entered rectum and colon. Instruct client to retain solution until the urge to defecate occurs, usually 2 to 5 minutes. ____ ____ ____ _____

18. Place layers of toilet tissue around tube at anus, and gently withdraw rectal tube. ____ ____ ____ _____

19. Explain to client that feeling of distention is normal. Ask client to retain solution as long as possible while lying quietly in bed. (For infant or young child, gently hold buttocks together for a few minutes.) ____ ____ ____ _____

20. Discard enema container and tubing in proper receptacle, or rinse out thoroughly with warm soap and water if reusing container. ____ ____ ____ _____

21. Assist client to bathroom, or help to position client on bedpan. ____ ____ ____ _____

22. Observe character of feces and solution (caution client against flushing toilet before inspection). ____ ____ ____ _____

23. Assist client as needed in washing anal area with warm soap and water (if administering perineal care, use gloves). ____ ____ ____ _____

24. Remove and discard gloves, and perform hand hygiene. ____ ____ ____ _____

25. Inspect color, consistency, amount of stool, and fluid passed. ____ ____ ____ _____

26. Assess condition of abdomen; cramping, rigidity, or distention indicates a serious problem. ____ ____ ____ _____

STUDENT: _____ DATE: _____

INSTRUCTOR: _____ DATE: _____

Skill 46-2 Inserting and Maintaining a Nasogastric Tube for Gastric Decompression

	S	U	NP	Comments
1. Inspect condition of client's nasal and oral cavity.	___	___	___	_____
2. Ask if client has had history of nasal surgery, and note if deviated nasal septum is present.	___	___	___	_____
3. Auscultate for bowel sounds. Palpate client's abdomen for distention, pain, and rigidity.	___	___	___	_____
4. Assess client's level of consciousness and ability to follow instructions.	___	___	___	_____
5. Determine if client has had a nasogastric (NG) tube insertion in the past and which naris was used.	___	___	___	_____
6. Check medical record for surgeon's order, type of NG tube to be placed, and whether tube is to be attached to suction or drainage bag.	___	___	___	_____
7. Prepare equipment at the bedside.	___	___	___	_____
8. Cut a piece of tape about 4 inches (10 cm) long, and split one end in half to form a V, or have NG tube fixator device available.	___	___	___	_____
9. Identify client, and explain procedure.	___	___	___	_____
10. Position client in high Fowler's position with pillows behind head and shoulders. Raise bed to a horizontal level comfortable for the nurse.	___	___	___	_____
11. Have client blow nose. Place bath towel over client's chest; give facial tissues to client. Place emesis basin within reach.	___	___	___	_____
12. Pull curtain around the bed, or close room door.	___	___	___	_____
13. Stand on client's right side if right-handed, left side if left-handed.	___	___	___	_____
14. Perform hand hygiene, and apply clean gloves.	___	___	___	_____
15. Measure distance to insert tube:				
A. Traditional method: Measure distance from tip of nose to earlobe to xiphoid process.	___	___	___	_____
B. Hanson method: First mark 50-cm point on tube, and then do traditional measurement. Tube insertion should be to midway point between 50 cm (20 inches) and traditional mark.	___	___	___	_____
16. Mark length of tube to be inserted with small piece of tape placed so it can easily be removed.	___	___	___	_____
17. Curve 10 to 15 cm (4 to 6 inches) of end of tube tightly around index finger, then release.	___	___	___	_____
18. Lubricate 7.5 to 10 cm (3 to 4 inches) of end of tube with water-soluble lubricating jelly.	___	___	___	_____
19. Alert client that procedure is to begin.	___	___	___	_____
20. Initially instruct client to extend neck back against pillow; insert tube gently and slowly through naris, aiming end of tube downward.	___	___	___	_____
21. Continue to pass tube along floor of nasal passage, aiming downward toward client's ear. If resistance is met, apply gentle downward pressure to advance tube. (Do not force past resistance.)	___	___	___	_____
22. If resistance is met, try to rotate the tube and see if it advances. If still resistant, withdraw tube, allow client to rest, relubricate tube, and insert into other naris.	___	___	___	_____
23. Continue insertion of tube until just past nasopharynx by gently rotating tube toward opposite nostril and then pass tube just above oropharynx.	___	___	___	_____

Continued

	S	U	NP	Comments

A. Stop tube advancement, allow client to relax, and provide tissues.

B. Explain to client that next step requires that client swallow. Give client glass of water unless contraindicated.

24. With tube just above oropharynx, instruct client to flex head forward, take a small sip of water, and swallow. Advance tube 2.5 to 5 cm (1 to 2 inches) with each swallow of water. If client is not allowed fluids, instruct to dry swallow or suck air through straw.

25. If client begins to cough, gag, or choke, withdraw tube slightly (do not remove the tube) and stop tube advancement. Instruct client to breathe easily and take sips of water.

26. If client continues to gag and cough or complains that tube feels as though it is coiling in the back of throat, check back of oropharynx using tongue blade. If tube has coiled, withdraw it until the tip is back in the oropharynx. Then reinsert with client swallowing.

27. After client relaxes, continue to advance tube with swallowing until tape or mark is reached. Temporarily anchor tube to client's cheek with a piece of tape until tube placement is checked.

28. Verify tube placement: (Check agency policy for preferred methods for checking NG tube placement.)
    A. Ask client to talk.
    B. Inspect posterior pharynx for presence of coiled tube.
    C. Attach Asepto or catheter-tipped syringe to end of tube, and aspirate gently back on syringe to obtain gastric contents, observing color.
    D. Measure pH of aspirate with color-coded pH paper with range of whole numbers greater than 11.
    E. Have ordered x-ray examination performed of chest/abdomen.
    F. If tube is not in stomach, advance another 2.5 to 5 cm (1 to 2 inches) and repeat Steps 28A through 28E to check tube position.

29. Anchoring tube:
    A. After tube is properly inserted and positioned, either clamp end or connect it to drainage bag or suction source.
    B. Tape tube to nose; avoid putting pressure on nares.
       (1) Apply small amount of tincture of benzoin to lower end of nose, and allow to dry (optional).
       (2) Apply tape to nose, leaving splint ends free. Be sure top end of tape over nose is secure.
       (3) Carefully wrap two split ends of tape around tube.
       (4) Alternative: Apply tube fixation device using shaped adhesive patch.
    C. Fasten end of NG tube to client's gown by looping rubber band around tube in slip knot. Pin rubber band to gown (provides slack for movement).

30. Unless health care provider orders otherwise, head of bed should be elevated 30 degrees.

31. Once placement is confirmed:
    A. Place a mark, either a red mark or tape, on the tube to indicate where the tube exists in the nose.
    B. Measure the tube length from nares to connector is an alternate method.
    C. Document the tube length in the client record.

Continued

336

	S	U	NP	Comments

32. Remove gloves, and wash hands.
33. Tube irrigation:
   A. Perform hand hygiene, and apply gloves.
   B. Check for tube placement in stomach (see Step 28). Reconnect NG tube to connecting tube.
   C. Draw up 30 mL of normal saline into Asepto or catheter-tipped syringe.
   D. Clamp NG tube. Disconnect from connection tubing, and lay end of connection tubing on towel.
   E. Insert tip of irrigating syringe into end of NG tube. Remove clamp. Hold syringe with tip pointed at floor, and inject saline slowly and evenly. Do not force solution.
   F. If resistance occurs, check for kinks in tubing. Turn client onto left side. Repeated resistance should be reported to the health care provider.
   G. After instilling saline, immediately aspirate or pull back slowly on syringe to withdraw fluid. If amount aspirated is greater than amount instilled, record the difference as output. If amount aspirated is less than amount instilled, record the difference as intake.
   H. Reconnect NG tube to drainage or suction. (If solution does not return, repeat irrigation.)
   I. Remove gloves, and perform hand hygiene.
34. Discontinuation of NG tube:
   A. Verify order to discontinue NG tube.
   B. Explain procedure to client, and reassure that removal is less distressing than insertion.
   C. Perform hand hygiene, and apply disposable gloves.
   D. Turn off suction, and disconnect NG tube from drainage bag or suction. Remove tape or fixation device from bridge of nose, and unpin tube from gown.
   E. Stand on client's right side if right-handed, left side if left-handed.
   F. Hand the client facial tissue; place clean towel across chest. Instruct client to take and hold a deep breath.
   G. Clamp or kink tubing securely, and then pull tube out steadily and smoothly into towel held in other hand while client holds breath.
   H. Measure amount of drainage, and note character of content. Dispose of tube and drainage equipment into proper container.
   I. Clean nares, and provide mouth care.
   J. Position client comfortably, and explain procedure for drinking fluids, if not contraindicated.
35. Clean equipment, and return to proper place. Place soiled linen in utility room or proper receptacle.
36. Remove gloves, and perform hand hygiene.
37. After tube removal, auscultate client's bowel sounds and periodically check for abdominal distention.

STUDENT: _____ DATE: _____

INSTRUCTOR: _____ DATE: _____

Skill 46-3 Pouching an Ostomy

	S	U	NP	Comments
1. Perform hand hygiene, and auscultate for bowel sounds.				
2. Apply gloves, and observe skin barrier and pouch for leakage and length of time in place.				
3. Observe stoma for color, swelling, trauma, and healing; stoma is normally moist and reddish-pink. Assess type of stoma. Stoma is flush with the skin or a budlike protrusion on the abdomen.				
4. Measure the stoma with each pouching change. Follow pouch manufacturer's directions and measuring guide as to which pouch to use based on client's stoma size.				
5. Observe abdominal incision (if present).				
6. Observe effluent from stoma, and keep a record of intake and output. Ask client about skin tenderness. Remove gloves, and perform hand hygiene.				
7. When assessing skin for irritation, check that pouching system is not leaking.				
8. Check existing bag for gas accumulation.				
9. Assess abdomen for best type of pouching system to use. Consider the following:				
A. Contour and peristomal plane.				
B. Presence of scars, incisions.				
C. Location and type of stoma.				
10. Select appropriate pouching system. Options include:				
A. One-piece pouch with skin barrier already attached.				
B. Pre-cut pouch and skin barrier.				
C. Two-piece pouch system which consists of pouch that detaches from skin barrier and remains around client's stoma for several days.				
11. To minimize skin irritation, avoid unnecessary changing of entire pouching system.				
12. Assess the client's self-care ability to determine the best type of pouching system to use.				
13. After skin barrier and pouch removal, assess skin around stoma, noting scars, folds, skin breakdown, and peristomal suture line, if present. Keep pouch loosely attached to stoma to collect any drainage while changing the system. Remove gloves, and perform hand hygiene.				
14. Determine client's emotional response and knowledge and understanding of an ostomy and its care.				
15. Explain procedure to client; encourage client's interaction and questions.				
16. Perform hand hygiene. Assemble equipment, and close room curtains or door.				
17. Position client either standing or supine, and drape. If seated, position either on or in front of the toilet. Perform hand hygiene, and apply clean gloves.				
18. Place towel or disposable waterproof barrier under the client.				
19. If not done in Step 2, completely remove used pouch and skin barrier gently by pushing the skin away from the barrier. Use an adhesive remover to facilitate removal of the skin barrier.				
20. Cleanse peristomal skin gently with warm tap water using gauze pads or clean washcloth; do not scrub the skin; dry completely by patting the skin with gauze or towel.				

Continued

338

21. Measure the stoma for correct size of pouching system needed, using the manufacturer's measuring guide.

22. Select appropriate pouch for client based on client assessment. With a custom cut-to-fit pouch, use an ostomy guide to cut opening on the pouch $1/16$ inch larger than stoma before removing backing. Prepare pouch by removing backing from barrier and adhesive. With ileostomy, apply thin circle of barrier paste around opening in pouch; allow to dry.

23. Apply the skin barrier and pouch. If creases next to stoma occur, use barrier paste to fill in; let dry 1 to 2 minutes.
    A. For one-piece pouching system:
       (1) Use skin sealant wipes on skin directly under adhesive skin barrier or pouch; allow to dry. Press the adhesive backing of the pouch and/or skin barrier smoothly against the skin, starting from the bottom and working up and around the sides.
       (2) Hold pouch by barrier, center over stoma, and press down gently on barrier; bottom of pouch should point toward client's knees.
       (3) Maintain gentle finger pressure around the barrier for 1 to 2 minutes.
    B. For two-piece pouching system:
       (1) Apply flange (barrier with adhesive) as in steps above for one-piece system. Then snap on pouch and maintain finger pressure.
    C. For both pouching systems gently tug on the pouch in a downward direction.

24. Gently press on the pectin or karaya flange to facilitate adhesion.

25. Although many ostomy pouches are odor-proof, some nurses and clients like to put a small amount of ostomy deodorant into the pouch. Do not use "home remedies," such as aspirin, to control ostomy odor.

26. Fold bottom of drainable open-ended pouches up once, and close using a closure device such as a clamp (or follow manufacturer's instructions for closure).

27. Properly dispose of old pouch and soiled equipment. Consider spraying deodorant in room if needed.

28. Remove gloves, and perform hand hygiene.

29. Ask if client feels discomfort around stoma.

30. Observe condition of skin barrier and adhesive.

31. Auscultate bowel sounds, and observe characteristics of stool.

32. Observe client's nonverbal behaviors while applying the pouch. Ask if client has any questions about pouching.

CHECKLIST
Skill 47-1 Moving and Positioning Clients in Bed

	S	U	NP	Comments
1. Assess client's body alignment and comfort level while client is lying down.				
2. Assess for risk factors that contribute to complications of immobility:				
A. Paralysis, hemiparesis, and/or decreased sensation.	___	___	___	_____
B. Impaired mobility from traction, arthritis, or other contributing disease processes.	___	___	___	_____
C. Impaired circulation.	___	___	___	_____
D. Age: very young, older adults.	___	___	___	_____
E. Level of consciousness and mental status.				
3. Refer to appropriate algorithm for repositioning client. Assess client's physical ability to help with moving and positioning:				
A. Age.	___	___	___	_____
B. Ability to understand instructions and cooperate with nursing staff.	___	___	___	_____
C. Disease process.	___	___	___	_____
D. Strength, coordination.	___	___	___	_____
E. Range of motion (ROM).	___	___	___	_____
4. Assess client's height, weight, and body shape.	___	___	___	_____
5. Assess health care provider's orders. Clarify whether any positions are contraindicated because of client's condition (e.g., spinal cord injury; respiratory difficulties, joint replacement, certain neurological conditions).	___	___	___	_____
6. Perform hand hygiene.	___	___	___	_____
7. Assess for the presence of tubes, incisions, drains, and equipment (e.g., traction).	___	___	___	_____
8. Assess ability and motivation of client, family members, and primary caregiver to participate in moving and positioning client in bed in anticipation of discharge to home.	___	___	___	_____
9. Raise level of bed to comfortable working height, and get extra help if needed.	___	___	___	_____
10. Explain procedure to client and what client is expected to do during procedure.	___	___	___	_____
11. Position client flat in bed if tolerated.	___	___	___	_____
12. Position client in bed:				
A. Move client up in bed				
(1) Put bed flat or in Trendelenburg's position with the side rail down.	___	___	___	_____
(2) Place height of bed at level appropriate for all staff.	___	___	___	_____
(3) For client able to move self without assistance instruct client to move self or offer positioning aid if needed.	___	___	___	_____
(4) For client partially able to move self:				
a. Ask appropriate number of staff to help with task. For clients less than 200 pounds, two to three caregivers are needed; for clients greater than 200 pounds, at least three caregivers are needed.	___	___	___	_____
b. Select appropriate friction-reducing device (e.g., friction-reducing slide sheet).	___	___	___	_____
c. Encourage client to assist using positioning aid if possible.	___	___	___	_____
d. Use friction-reducing device per manufacturer's guidelines with appropriate number of help, and move client up in	___	___	___	_____

Continued

	S	U	NP	Comments

bed. Instruct client to flex the knees and push on the count of three if the client is able to help.

(5) For client unable to assist:

    a. Ask appropriate number of staff to help with repositioning; at least two caregivers are needed. ____ ____ ____ _____

    b. Select appropriate safe-client-handling device (e.g., full-body sling, friction-reducing device). ____ ____ ____ _____

    c. Use friction-reducing device or full-body sling per manufacturer's guidelines with appropriate number of help, and move client up in bed. ____ ____ ____ _____

B. Position client in supported Fowler's position:

(1) Elevate head of bed 45 to 60 degrees. ____ ____ ____ _____

(2) Rest head against mattress or on small pillow. ____ ____ ____ _____

(3) Use pillows to support arms and hands if client does not have voluntary control or use of hands and arms. ____ ____ ____ _____

(4) Position pillow at lower back. ____ ____ ____ _____

(5) Place small pillow or roll under thigh. ____ ____ ____ _____

(6) Place small pillow or roll under ankles. ____ ____ ____ _____

C. Position client with hemiplegia in supported Fowler's position:

(1) Elevate head of bed 45 to 60 degrees. ____ ____ ____ _____

(2) Position client in sitting position as straight as possible. ____ ____ ____ _____

(3) Position head on small pillow with chin slightly forward. If client is totally unable to control head movement, avoid hyperextension of the neck. ____ ____ ____ _____

(4) Flex knees and hips by using pillow or folded blanket under knees. ____ ____ ____ _____

(5) Support feet in dorsiflexion with firm pillow or footboard. ____ ____ ____ _____

D. Position client in supine position:

(1) Be sure client is comfortable on back with head of bed flat. ____ ____ ____ _____

(2) Place small rolled towel under lumbar area of back. ____ ____ ____ _____

(3) Place pillow under upper shoulders, neck, or head. ____ ____ ____ _____

(4) Place trochanter rolls or sandbags parallel to lateral surface of client's thighs. ____ ____ ____ _____

(5) Place small pillow or roll under ankle to elevate heels. ____ ____ ____ _____

(6) Place footboard or firm pillows against bottom of client's feet. ____ ____ ____ _____

(7) Place foot splints or high-top sneakers on client's feet if ordered. ____ ____ ____ _____

(8) Place pillows under pronated forearms, keeping upper arms parallel to client's body ____ ____ ____ _____

(9) Place hand rolls in client's hands. Consider physical therapy referral for use of hand splints. ____ ____ ____ _____

E. Position client with hemiplegia in supine position:

(1) Place head of bed flat. ____ ____ ____ _____

(2) Place folded towel or small pillow under shoulder or affected side. ____ ____ ____ _____

(3) Keep affected arm away from body with elbow extended and palm up. (Alternative is to place arm out to side, with elbow bent and hand toward head of bed.) ____ ____ ____ _____

(4) Place folded towel under hip of involved side. ____ ____ ____ _____

(5) Flex affected knee 30 degrees by supporting it on pillow or folded blanket. ____ ____ ____ _____

(6) Support feet with soft pillows at right angle to leg. ____ ____ ____ _____

Continued

	S	U	NP	Comments

F. Position client in prone position:
   (1) Determine need for assistance from other caregivers.
   (2) With client supine, roll client over arm positioned close to body, with elbow straight and hand under hip. Position on abdomen in center of bed.
   (3) Turn client's head to one side, and support head with small pillow.
   (4) Place small pillow under client's abdomen below level of diaphragm.
   (5) Support arms in flexed position level at shoulders.
   (6) Support lower legs with pillows to elevate toes.

G. Position client with hemiplegia in prone position:
   (1) Determine need for friction-reducing device or full-body sling and number of people needed to help with repositioning.
   (2) Move client toward unaffected side using assistance and safe-client-handling equipment following manufacturer's guidelines.
   (3) Roll client onto side.
   (4) Place pillow on client's abdomen.
   (5) Roll client onto abdomen by positioning involved arm close to client's body, with elbow straight and hand under hip. Roll client carefully over arm.
   (6) Turn head toward involved side.
   (7) Position involved arm out to side, with elbow bent, hand toward head of bed, and fingers extended (if possible).
   (8) Flex knees slightly by placing pillow under legs from knees to ankles.
   (9) Keep feet at right angle to legs by using pillow high enough to keep toes off mattress.

H. Position client in lateral (side-lying) position:
   (1) Obtain assistance from at least one or two other people.
   (2) Lower head of bed completely or as low as client is able to tolerate.
   (3) Position client to side of bed. Use friction-reducing device or mechanical lift per manufacturer's guidelines if client cannot assist with rolling or is obese.
   (4) Prepare to turn client onto side. Flex client's knee that will not be next to mattress. Place one hand on client's hip and one hand on client's shoulder.
   (5) Roll client onto the side opposite of the flexed knee.
   (6) Place pillow under client's head and neck.
   (7) Bring shoulder blade forward.
   (8) Position both arms in slightly flexed position. Upper arm is supported by pillow level with shoulder; other arm, by mattress.
   (9) Place tuck-back pillow behind client's back. (Make by folding pillow lengthwise. Smooth area is slightly tucked under client's back.)
   (10) Place pillow under semiflexed upper leg level at hip from groin to foot.
   (11) Place sandbag parallel to plantar surface of dependent foot.

I. Position client in Sims' (semiprone) position:
   (1) Obtain assistance from at least one or two other people.
   (2) Lower head of bed completely.

Continued

	S	U	NP	Comments

(3) Be sure client is comfortable in supine position. _____ _____ _____ _____

(4) Position client in lateral position, with dependent arm straight along client's body and with client lying partially on abdomen. _____ _____ _____ _____

(5) Carefully lift client's dependent shoulder, and bring arm back behind client. _____ _____ _____ _____

(6) Place small pillow under client's head. _____ _____ _____ _____

(7) Place pillow under flexed upper arm, supporting arm level with shoulder. _____ _____ _____ _____

(8) Place pillow under flexed upper legs, supporting leg level with hip. _____ _____ _____ _____

(9) Place sandbags parallel to plantar surface of foot. _____ _____ _____ _____

J. Logrolling the client:

(1) Obtain assistance from at least two or three other people. _____ _____ _____ _____

(2) Place pillow between client's knees. _____ _____ _____ _____

(3) Cross client's arms on chest. _____ _____ _____ _____

(4) Position two nurses or other staff members on side of bed to which the client will be turned. Position third nurse or staff member on the other side of bed. If needed, four nurses are used; fourth nurse stands on same side as third nurse. _____ _____ _____ _____

(5) Fanfold or roll the drawsheet or pull sheet. _____ _____ _____ _____

(6) Move the client as one unit in a smooth, continuous motion on the count of three. _____ _____ _____ _____

(7) Nurse on the opposite side of the bed places pillows along the length of the client. _____ _____ _____ _____

(8) Gently lean the client as a unit back toward the pillows for support. _____ _____ _____ _____

13. Perform hand hygiene.

14. Evaluate client's level of comfort and ability to assist in position change. _____ _____ _____ _____

15. Following each position change, evaluate client's body alignment, positioning, and presence of any pressure areas. _____ _____ _____ _____

16. Document repositioning or turn and observations during procedure (e.g., condition of skin, joint movement, client's ability to assist with positioning) in nurses' notes. _____ _____ _____ _____

17. Report observations at change of shift. _____ _____ _____ _____

STUDENT: _____ DATE: _____

INSTRUCTOR: _____ DATE: _____

CHECKLIST
Skill 47-2 Using Safe and Effective Transfer Techniques

	S	U	NP	Comments
1. Assess the client for the following:				
A. Muscle strength (legs and upper arms).				
B. Joint mobility and contracture formation.				
C. Paralysis or paresis (spastic or flaccid).				
D. Orthostatic hypotension.				
E. Activity tolerance.				
F. Level of comfort.				
G. Vital signs.				
2. Assess client's sensory status:				
A. Adequacy of central and peripheral vision.				
B. Adequacy of hearing.				
C. Loss of peripheral sensation.				
3. Assess client's cognitive status.				
4. Assess client's level of motivation:				
A. Is client eager or unwilling to be mobile?				
B. Does client avoid activity and offer excuses?				
5. Refer to appropriate safe-client-handling algorithm, and assess previous mode of transfer (if applicable).				
6. Assess client's specific risk for falling when transferred.				
7. Perform hand hygiene, and ensure bed's brakes are locked.				
8. Explain procedure to client and what client is expected to do during the procedure.				
9. Determine number of people needed to assist with transfer; do not start procedure until all required caregivers are available.				
10. Transfer client:				
A. Assist cooperative client who can partially bear weight to sitting position with bed at waist level:				
(1) Place client in supine position. Use assistance of additional caregiver if necessary.				
(2) Face head of bed at a 45-degree angle, and remove pillows.				
(3) Place feet apart with foot nearer bed behind other foot, continuing at a 45-degree angle to the head of the bed.				
(4) Place hand farther from client under shoulders, supporting client's head and cervical vertebrae.				
(5) Place other hand on bed surface.				
(6) Raise client to sitting position by shifting weight from front to back leg.				
(7) Push against bed using arm that is on bed surface.				
B. Assist cooperative client who can partially bear weight to sitting position on side of bed with bed in low position:				
(1) Turn client to side, using assistance of another caregiver if necessary; client needs to face nurse on side of bed that client will be sitting.				
(2) With client in supine position, raise head of bed 30 degrees.				
(3) Stand opposite client's hips. Turn diagonally so you face client and far corner of foot of bed.				
(4) Place feet apart with foot closer to head of bed in front of other foot.				
(5) Place arm nearer head of bed under client's shoulders, supporting head and neck.				

Continued

	S	U	NP	Comments

(6) Place other arm over client's thighs. ___ ___ ___ _____

(7) Move client's lower legs and feet over side of bed. Pivot toward rear leg, allowing client's upper legs to swing downward. ___ ___ ___ _____

(8) At same time, shift weight to rear leg and elevate client. ___ ___ ___ _____

C. Transfer cooperative client who is partially weight-bearing from bed to chair with bed in low position:

  (1) Assist client to sitting position on side of bed. Have chair in position at 45-degree angle to bed. ___ ___ ___ _____

  (2) Apply transfer or gait belt. ___ ___ ___ _____

  (3) Ensure that client has stable nonskid shoes. Weight-bearing or strong leg is forward, with weak foot back. ___ ___ ___ _____

  (4) Spread feet apart.

  (5) Flex hips and knees, aligning knees with client's knees. ___ ___ ___ _____

  (6) Grasp transfer belt from underneath. ___ ___ ___ _____

  (7) Rock client up to standing position on count of three while straightening hips and legs and keeping knees slightly flexed. Unless contraindicated, instruct client to use hands to push up. ___ ___ ___ _____

  (8) Maintain stability of client's weak or paralyzed leg with knee. ___ ___ ___ _____

  (9) Pivot on foot farther from chair. ___ ___ ___ _____

  (10) Instruct client to use armrests on chair for support, and ease into chair. ___ ___ ___ _____

  (11) Flex hips and knees while lowering client into chair. ___ ___ ___ _____

D. Transfer cooperative client who cannot bear weight but who has upper extremity strength from bed to chair with bed in low position:

  (1) Remove arms from chair, or move them out of the way. ___ ___ ___ _____

  (2) Assist client to sitting position on side of bed. Have chair in position at 45-degree angle to bed. Apply transfer or gait belt until client is able to transfer independently with ease. ___ ___ ___ _____

  (3) Using seated transfer aid, have client use upper body to slide from bed to chair. Follow manufacturer's directions for use of the transfer aid. ___ ___ ___ _____

E. Use mechanical lift and full-body sling to transfer uncooperative client who can bear partial weight or client who cannot bear weight and is either uncooperative or does not have upper body strength into chair:

  (1) Position lift properly at bedside. ___ ___ ___ _____

  (2) Position chair near bed, and allow adequate space to maneuver lift. ___ ___ ___ _____

  (3) Raise bed to high position with mattress flat. Lower side rail. ___ ___ ___ _____

  (4) Roll client to side.

  (5) Place sling under client. Place lower edge under client's knees (wide piece), and upper edge under client's shoulders (narrow piece). ___ ___ ___ _____

  (6) Roll client to opposite side, and pull body sling through. ___ ___ ___ _____

  (7) Roll client supine onto canvas seat. ___ ___ ___ _____

  (8) Remove client's glasses, if appropriate. ___ ___ ___ _____

  (9) If using transportable Hoyer lift, place lift's horseshoe-shaped base under side of bed (on side with chair). ___ ___ ___ _____

  (10) Lower upper horizontal bar to sling level following manufacturer's directions. Some lifts require valve to be locked. ___ ___ ___ _____

Continued

	S	U	NP	Comments

(11) Attach hooks on strap to holes in sling. Short straps hook to top holes of sling; longer straps hook to bottom of sling.

(12) Elevate head of bed.

(13) Fold client's arms over chest.

(14) Use lift to raise client off bed.

(15) Move lift to chair.

(16) Position client, and lower slowly into chair following manufacturer's guidelines.

(17) Remove straps and mechanical/hydraulic lift.

(18) Check client's sitting alignment, and correct if necessary.

F. Transfer client from bed to stretcher (bed at stretcher level):

(1) Place bed flat, and position at same level as stretcher. Ensure bed brakes are locked.

(2) Lower side rails. Two caregivers stand on the side where the stretcher will be while third caregiver stands on the other side.

(3) Two caregivers help client roll onto side toward one caregiver.

(4) Caregivers work together to position friction-reducing device properly under client's back following manufacturer's guidelines.

(5) Roll stretcher along the side of the bed. Lock wheels of stretcher once it is in place. Instruct the client not to move.

(6) All three caregivers place feet widely apart with one slightly in front of the other, and grasp the friction-reducing device.

(7) On the count of three, caregivers pull the client from the bed onto the stretcher using the friction-reducing device and shifting weight from front foot to back foot.

(8) Put up side rail of stretcher on side where caregivers are, then roll stretcher away from side of bed and put side rails up on that side.

(9) Cover client with sheet or blanket.

11. Perform hand hygiene.

12. With each transfer evaluate client's tolerance and level of fatigue and comfort. Praise the client's progress, effort, or performance.

13. Following each transfer, evaluate client's body alignment.

14. Record procedure, including pertinent observations: weakness, ability to follow directions, weight-bearing ability, balance, ability to pivot, number of personnel needed to assist, and amount of assistance (muscle strength) required in nurses' notes.

15. Report any unusual occurrence to nurse in charge. Report transfer ability and assistance needed to next shift or other caregivers. Report progress or remission to rehabilitation staff (physical therapist or occupational therapist).

STUDENT: _____ DATE: _____

INSTRUCTOR: _____ DATE: _____

Skill 48-1 Assessment for Risk for Pressure Ulcer Development

	S	U	NP	Comments
1. Identify at-risk individuals needing prevention and the specific factors placing them at risk:				
A. Use a validated risk assessment tool such as the Braden Scale or Norton Scale.	____	____	____	_____
B. Assess the client upon admission to acute care, rehabilitation hospitals, nursing homes, home care programs, and other health care facilities.	____	____	____	_____
C. Inspect the condition of the client's skin at least once a day, and examine all bony prominences, noting skin integrity. (Check agency policy for reassessment, and reassess at periodic intervals.) If you notice redness or discoloration, use thumb to gently palpate area of redness. The discoloration often varies from pink to deep red.	____	____	____	_____
D. Observe all assistive devices, such as braces or casts, and medical equipment, such as nasogastric tubes and catheters, for pressure points.	____	____	____	_____
2. Determine the client's ability to respond meaningfully to pressure-related discomfort (sensory perception).	____	____	____	_____
3. Assess the degree to which the client's skin is exposed to moisture.	____	____	____	_____
4. Evaluate the client's activity level:				
A. Determine the client's ability to change and control body position (mobility).	____	____	____	_____
B. Determine client's preferred positions.	____	____	____	_____
5. Assess the client's usual food intake pattern (nutrition):				
A. Review weight pattern and nutritional laboratory values.	____	____	____	_____
B. Complete fluid intake assessment.	____	____	____	_____
6. Evaluate the presence of friction and/or shear.	____	____	____	_____
7. Document the risk assessment. (NOTE: Numerical values in Steps A through F refer to the Braden Scale.):				
A. As the Braden Scale scores become lower, predicted risk becomes higher.	____	____	____	_____
B. Link the risk assessment to preventative protocols.	____	____	____	_____
C. Institute at-risk interventions (score of 15 to 18). Consider instituting frequent turning, protection of client's heels, use of a pressure-redistribution surface, and managing moisture.	____	____	____	_____
D. Institute moderate-risk interventions (score of 13 to 14). Consider a protocol of frequent turning, protect client's heels, provide a pressure-redistribution surface, provide foam wedges for 30-degree lateral positioning, and manage moisture, shear, and friction.	____	____	____	_____
E. Institute high-risk interventions (score of 10 to 12). Consider a protocol that increases the frequency of turning, supplements turning with small shifts in position, facilitates maximal remobilization, protects the client's heels, provides a pressure-redistribution surface, provides foam wedges for 30-degree lateral positioning, and manages moisture, friction,	____	____	____	_____

Continued

	S	U	NP	Comments

and shear. If needed, institute nutritional
interventions to reduce risk for pressure ulcer
development.

F. Institute very-high-risk interventions (score
of 9 or below). Consider a protocol that
incorporates the points for high-risk clients
plus uses a pressure-redistribution surface if the
client has intractable pain, severe pain
exacerbated by turning.

8. Provide education to client and family regarding
pressure ulcer risk and prevention.

9. Evaluate measures to reduce pressure ulcer
development:
   A. Observe client's skin for areas at risk.
   B. Observe tolerance of client for positioning.
   C. Monitor the success of a toileting program
   or other measures to reduce the frequency
   of incontinence of urine or stool.
   D. Evaluate nutrition laboratory values.

10. Record client's risk score.

11. Describe position, turning intervals,
pressure-redistribution devices, and other
prevention strategies.

12. Report any need for additional consultations
for the high-risk client.

STUDENT: _____ DATE: _____

INSTRUCTOR: _____ DATE: _____

Skill 48-2 Treating Pressure Ulcers

	S	U	NP	Comments
1. Assess client's level of comfort using a pain scale of 0 to 10 and their need for pain medication before beginning procedure.	____	____	____	_____
2. Determine if client has allergies to topical agents.	____	____	____	_____
3. Review order for topical agent or dressing.	____	____	____	_____
4. Close room door or bedside curtains. Position client to allow dressing removal.	____	____	____	_____
5. Perform hand hygiene, and apply clean gloves. Remove dressing, and place in plastic bag.	____	____	____	_____
6. Assess pressure ulcer(s). All pressure ulcers need individual assessments.				
A. Note color, type, and percentage of tissue present in the wound base.	____	____	____	_____
B. Measure width and length of the ulcer(s). Determine width by measuring the dimension from left to right, and the length from top to bottom.	____	____	____	_____
C. Measure depth of pressure ulcer using sterile cotton-tipped applicator or other device that will allow measurement of wound depth.	____	____	____	_____
D. Measure depth of undermining using a cotton-tipped applicator and gently probing under skin edges.	____	____	____	_____
E. Assess the periwound skin; check for maceration, redness, denuded area.	____	____	____	_____
7. Change to sterile gloves (check agency policy).	____	____	____	_____
8. Cleanse ulcer thoroughly with normal saline or cleansing agent. Use irrigating syringe for deep ulcers.	____	____	____	_____
9. Apply topical agents, as prescribed:				
A. Enzymes				
(1) Apply thin, even layer of ointment over necrotic areas of ulcer only. Do not apply enzyme to surrounding skin.	____	____	____	_____
(2) Apply gauze dressing directly over ulcer.	____	____	____	_____
(3) Tape securely in place.	____	____	____	_____
B. Hydrogel				
(1) Cover surface of ulcer with hydrogel using applicator or gloved hand.	____	____	____	_____
(2) Apply dry gauze, hydrocolloid, or transparent film dressing over wound, and adhere to intact skin.	____	____	____	_____
C. Calcium alginate				
(1) Pack wound with alginate using applicator or gloved hand.	____	____	____	_____
(2) Apply dry gauze or foam over alginate. Tape in place.	____	____	____	_____
10. Remove gloves, and dispose of soiled supplies. Perform hand hygiene.	____	____	____	_____
11. Assess the pressure ulcer at each dressing change or sooner if the wound or client's condition deteriorates. Utilize the agency's tool for wound assessment. Compare wound assessment to the identified plan of care, and if the wound is not progressing toward healing as indicated by an increase in size, increased presence of pain, foul-smelling drainage, or increase in devitalized tissue, discuss findings with the health care team.	____	____	____	_____
12. Record assessment of ulcer in client's record.	____	____	____	_____
13. Describe type of topical agent used, dressing applied, and client's response.	____	____	____	_____
14. Report any deterioration in ulcer appearance.	____	____	____	_____

STUDENT: _____ DATE: _____

INSTRUCTOR: _____ DATE: _____

CHECKLIST
Skill 48-3 Applying Dry and Moist Dressings

	S	U	NP	Comments
1. Perform hand hygiene. Obtain information about size and location of wound.	___	___	___	_____
2. Assess client's level of comfort.	___	___	___	_____
3. Review orders for dressing change procedure.	___	___	___	_____
4. Identify client with two client identifiers.	___	___	___	_____
5. Explain procedure to client, and instruct client not to touch wound area or sterile supplies.	___	___	___	_____
6. Close room or cubicle curtains and windows.	___	___	___	_____
7. Position client comfortably, and drape with bath blanket to expose only wound site.	___	___	___	_____
8. Place disposable bag within reach of work area. Fold top of bag to make cuff.	___	___	___	_____
9. Apply face mask and protective eyewear, if splashing occurs.	___	___	___	_____
10. Put on clean, disposable gloves, and remove tape, bandage, or ties.	___	___	___	_____
11. Remove tape: pull parallel to skin toward dressing; remove remaining adhesive from skin.	___	___	___	_____
12. With gloved hand carefully remove gauze dressings one layer at a time, taking care not to dislodge drains or tubes. (If dressing sticks on a wet-to-dry dressing, do not moisten it; instead gently free dressing and alert client of potential discomfort.)	___	___	___	_____
13. Observe character and amount of drainage on dressing and appearance of wound.	___	___	___	_____
14. Fold dressings with drainage contained inside, and remove gloves inside out. With small dressings, remove gloves inside out over dressing. Dispose of gloves and soiled dressings in disposable bag. Perform hand hygiene.	___	___	___	_____
15. Open sterile dressing tray or individually wrapped sterile supplies. Place on bedside table.	___	___	___	_____
16. If ordered, cleanse wound:				
A. Pour ordered solution into sterile irrigation container.	___	___	___	_____
B. Using syringe, gently allow solution to flow over wound.	___	___	___	_____
C. Continue until the irrigation flow is clear.	___	___	___	_____
D. Dry surrounding skin.	___	___	___	_____
17. Apply dressing:				
A. Dry dressing:				
(1) Apply sterile gloves.	___	___	___	_____
(2) Inspect wound for appearance, drains, drainage, and integrity.	___	___	___	_____
(3) Cleanse wound with solution. (Clean from least-contaminated area to most-contaminated area.)	___	___	___	_____
(4) Dry area.	___	___	___	_____
(5) Apply sterile dry dressing covering wound.	___	___	___	_____
(6) Apply topper dressing if indicated.	___	___	___	_____
B. Moist dressing:				
(1) Apply clean gloves.	___	___	___	_____
(2) Remove old dressings; discard.	___	___	___	_____
(3) Assess surrounding skin. Discard gloves.	___	___	___	_____
(4) Apply sterile gloves.	___	___	___	_____
(5) Cleanse wound base with normal saline or commercially prepared wound cleanser. Assess wound base.	___	___	___	_____
(6) Moisten gauze with prescribed solution. Gently wring out excess solution. Unfold.	___	___	___	_____

Continued

350

	S	U	NP	Comments

(7) Apply gauze as a single layer directly onto the wound surface. If wound is deep, gently pack dressing into wound base by hand or forceps until all wound surfaces are in contact with the gauze. If tunneling is present, use a cotton-tipped applicator to place gauze into tunneled area. Be sure gauze does not touch the surrounding skin. ____ ____ ____ _____

(8) Cover with sterile dry gauze and topper dressing. ____ ____ ____ _____

18. Secure dressing:
   A. Tape: Apply nonallergenic tape to secure dressing in place. ____ ____ ____ _____
   B. Montgomery ties:
      (1) Expose adhesive surface of tape on end of each tie. ____ ____ ____ _____
      (2) Place ties on oppositesides of dressing. ____ ____ ____ _____
      (3) Place adhesive directly on skin, or use skin barrier. ____ ____ ____ _____
      (4) Secure dressing by lacing ties across it. ____ ____ ____ _____
   C. For dressings on an extremity, secure dressing with rolled gauze or an elastic net. ____ ____ ____ _____
19. Remove gloves, and dispose of in bag. Remove any mask or eyewear. ____ ____ ____ _____
20. Dispose of supplies, and perform hand hygiene. ____ ____ ____ _____
21. Assist client to comfortable position. ____ ____ ____ _____
22. Report brisk, bright red bleeding or evidence of wound dehiscence or evisceration to health care provider immediately. ____ ____ ____ _____
23. Report wound and periwound tissue appearance, color, and tissue type and presence and characteristics of exudate, type and amount of dressings used, and tolerance of client to procedure. ____ ____ ____ _____
24. Record client's level of comfort. ____ ____ ____ _____
25. Write date and time dressing applied on tape in ink (not marker). ____ ____ ____ _____

STUDENT: _____ DATE: _____

INSTRUCTOR: _____ DATE: _____

Skill 48-4 Implementation of Negative Pressure Wound Closure

	S	U	NP	Comments
1. Identify client with two client identifiers.	___	___	___	_____
2. Perform hand hygiene. Assemble supplies.	___	___	___	_____
3. Position client comfortably, and drape to expose only wound site. Instruct client not to touch wound or sterile supplies.	___	___	___	_____
4. Place disposable waterproof bag within reach of work area with top folded to make a cuff.	___	___	___	_____
5. When Vacuum Assisted Closure (V.A.C.) is in place, push therapy on/off button.				
A. Keeping tube connectors with V.A.C. unit, disconnect tubes from each other to drain fluids into canister.	___	___	___	_____
B. Before lowering, tighten clamp on canister tube.	___	___	___	_____
6. With dressing tube unclamped, introduce 10 to 30 mL of normal saline, if ordered, into tubing to soak underneath foam.	___	___	___	_____
7. Gently stretch transparent film horizontally, and slowly pull away from the skin.	___	___	___	_____
8. Remove old V.A.C. dressing, observing appearance and drainage on dressing. Use caution to avoid tension on any drains that are present. Discard dressing, and remove gloves.	___	___	___	_____
9. Apply sterile or clean gloves. Irrigate the wound with normal saline or other solution ordered by the health care provider.	___	___	___	_____
10. Measure wound as ordered: at baseline, first dressing change, weekly, and discharge from therapy. Remove and discard gloves.	___	___	___	_____
11. Depending on the type of wound, apply sterile gloves or new clean gloves.	___	___	___	_____
12. Prepare V.A.C. foam.				
A. Select appropriate foam.	___	___	___	_____
B. Using sterile scissors, cut foam to wound size. Dressing must fit the size and shape of the wound including tunnels and undermined areas.	___	___	___	_____
13. Gently place foam in wound; be sure that the foam is in contact with entire wound base and margins and tunneled and undermined areas.	___	___	___	_____
14. Apply wrinkle-free transparent dressing over foam, and secure tubing to the unit.	___	___	___	_____
15. Apply V.A.C. adhesive transparent drape to cover the foam dressing, and overlap onto intact periwound skin. Secure tubing to transparent film, aligning drainage holes to ensure an occlusive seal. Do not apply tension to drape and tubing.	___	___	___	_____
16. Secure tubing several centimeters away from the dressing.	___	___	___	_____
17. Once you have completely covered the wound, connect the tubing from the dressing to the tubing from the canister and V.A.C. unit.				
A. Remove canister from sterile packaging, and push into V.A.C. unit until you hear a click. NOTE: **an alarm will sound if the canister is not properly engaged.**	___	___	___	_____
B. Connect the dressing tubing to the canister tubing. Make sure both clamps are open.	___	___	___	_____
C. Place V.A.C. unit on a level surface, or hang from the foot of the bed. NOTE: **The V.A.C. unit will alarm and deactivate therapy if the unit is tilted beyond 45 degrees.**	___	___	___	_____

Continued

	S	U	NP	Comments
D. Press in green-lit power button, and set pressure as ordered.	____	____	____	_____
18. Discard old dressing materials; remove gloves, and perform hand hygiene.	____	____	____	_____
19. Inspect V.A.C. system to verify that negative pressure is achieved.				
A. Verify that display screen reads THERAPY ON.	____	____	____	_____
B. Be sure clamps are open and tubing is patent.	____	____	____	_____
C. Identify air leaks by listening with stethoscope or by moving hand around edges of wound while applying light pressure.	____	____	____	_____
D. If a leak is present, use strips of transparent film to patch areas.	____	____	____	_____
20. Compare wound with baseline wound assessment.	____	____	____	_____
21. Verify airtight dressing seal and proper negative pressure.	____	____	____	_____
22. Record appearance of wound, color, characteristics of any drainage, presence of wound healing augmentation.	____	____	____	_____
23. Record pressure setting of V.A.C.	____	____	____	_____
24. Record date and time of dressing change.	____	____	____	_____
25. Report brisk, bright bleeding, evidence of poor wound healing, and possible wound infection.	____	____	____	_____

STUDENT: _____ DATE: _____

INSTRUCTOR: _____ DATE: _____

CHECKLIST
Skill 48-5 Performing Wound Irrigation

	S	U	NP	Comments
1. Assess client's level of pain. Administer prescribed analgesic 30 to 45 minutes before starting wound irrigation procedure.	___	___	___	_____
2. Review medical record for health care provider's prescription for irrigation of open wound and type of solution to be used.	___	___	___	_____
3. Identify client using two client identifiers.	___	___	___	_____
4. Assess recent recording of signs and symptoms related to client's open wound:				
A. Condition of skin and wound.	___	___	___	_____
B. Elevation of body temperature.	___	___	___	_____
C. Drainage from wound (amount, color).	___	___	___	_____
D. Odor.	___	___	___	_____
E. Consistency of drainage.	___	___	___	_____
F. Size of wounds, including depth, length, and width.	___	___	___	_____
5. Explain procedure of wound irrigation and cleansing.	___	___	___	_____
6. Perform hand hygiene.	___	___	___	_____
7. Position client comfortably to permit gravitational flow of irrigating solution through wound and into collection receptacle. Position client so that wound is vertical to collection basin.	___	___	___	_____
8. Warm irrigation solution to approximate body temperature.	___	___	___	_____
9. Form cuff on waterproof bag, and place it near bed.	___	___	___	_____
10. Close room door or bed curtains.	___	___	___	_____
11. Apply gown and goggles if needed.	___	___	___	_____
12. Put on clean gloves, and remove soiled dressing and discard in waterproof bag. Discard gloves.	___	___	___	_____
13. Prepare equipment; open sterile supplies.	___	___	___	_____
14. Put on sterile gloves.	___	___	___	_____
15. To irrigate wound with wide opening:				
A. Fill 35-mL syringe with irrigation solution.	___	___	___	_____
B. Attach 19-gauge needle or angiocatheter.	___	___	___	_____
C. Hold syringe tip 2.5 cm (1 inch) above upper end of wound and over area being cleansed.	___	___	___	_____
D. Using continuous pressure, flush wound; repeat Steps 15A, B, and C until solution draining into basin is clear.	___	___	___	_____
16. To irrigate deep wound with very small opening:				
A. Attach soft angiocatheter to filled irrigating syringe.	___	___	___	_____
B. Lubricate tip of catheter with irrigating solution; then gently insert tip of catheter, and pull out about 1 cm (½ inch).	___	___	___	_____
C. Using slow, continuous pressure, flush wound. CAUTION: Splashing sometimes occurs during this step.	___	___	___	_____
D. Pinch off catheter just below syringe while keeping catheter in place.	___	___	___	_____
E. Remove and refill syringe. Reconnect to catheter, and repeat until solution draining into basin is clear.	___	___	___	_____
17. Obtain cultures, if needed, after cleansing with nonbacteriostatic saline.	___	___	___	_____
18. Dry wound edges with gauze.	___	___	___	_____
19. Apply appropriate dressing.	___	___	___	_____
20. Remove gloves and, if worn, mask, goggles, and gown.	___	___	___	_____

Continued

	S	U	NP	Comments
21. Dispose of equipment and soiled supplies. Perform hand hygiene.	___	___	___	_____
22. Assist client to comfortable position.	___	___	___	_____
23. Assess type of tissue in the wound bed.	___	___	___	_____
24. Inspect dressing periodically.	___	___	___	_____
25. Evaluate skin integrity.	___	___	___	_____
26. Observe client for signs of discomfort.	___	___	___	_____
27. Observe for presence of retained irrigant.	___	___	___	_____
28. Record wound irrigation and client response on progress notes.	___	___	___	_____
29. Immediately report any evidence of fresh bleeding, sharp increase in pain, retention of irrigant, or signs of shock to attending health care provider.	___	___	___	_____
30. At change of shift, report expected and unexpected outcomes that have actually occurred.	___	___	___	_____

STUDENT: _____ DATE: _____

INSTRUCTOR: _____ DATE: _____

Skill 48-6 Applying an Abdominal Binder

	S	U	NP	Comments
1. Observe client with need for support of thorax or abdomen. Observe ability to breathe deeply and cough effectively.	___	___	___	_____
2. Review medical record if medical prescription for particular binder is required and reasons for application.	___	___	___	_____
3. Identify client with two client identifiers.	___	___	___	_____
4. Inspect skin for actual or potential alterations in integrity. Observe for irritation, abrasion, skin surfaces that rub against each other, or allergic response to adhesive tape used to secure dressing.	___	___	___	_____
5. Inspect any surgical dressing.	___	___	___	_____
6. Assess client's comfort level, using analog scale of 0 to 10 and noting any objective signs and symptoms.	___	___	___	_____
7. Gather necessary data regarding size of client and appropriate binder.	___	___	___	_____
8. Explain procedure to client.	___	___	___	_____
9. Teach skill to client or significant other.	___	___	___	_____
10. Perform hand hygiene, and apply gloves (if likely to contact wound drainage).	___	___	___	_____
11. Close curtains or room door.	___	___	___	_____
12. Apply binder.				
A. Abdominal binder:				
(1) Position client in supine position with head slightly elevated and knees slightly flexed.	___	___	___	_____
(2) Fanfold far side of binder toward midline of binder.	___	___	___	_____
(3) Instruct and help client to roll away from nurse toward raised side rail while firmly supporting abdominal incision and dressing with hands.	___	___	___	_____
(4) Place fanfolded ends of binder under client.	___	___	___	_____
(5) Instruct or assist client to roll over folded ends.	___	___	___	_____
(6) Unfold and stretch ends out smoothly on far side of bed.	___	___	___	_____
(7) Instruct client to roll back into supine position.	___	___	___	_____
(8) Adjust binder so that supine client is centered over binder using symphysis pubis and costal margins as lower and upper landmarks.	___	___	___	_____
(9) Close binder. Pull one end of binder over center of client's abdomen. While maintaining tension on that end of binder, pull opposite end of binder over center and secure with Velcro closure tabs, metal fasteners, or horizontally placed safety pins.	___	___	___	_____
B. Breast binder:				
(1) Assist client in placing arms through binder's armholes.	___	___	___	_____
(2) Assist client to supine position in bed.	___	___	___	_____
(3) Pad area under breasts if necessary.	___	___	___	_____
(4) Using Velcro closure tabs or horizontally placed safety pins, secure binder at nipple level first. Continue closure process above and then below nipple line until entire binder is closed.	___	___	___	_____
(5) Make appropriate adjustments, including individualizing fit of shoulder straps and pinning waistline darts to reduce binder size.	___	___	___	_____

Continued

	S	U	NP	Comments
(6) Instruct and observe skill development in self-care related to reapplying breast binder.	___	___	___	_____
13. Assess client's comfort level.	___	___	___	_____
14. Adjust binder as necessary.	___	___	___	_____
15. Remove gloves, and perform hand hygiene.	___	___	___	_____
16. Observe site for skin integrity, circulation, and characteristics of the wound. (Periodically remove binder and surgical dressing to assess wound characteristics.)	___	___	___	_____
17. Assess comfort level of client, using analog scale of 0 to 10 and noting any objective signs and symptoms.	___	___	___	_____
18. Assess client's ability to ventilate properly, including deep breathing and coughing.	___	___	___	_____
19. Identify client's need for assistance with activities such as hair combing, dressing, and ambulating.	___	___	___	_____
20. Report any skin irritation to nurse at between-shift report.	___	___	___	_____
21. Record application of binder, condition of skin, circulation, integrity of dressing, and client's comfort level.	___	___	___	_____
22. Report ineffective lung expansion to health care provider immediately.	___	___	___	_____

STUDENT: _____ DATE: _____

INSTRUCTOR: _____ DATE: _____

Skill 48-7 Applying an Elastic Bandage

	S	U	NP	Comments
1. Perform hand hygiene, and apply gloves if needed. Inspect skin for alterations in integrity as indicated by abrasions, discoloration, chafing, or edema. (Look carefully at bony prominences.)	____	____	____	_____
2. Inspect surgical dressing. Remove gloves, and perform hand hygiene.	____	____	____	_____
3. Observe adequacy of circulation (distal to bandage) by noting surface temperature, skin color, and sensation of body parts to be wrapped.	____	____	____	_____
4. Review medical record for specific orders related to application of elastic bandage. Note area to be covered, type of bandage required, frequency of change, and previous response to treatment.	____	____	____	_____
5. Identify client using two client identifiers.	____	____	____	_____
6. Identify client's and primary caregiver's present knowledge level of skill if bandaging will be continued at home.	____	____	____	_____
7. Explain procedure to client.	____	____	____	_____
8. Teach skill to client or significant other.	____	____	____	_____
9. Perform hand hygiene, and apply gloves if drainage is present.	____	____	____	_____
10. Close room door or curtains.	____	____	____	_____
11. Help client to assume comfortable, anatomically correct position.	____	____	____	_____
12. Hold roll of elastic bandage in dominant hand, and use other hand to lightly hold beginning of bandage at distal body part. Continue transferring roll to dominant hand as bandage is wrapped.	____	____	____	_____
13. Apply bandage from distal point toward proximal boundary using variety of turns to cover various shapes of body parts. A spiral dressing is often used to cover cylindrical body parts such as wrist or upper arms. Bandage in an ascending motion, overlapping the previous bandage by one-half or two-thirds width of bandage. Use a figure-eight dressing to cover joint because the snug fit provides excellent immobilization. To apply: Overlap turns alternately ascending and descending over bandaged part, each turn crossing previous one to form figure eight.	____	____	____	_____
14. Unroll and very slightly stretch bandage.	____	____	____	_____
15. Overlap turns by one-half to two-thirds width of bandage roll.	____	____	____	_____
16. Secure first bandage with clip or tape before applying additional rolls. (Apply additional rolls without leaving any uncovered skin surface. Secure last bandage applied.)	____	____	____	_____
17. Remove gloves if worn, and perform hand hygiene.	____	____	____	_____
18. Assess distal circulation when bandage application is complete and at least twice during 8-hour period:				
A. Observe skin color for pallor or cyanosis.	____	____	____	_____
B. Palpate skin for warmth.	____	____	____	_____
C. Palpate pulses, and compare bilaterally.	____	____	____	_____
D. Ask if client is aware of pain, numbness, tingling, or other discomfort.	____	____	____	_____
E. Observe mobility of extremity.	____	____	____	_____
19. Have client demonstrate bandage application.	____	____	____	_____
20. Document condition of wound, integrity of dressing, application of bandage, circulation, and client's comfort level.	____	____	____	_____
21. Report any changes in neurological or circulatory status to nurse in charge or health care provider.	____	____	____	_____

CHECKLIST

Skill 48-8 Applying a Warm, Moist Compress to an Open Wound

	S	U	NP	Comments
1. Refer to health care provider's order for type of compress, location and duration of application, desired temperature, and institutional policies regarding temperature of compress.	____	____	____	_____
2. Refer to medical record to identify any systemic contraindications to heat application.	____	____	____	_____
3. Identify client using two client identifiers.	____	____	____	_____
4. Perform hand hygiene.	____	____	____	_____
5. Inspect condition of exposed skin and wound where you will apply compress.	____	____	____	_____
6. Assess client's extremities for sensitivity to temperature and pain by measuring light touch, pinprick, and temperature sensation.	____	____	____	_____
7. Assemble equipment and supplies.	____	____	____	_____
8. Explain steps of procedure and purpose to client. Describe sensations to be felt, such as decreasing warmth and wetness. Explain precautions to prevent burning.	____	____	____	_____
9. Close door and bedside curtains.	____	____	____	_____
10. Assist client in assuming comfortable position in proper body alignment, and place waterproof pad under area you will treat.	____	____	____	_____
11. Expose body part you will treat with compress, and drape client with bath blanket.	____	____	____	_____
12. Prepare compress:				
A. Pour solution into sterile container.	____	____	____	_____
B. If using portable heating source, warm solution. Commercially prepared compresses remain under infrared lamp until just before use. Open sterile packages, and drop gauze into container to become immersed in solution. Note: You must test the temperature by applying sterile solution to your forearm (without contaminating solution).	____	____	____	_____
C. Adjust temperature of aquathermia pad (if needed).	____	____	____	_____
13. Apply disposable gloves. Remove any existing dressing covering wound. Dispose of gloves and dressings in proper receptacle.	____	____	____	_____
14. Assess condition of wound and surrounding skin. Inflamed wound appears reddened, but surrounding skin is less red in color.	____	____	____	_____
15. Apply sterile gloves.	____	____	____	_____
16. Pick up one layer of immersed gauze, wring out any excess solution, and apply it lightly to open wound.	____	____	____	_____
17. In a few seconds, lift edge of gauze to assess for redness.	____	____	____	_____
18. If client tolerates compress, pack gauze snugly against the wound. Be sure all wound surfaces are covered by warm compress.	____	____	____	_____
19. Cover moist compress with dry sterile dressing and bath towel. If necessary, pin or tie in place. Remove sterile gloves.	____	____	____	_____
20. Apply aquathermia or waterproof heating pad over towel (optional). Keep it in place for desired duration of application.	____	____	____	_____
21. If you are not using an aquathermia pad to maintain temperature of application, change warm compress using sterile technique every 5 minutes or as ordered during duration of therapy.	____	____	____	_____

Continued

	S	U	NP	Comments

22. After prescribed time, apply disposable gloves and remove pad, towel, and compress. Reassess wound and condition of skin, and replace dry sterile dressing as ordered.

23. Assist client to preferred comfortable position.

24. Dispose of equipment and soiled compress. Perform hand hygiene.

25. Inspect affected area covered by compress and heating pad every 5 to 10 minutes.

26. Ask every 5 to 10 minutes if client notices any unusual burning sensation not felt before application.

27. Have client explain and demonstrate application.

28. Record type, location, and duration of application. Note solution and temperature.

29. Describe condition of wound and skin before and after treatment, as well as client's response to therapy.

30. Describe any instructions given and client's ability to explain and perform procedure.

31. Report unusual findings to nurse in charge or health care provider.

STUDENT: _____ DATE: _____

INSTRUCTOR: _____ DATE: _____

Skill 50-1 Demonstrating Postoperative Exercises

	S	U	NP	Comments
1. Assess client's risk for postoperative respiratory complications. Review medical history to identify presence of chronic pulmonary conditions (e.g., emphysema, asthma), any condition that affects chest wall movement, history of smoking, or presence of reduced hemoglobin.	____	____	____	_____
2. Assess ability to cough and deep breathe by having client take deep breath, and observe movement of shoulders and chest wall. Measure chest excursion during deep breath. Ask client to cough after taking deep breath.	____	____	____	_____
3. Assess risk for postoperative thrombus formation (e.g., older clients, those with active cancer, and clients immobilized for more than 3 days). Observe for localized tenderness along the distribution of the venous system, swollen calf or thigh, calf swelling more than 3 cm compared with asymptomatic leg, pitting edema in symptomatic leg, and collateral superficial veins. If any of these signs are present, notify the health care provider.	____	____	____	_____
4. Assess client's ability to move independently while in bed.	____	____	____	_____
5. Explain postoperative exercises to client, including importance to recovery and physiological benefits.	____	____	____	_____
6. Demonstrate exercises:				
A. Diaphragmatic breathing:				
(1) Assist client to comfortable sitting position on side of bed or in chair or standing position.	____	____	____	_____
(2) Stand or sit facing client.	____	____	____	_____
(3) Instruct client to place palms of hands across from each other, down and along lower borders of anterior rib cage. Place tips of third fingers lightly together. Demonstrate for client.	____	____	____	_____
(4) Have client take slow, deep breaths, inhaling through nose and push abdomen against hands. Tell client to feel middle fingers separate during inhalation. Demonstrate.	____	____	____	_____
(5) Explain that client will feel normal downward movement of diaphragm during inspiration. Explain that abdominal organs descend and chest wall expands.	____	____	____	_____
(6) Avoid using chest and shoulders while inhaling, and instruct client in same manner.	____	____	____	_____
(7) Have client hold slow, deep breath for count of three and then slowly exhale through mouth as if blowing out a candle (pursed lips). Tell client middle fingertips will touch as chest wall contracts.	____	____	____	_____
(8) Repeat breathing exercise three to five times.	____	____	____	_____
(9) Instruct client to take 10 slow, deep breaths every hour while awake during postoperative period until mobile.	____	____	____	_____
B. Incentive spirometry (IS):				
(1) Perform hand hygiene.	____	____	____	_____
(2) Instruct client to assume semi-Fowler's or high-Fowler's position.	____	____	____	_____
(3) For the bariatric client, consider the reverse Trendelenburg's position.	____	____	____	_____

Continued

	S	U	NP	Comments

(4) Either set or indicate to client on the IS device scale the volume level to be attained with each breath.

(5) Demonstrate to client how to place mouthpiece of IS so that lips completely cover mouthpiece.

(6) Instruct client to inhale slowly and maintain constant flow through unit, attempting to reach goal volume. When client reaches maximal inspiration, have client hold breath for 3 to 5 seconds and then exhale slowly. Ensure number of breaths does not exceed 10 to 12 per session.

(7) Instruct client to breathe normally for short period between the 10 breaths on IS.

(8) Have client repeat maneuver until goals are achieved.

(9) Have client end with two coughs after end of 10 IS breaths.

(10) Perform hand hygiene.

C. Controlled coughing:

(1) Explain importance of maintaining upright position.

(2) Demonstrate coughing. Take two slow, deep breaths, inhaling through nose and exhaling through mouth.

(3) Inhale deeply third time, and hold breath to count of three. Cough fully for two or three consecutive coughs without inhaling between coughs. (Tell client to push all air out of lungs.)

(4) Caution client against just clearing throat instead of coughing. Explain that coughing will not cause injury to incision when done correctly.

(5) If surgical incision will be abdominal or thoracic, teach client to place one hand over incisional area and other hand on top of first. During breathing and coughing exercises, client presses gently against incisional area to splint or support it. Pillow over incision is optional.

(6) Client continues to practice coughing exercises, splinting imaginary incision. Instruct client to cough two to three times every 2 hours while awake.

(7) Instruct client to examine sputum for consistency, odor, amount, and color changes.

D. Turning:

(1) Instruct client to assume supine position and move to side of bed if permitted by surgery. Have client move by bending knees and pressing heels against the mattress to raise and move buttocks. Top side rails on both sides of bed should be in up position.

(2) Instruct client to place right hand over incisional area to splint it.

(3) Instruct client to keep right leg straight and flex left knee up. If back or vascular surgery was performed, client will need to logroll or will require assistance with turning.

(4) Have client grab right side rail with left hand, pull toward right, and roll onto right side.

(5) Instruct client to turn every 2 hours while awake.

Continued

	S	U	NP	Comments

E. Leg exercises:
   (1) Have client assume supine position in bed. Demonstrate leg exercises by performing passive range-of-motion exercises and simultaneously explaining exercise.

   (2) Rotate each ankle in complete circle. Instruct client to draw imaginary circles with big toe. Repeat five times.

   (3) Alternate dorsiflexion and plantar flexion of both feet. Direct client to feel calf muscles contract and relax alternately. Repeat five times.

   (4) Perform quadriceps setting by tightening thigh and bringing knee down toward mattress, then relaxing. Repeat five times.

   (5) Have client alternately raise each leg straight up from bed surface, keeping legs straight, and then have client bend leg at hip and knee Repeat five times.

7. Have client perform exercises at least every 2 hours while awake. Instruct client to coordinate turning and leg exercises with diaphragmatic breathing, incentive spirometry, and coughing exercises.

8. Observe client's ability to perform all five exercises independently.

9. Record exercises demonstrated and whether client is able to perform them independently.

10. Report any problems client has in practicing exercises to nurse assigned to client on next shift for follow-up.

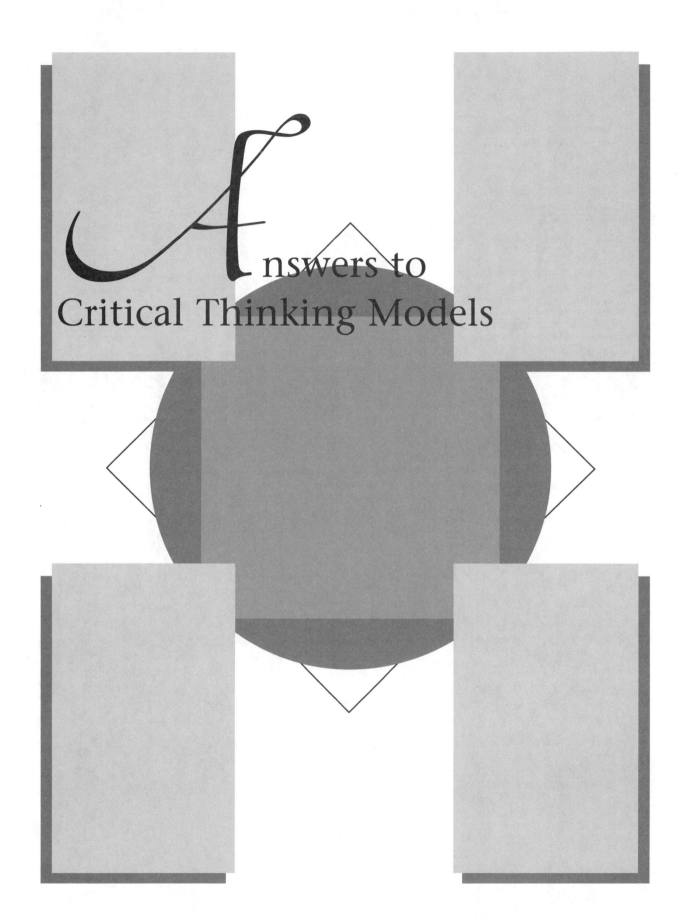

Answers to
Critical Thinking Models

KNOWLEDGE

- Components of self-concept (identity, body image, self-esteem, role performance)
- Self-concept stressors related to identity, body image, self-esteem, role
- Therapeutic communication principles, nonverbal indicators of distress
- Cultural factors that influence self-concept
- Growth and development (middle-age adult)
- Pharmacologic effects of medicine (pain medication)

EXPERIENCE

- Caring for a client who had an alteration in body image, self-esteem, role, or identity
- Susan's own personal experience of threat to self-concept

Assessment

- Observe Mrs. Johnson's behaviors that suggest an alteration in self-concept
- Assess the Mrs. Johnson's cultural background
- Assess the Mrs. Johnson's coping skills and resources
- Converse with Mrs. Johnson to determine her feelings, perceptions about changes in body image, self-esteem, or role
- Assess the quality of Mrs. Johnson's relationships

STANDARDS

- Support Mrs. Johnson's autonomy to make choices and express values that support positive self-concept
- Apply intellectual standards of relevance and plausibility for care to be acceptable to Mrs. Johnson
- Susan needs to safeguard Mrs. Johnson's right to privacy by judiciously protecting information of a confidential nature

ATTITUDES

- Display curiosity in considering why Mrs. Johnson might be behaving or responding in this manner
- Susan needs to display integrity when her beliefs and values differ from Mrs. Johnson's; admit to any inconsistencies between her values and his
- Risk taking may be necessary in developing a trusting relationship with Mrs. Johnson

CHAPTER 27   *Critical Thinking Model for Nursing Care Plan* (page 89)

KNOWLEDGE

- A basic understanding of sexual development, sexual orientation, sociocultural dimensions, the imapct of self-concept, STDs, safe sex practices
- Ways to phrase questions regarding sexuality and functioning
- Disease conditions that affect sexual functioning
- How interpersonal relationship factors may affect sexual functioning

EXPERIENCE

- Explore discomfort with discussing topics related to sexuality and develop a plan for addressing these discomforts
- Reflect on personal sexual experiences and how he has responded

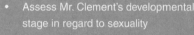

Assessment

- Assess Mr. Clement's developmental stage in regard to sexuality
- Consider self-concept as a factor that will influence sexual satisfaction and functioning
- Physical assessment of urogenital area
- Determine Mr. Clement's sexual concerns
- Assess safe sex practices and the use of contraception
- Assess the medical conditions and medications which may be affecting his sexual functioning
- Assess the impact of high-risk behaviors on sexual health

STANDARDS

- Apply intellectual standards of relevance and plausibility for care to be acceptable to Mr. Clement
- Safeguard Mr. Clement's right to privacy by judiciously protecting information of a confidential nature
- Apply the principles of ethic of care

ATTITUDES

- Display curiosity, consider why Mr. Clement might behave or respond in a particular manner
- Display integrity; his beliefs and values may differ from Mr. Clement's
- Admit to any inconsistencies in his and Mr. Clement's values
- Risk taking: Be willing to explore both personal and Mr. Clement's sexual issues and concerns

CHAPTER 28   *Critical Thinking Model for Nursing Care Plan* (page 93)

KNOWLEDGE

- The concepts of faith, hope, spiritual well-being and religion
- Caring practices in the individual approach to a client
- Available services in the community (health care providers and agencies)

EXPERIENCE

- Leah's past experience in selecting interventions that support client's spiritual well-being

Planning

- Leah needs to collaborate with Jose and his family on choice of interventions
- Consult with pastoral care or other clergy, holy leaders as appropriate
- Continue appropriate religious rituals specific to Jose
- Ask if the client's expectations have been met

STANDARDS

- Standards of autonomy and self determination to support Jose's decisions about the plan

ATTITUDES

- Leah will exhibit confidence in her skills and know to develop a trusting relationship with Jose
- Be open to any possible CONFLICT between the client's opinion and Leah's; decide how to reach mutually beneficial outcomes

CHAPTER 29   *Critical Thinking Model for Nursing Care Plan* (page 98)

KNOWLEDGE

- Characteristics of a resolution of grief
- Clinical symptoms of an improved level of comfort (applicable for the terminally ill)
- Principles of palliative care

EXPERIENCE

- Previous client responses to planned nursing interventions for management or the loss of a significant other

Evaluation

- Evaluate signs and symptoms of Mr. Stevens' grief and his wife's
- Evaluate his wife's ability to provide supportive care
- Evaluate Mr. Stevens' level of comfort and symptom relief
- Ask if the client/family's expectations are being met

STANDARDS

- Use established expected outcomes to evaluate Mr. Stevens' plan of care (participation in life review)
- Evaluate Mr. Stevens' role in end-of-life decisions and (or the grieving) process

ATTITUDES

- Persevere in seeking successful comfort measures for Mr. Stevens

CHAPTER 30 *Critical Thinking Model for Nursing Care Plan* (page 103)

KNOWLEDGE

- Characteristics of adaptive behaviors
- Characteristics of continuing stress response
- Differentiation of stress and trauma

EXPERIENCE

- Previous client responses to planned nursing interventions

Evaluation

- Reassess Carl for the presence of new or recurring stress related problems or symptoms (fatigue, changes in energy level, weight, or eating habits)
- Determine if change in care promoted Carl's adaptation to stress
- Evaluate if Carl's expectations have been achieved

STANDARDS

- Use of established expected outcomes to evaluate Carl's plan of care (rest and relaxation, stable weight, positive feelings about wife and their relationship)
- Apply the intellectual standard of relevance; be sure that Carl achieves goals relevant to his needs

ATTITUDES

- Janet needs to demonstrate perseverance in redesigning interventions to promote Carl's adaptation to stress
- Janet needs to display integrity in accurately evaluating nursing interventions

CHAPTER 31   *Critical Thinking Model for Nursing Care Plan* (page 107)

KNOWLEDGE

- The role of physical therapist and exercise trainers in improving Mrs. Smith's activity and exercise program
- Determine Mrs. Smith's ability to increase her level of activity
- Impact of medication on Mrs. Smith's activity tolerance

EXPERIENCE

- Consider previous client and personal experiences to therapies designed to improve exercise and activity tolerance
- Consider personal experience with exercise regimens

Planning

- Consult and collaborate with members of the health team to increase Mrs. Smith's activity
- Involve Mrs. Smith and her family in designing her activity and exercise plan
- Consider Mrs. Smith's ability to increase her activity level and follow an exercise program

STANDARDS

- Therapies need to be individualized to Mrs. Smith's activity tolerance
- Apply the goals of the American College of Sports Medicine in the application

ATTITUDES

- Be responsible and creative in designing interventions to improve Mrs. Smith's activity tolerance

CHAPTER 37   *Critical Thinking Model for Nursing Care Plan* (page 148)

KNOWLEDGE

- Basic human needs
- The potential risks to a client's safety from physical and environmental hazards
- The influence of developmental stage on safety needs (older adult)
- The influence of illness and medications on Ms. Cohen's safety (immobilization and visual impairment)

EXPERIENCE

- Past experiences of Mr. Key in caring for clients with mobility or sensory impairments that threaten safety
- Personal experiences in caring for the older adult

Assessment

- Identification of actual and potential threats to Ms. Cohen's safety
- Determine the impact of Ms. Cohen's underlying disease on her safety
- The presence of risks for Ms. Cohen's developmental stage

STANDARDS

- Mr. Key needs to apply intellectual standards of accuracy, significance, completeness, and fairness when assessing for threats to Ms. Cohen's safety
- ANA standards of nursing practice
- Fall prevention protocols (Practice Standards)

ATTITUDES

- Perseverance is needed when identifying all threats to Ms. Cohen's safety
- Responsibility for collecting unbiased accurate data regarding Ms. Cohen's threat to safety
- Fairness is appropriate to objectively evaluate the risk to Ms. Cohen's safety within the home and the community

CHAPTER 38   *Critical Thinking Model for Nursing Care Plan* (page 153)

KNOWLEDGE

- Principles of comfort and safety
- Adult learning principles to apply when educating the client and family
- Services available through community agencies

EXPERIENCE

- Care of previous clients that required adaptation of hygiene approaches

Planning

- Involve Mrs. Wyatt and her family in planning and adapting approaches as well as in hygiene instruction
- Know community resources applicable to Mrs. Wyatt's needs
- Consider the timing of other care activities when choosing the best time for hygienic care

STANDARDS

- Individualize the hygiene care to meet Mrs. Wyatt's preferences
- Apply standards of safety and promotion of client dignity

ATTITUDES

- Jeanette needs to be creative when adapting approaches to any self-care limitations that Mrs. Wyatt might have
- Jeanette needs to take responsibility for following standards of good hygiene practice

CHAPTER 39 *Critical Thinking Model for Nursing Care Plan* (page 160)

KNOWLEDGE

- Cardiac and respiratory anatomy and physiology
- Cardiopulmonary pathophysiology
- Clinical signs and symptoms of altered oxygenation
- Developmental factors affecting oxygenation
- Impact on lifestyle
- Environmental impact

EXPERIENCE

- Caring for clients with impaired oxygenation, activity intolerance, and respiratory infections
- Observations of changes in client respiratory patterns made during poor air quality days
- Personal experience with how a change in altitudes or physical conditioning affects respiratory patterns
- Personal experience with respiratory infections or cardiopulmonary alterations

Assessment

- Identify recurring and present signs and symptoms associated with Mr. Edwards impaired oxygenation
- Determine the presence of risk factors that apply to Mr. Edwards
- Ask Mr. Edwards about the use of medication
- Determine Mr. Edwards activity status
- Determine Mr. Edwards tolerance to activity

STANDARDS

- Apply intellectual standards of clarity, precision, specificity, and accuracy when obtaining a health history for a client with cardiopulmonary alterations

ATTITUDES

- Carry out the responsibility of obtaining correct information about Mr. Edwards and explaining risk factors, health promotion and disease prevention activities, and therapies for disease/symptom management
- Display confidence in assessing Mr. Edwards management of illness

CHAPTER 40 *Critical Thinking Model for Nursing Care Plan* (page 168)

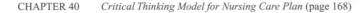

KNOWLEDGE

- Consider the other health care professionals caring for Mrs. Bottomley
- The impact of specific fluid regimens on the Mrs. Bottomley's fluid balance
- The impact of new medications on Mrs. Bottomley's fluid balance

EXPERIENCE

- Consider the previous clinical assignments you have had and how those clients responded to nursing therapies (what worked and what didn't?)

Planning

- Select nursing interventions to promote fluid, electrolyte and acid-base balance
- Consult with pharmacists and nutritionists
- Involve Mrs. Bottomley and her family in designing the interventions

STANDARDS

- Therapies need to be individualized to Mrs. Bottomley's fluid balance and acid-base requirements

ATTITUDES

- Use creativity to plan interventions that will achieve an effective airway and integrate those into Mrs. Bottomley's activities of daily living
- Be responsible in planning nursing interventions consistent with the client's fluid balance and acid-base requirements

CHAPTER 41   *Critical Thinking Model for Ineffective Airway Clearance/Risk* (page 178)

KNOWLEDGE

- The characteristics of a desirable sleep pattern
- Basis for the expected outcomes in the plan of care

EXPERIENCE

- Previous client's responses to planned nursing interventions for promoting sleep
- Previous experience in adapting sleep therapies to personal needs

Evaluation

- Evaluate signs and symptoms of Julie's sleep disturbance
- Review Julie's sleep pattern
- Have sleep partner report Julie's response to therapies
- The expected outcomes developed during the plan of care serve as the standards to evaluate its success
- Ask client if expectations of care are being met

STANDARDS

- Use of established expected outcomes to evaluate Julie's plan of care (improved duration of sleep, fewer awakenings)

ATTITUDES

- Humility may apply if an intervention is unsuccessful; rethink the approach
- In the case of chronic sleep problems, perseverance is needed in staying with the plan of care or in trying new approaches

CHAPTER 42   *Critical Thinking Model for Nursing Care Plan* (page 183)

KNOWLEDGE

- Physiology of pain
- Factors that potentially increase or decrease responses to pain
- Pathophysiology of conditions causing pain
- Awareness of biases affecting pain assessment and treatment
- Cultural variations in how pain is expressed
- Knowledge of nonverbal communication

EXPERIENCE

- Caring for clients with acute, chronic, and cancer pain
- Caring for clients who experienced pain as a result of a health care therapy
- Personal experience with pain

Assessment

- Determine Mrs. May's perspective of pain including history of pain, its meaning, and physical, emotional, and social effects
- Objectively measure the characteristics of Mrs. May's pain
- Review potential factors affecting Mrs. May's pain

STANDARDS

- Refer to AHCPR guidelines for acute pain management
- Apply intellectual standards (clarity, specificity, accuracy, and completeness) when gathering assessment
- Apply relevance when letting Mrs. May explore the pain experience

ATTITUDES

- Persevere in exploring causes and possible solutions for chronic pain
- Display confidence when assessing pain to relieve Mrs. May's anxiety
- Display integrity and fairness to prevent prejudice from affecting assessment

CHAPTER 43   *Critical Thinking Model for Nursing Care Plan* (page 189)

KNOWLEDGE

- Roles of dietitians and nutritionists in caring for clients with altered nutrition
- Impact of community support groups and other resources in assisting clients to manage nutrition
- Impact of bad diets on client's overall nutritional status

EXPERIENCE

- Previous client responses to nursing interventions for altered nutrition
- Personal experiences with dietary change strategies (what worked and what didn't)

Planning

- Select nursing interventions to promote optimal nutrition
- Select nursing interventions consistent with therapeutic diets
- Consult with other health care professinonals (dietitians, nutritionists, physicians, pharmacists, and physical and occupational therapists) to adopt interventions that reflect Mrs. Cooper's needs
- Involve the family when designing interventions

STANDARDS

- Refer to AHCPR guidelines for acute pain management
- Apply intellectual standards (clarity, specificity, accuracy, and completeness) when gathering assessment
- Apply relevance when letting Mrs. Cooper explore the pain experience

ATTITUDES

- Persevere in exploring causes and possible solutions for chronic pain
- Display confidence when assessing pain to relieve Mrs. Cooper's anxiety
- Display integrity and fairness to prevent prejudice from affecting assessment

CHAPTER 44   *Critical Thinking Model for Nursing Care Plan* (page 197)

KNOWLEDGE

- Physiology of fluid balance
- Anatomy and physiology of normal urine production and urination
- Pathophysiology of selected urinary alterations
- Factors affecting urination
- Principles of communication used to address issues related to self-concept and sexuality

EXPERIENCE

- Caring for clients with alterations in urinary elimination
- Caring for clients at risk for urinary infection
- Personal experience with changes in urinary elimination

Assessment

- Gather nursing history of the urination pattern, symptoms, and factors affecting urination
- Conduct a physical assessment of body systems potentially affected by urinary change
- Assess the characteristics of urine
- Assess perception of urinary problems as it affects self-concept and sexuality

STANDARDS

- Maintain privacy and dignity
- Apply intellectual standards to ensure history and assessment are complete and in depth
- Apply professional standards of care from professional organizations such as ANA and AHCPR

ATTITUDES

- Display humility in recognizing limitations in knowledge

CHAPTER 45   *Critical Thinking Model for Nursing Care Plan* (page 203)

KNOWLEDGE

- Role of the other health care professionals in returning the client's bowel elimination pattern to normal
- Impact of specific therapeutic diets and medication on bowel elimination patterns
- Expected results of cathartics, laxatives, and enemas on bowel elimination

EXPERIENCE

- Previous client response to planned nursing therapies for improving bowel elimination (what worked and what didn't)

Planning

- Javier needs to select nursing interventions to promote normal bowel elimination
- Consult with nurtitionists and enteral stoma therapists
- Involve Larry and his family in designing nursing interventions

STANDARDS

- Individualize therapies to Larry's bowel elimination needs
- Select therapies consistent within wound and ostomy professional practice standards

ATTITUDES

- Javier needs to be creative when planning interventions for Larry to achieve normal bowel elimination patterns
- Display independence when integrating interventions from other disciplines in Larry's plan of care
- Act responsibly by ensuring that interventions are consistent within standards

CHAPTER 46   *Critical Thinking Model for Nursing Care Plan* (page 210)

KNOWLEDGE

- Characteristics of improved mobility status on all physio-logical systems and the client's psychosocial and developmental status

EXPERIENCE

- Previous client responses to planned mobility interventions.

Evaluation

- Reassess Ms. Adams for signs and symptoms of improved or decreased mobility status
- Ask for Ms. Adams' perception of mobility status after intervention
- Evaluate whether or not Ms. Adams' expectations of care have been met

STANDARDS

- Use established expected out-comes for Ms. Adams' plan of care (lung fields remain clear) to evaluate her response to care

ATTITUDES

- Display humility when identi-fying those interventions that were not successful
- Use creativity when redesign-ing new interventions to improve Ms. Adams' mobility status

CHAPTER 47   *Critical Thinking Model for Nursing Care Plan* (page 215)

KNOWLEDGE

- Pathogenesis of pressure ulcers
- Factors contributing to pressure ulcer formation or poor wound healing
- Factors contributing to wound healing
- Impact of underlying disease process of skin integrity
- Impact of medication on skin integrity and wound healing

EXPERIENCE

- Caring for clients with inpaired skin integrity or wounds
- Observation of normal wound healing

Assessment

- Identify the risk for developing impaired skin integrity
- Identify signs and symptoms associated with impaired skin integrity or poor wound healing
- Examine Mrs. Stein's skin for actual impairment in skin integrity

STANDARDS

- Apply intellectual standards of accuracy, relevance, completeness, and precision when obtaining health history regarding skin integrity and wound management
- Knowledge of AHCPR standards for prevention or pressure ulcers

ATTITUDES

- Use discipline to obtain complete and correct assessment data regarding Mrs. Stein's skin and or/wound integrity
- Demonstrate responsibility for collecting appropriate specimens for diagnostic and laboratory tests related to wound management

CHAPTER 48   *Critical Thinking Model for Nursing Care Plan* (page 222)

KNOWLEDGE

- Understand how a sensory deficit can affect the client's functional status
- Role other health professionals might have in sensory function management
- Services of community resources
- Adult learning principles to apply when educating the client and family

EXPERIENCE

- Previous client responses to planned nursing interventions to promote sensory function

Planning

- Select strategies that assist Judy to remain functional in her home
- Adapt therapies based on short- or long-term sensory deficit
- Involve the family in helping Judy adjust to her limitations
- Refer Judy to appropriate health care professional and/or community agency

STANDARDS

- Individualize therapies that allow the client to adapt to sensory loss in any setting
- Apply standards of safety

ATTITUDES

- Use creativity to find interventions that help Judy adapt to the home environment

CHAPTER 49   *Critical Thinking Model for Nursing Care Plan* (page 228)

KNOWLEDGE

- Behaviors that demonstrate learning
- Characteristics of anxiety and/or fear
- Signs and symptoms or conditions that contraindicate surgery

EXPERIENCE

- Previous client responses to planned preoperative care
- Any personal experience with surgery

Evaluation

- Evaluate Mrs. Campana's knowledge of surgical procedure and planned postoperative care
- Have Mrs. Campana demonstrate postoperative exercises
- Observe behaviorus or nonverbal expressions of anxiety or fea
- Ask if client's expectation are being met

STANDARDS

- Use established expected outcomes to evaluate Mrs. Campana's plan of care (ability to perform postoperative exercises)

ATTITUDES

- Demonstrate perseverance when Mrs. Campana has difficulty performing postoperative exercises

CHAPTER 50   *Critical Thinking Model for Nursing Care Plan* (page 238)